Cli
Pharmacology

BI 3

D0308853

UCE
Birmingham

LECTURE NOTES ON

Clinical Pharmacology

JOHN L. REID
DM FRCP FRSE
Regius Professor of Medicine and Therapeutics
University of Glasgow

PETER C. RUBIN
DM FRCP
Professor of Therapeutics
Dean of Medicine and Health Sciences
University of Nottingham

BRIAN WHITING
MD FRCP FAMS
Emeritus Professor of Clinical Pharmacology
University of Glasgow

Sixth Edition

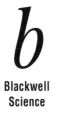

Blackwell
Science

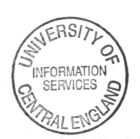

© 1982, 1985, 1989, 1992, 1996, 2001
by
Blackwell Science Ltd
Editorial Offices:
Osney Mead, Oxford OX2 0EL
25 John Street, London WC1N 2BS
23 Ainslie Place, Edinburgh EH3 6AJ
350 Main Street, Malden
  MA 02148–5018, USA
54 University Street, Carlton
  Victoria 3053, Australia
10, rue Casimir Delavigne
  75006 Paris, France

Other Editorial Offices:
Blackwell Wissenschafts-Verlag
  GmbH
Kurfürstendamm 57
10707 Berlin, Germany

Blackwell Science KK
MG Kodenmacho Building
7–10 Kodenmacho Nihombashi
Chuo-ku, Tokyo 104, Japan

Iowa State University Press
A Blackwell Science Company
2121 S. State Avenue
Ames, Iowa 50014-8300, USA

First published 1982
Second edition 1985
Reprinted 1987, 1988
Third edition 1989
Reprinted 1990, 1991
Fourth edition 1992
Reprinted 1993, 1994 (twice), 1995
Four Dragons edition 1992
Reprinted 1993, 1994 (twice)
Fifth edition 1996
Reprinted 1997, 1998, 2000
Sixth edition 2001

Set by Kolam Information Services
Pvt. Ltd., India
Printed and bound in Great Britain by
MPG Books Ltd., Bodmin, Cornwall

The Blackwell Science logo is a trade
mark of Blackwell Science Ltd,
registered at the United Kingdom
Trade Marks Registry

A catalogue record for this title is
available from the British Library

ISBN 0-632-05077-2

Library of Congress
Cataloging-in-Publication Data

Reid, John L.
  Lecture notes on clinical
pharmacology
  John L. Reid, Peter C. Rubin,
Brian Whiting – 6th ed.
    p.;   cm.
  Includes bibliographical
references and index.
  ISBN 0-632-05077-2
  1. Clinical pharmacology.
  I. Rubin, Peter C.
  II. Whiting, Brian.
  III. Title.
  [DNLM: 1. Pharmacology,
Clinical. QV 38 R356L 2001]
RM301.28 .R45 2001
615′.1—dc21
                    00-051903

DISTRIBUTORS
  Marston Book Services Ltd
  PO Box 269
  Abingdon, Oxon OX14 4YN
  (Orders: Tel: 01235 465500
          Fax: 01235 465555)

USA
  Blackwell Science, Inc.
  Commerce Place
  350 Main Street
  Malden, MA 02148–5018
  (Orders: Tel: 800 759 6102
          781 388 8250
          Fax: 781 388 8255)

Canada
  Login Brothers Book Company
  324 Saulteaux Crescent
  Winnipeg, Manitoba R3J 3T2
  (Orders: Tel: 204 837 2987)

Australia
  Blackwell Science Pty Ltd
  54 University Street
  Carlton, Victoria 3053
  (Orders: Tel: 3 9347 0300
          Fax: 3 9347 5001)

For further information on
Blackwell Science, visit our website:
www.blackwell-science.com

Contents

Section 3: Drug Use, Misuse and Regulation

Contributors

The following contributed substantially to the writing, revision and rewriting of chapters in the 6th edition of *Lecture Notes in Clinical Pharmacology.*

RICHARD DONNELLY, School of Medical and Surgical Sciences, University of Nottingham [Chapter 8, Hypertension and Hyperlipidaemia]

IAIN McINNES, Department of Medicine, University of Glasgow [Chapter 13, Cytotoxic Drugs and Immunopharmacology]

DAVID McKILLOP, Drug Metabolism and Pharmacokinetics, AstraZeneca, Alderley Park [Chapter 1, Principles of Clinical Pharmacology]

JOHN McMURRAY, Department of Medicine and Therapeutics, University of Glasgow [Chapter 7, Heart Failure and Angina Pectoris]

ROBIN SPILLER, School of Medical and Surgical Sciences, University of Nottingham [Chapter 3, Influence of Disease on Pharmacokinetics and Pharmacodynamics]

HUGH WILLISON, Department of Neurology, University of Glasgow [Chapter 20, Drugs and Neurological Disease]

ERIC WALKER, Scottish Centre for Infection and Environmental Health, Glasgow [Chapter 22, Travel Medicine and Tropical Disease]

Preface

Clinical pharmacology bridges the gap between laboratory science and the practice of medicine. Its primary aim is the promotion of safe and effective drug use: to optimize benefits and minimize risks. In the third millenium, there are increased responsibilities on the medical profession to base therapeutic decisions on clinical evidence and justify choices and actions, both to colleagues and patients.

Developments in medicine, pharmacology and physiology have led to a better understanding of diseaese processes and a more rational use of drugs. Many drugs are designed to interact with specific receptors or enzyme systems. In addition, the application of genetic, biochemical and immunological techniques has led to a clearer appreciation of the mechanisms involved in drug action.

For many years we have taught clinical pharmacology to medical practitioners and undergraduate students. We were persuaded by our students that there was a need for a brief, clearly written and up-to-date review of clinical pharmacology. *Lecture Notes on Clinical Pharmacology* was prepared to meet this need in 1982 and now enters its sixth edition. The new edition has been extensively revised and updated: several chapters have been rewritten. We have not attempted to be comprehensive, but have tried to emphasize the principles of clinical pharmacology, areas which are developing rapidly and topics which are of particular clinical importance. The book was based on a course of lectures and seminars in clinical pharmacology and therapeutics for medical students at the University of Glasgow. In addition, we have drawn on our experience of organizing courses for postgraduate students, general practitioners and medical specialists. Thus, while intended primarily for medical students, we believe this book will also be of use to those preparing for higher examinations and doctors in established practice who wish to remain well-informed of current concepts and new developments in clinical pharmacology.

For the sixth edition we have followed the policy of the British Pharmacopoeia and in most instances used the Recommended Non-proprietary Name (rINN) for drugs. Thus, lignocaine has become lidocaine. These changes have been introduced in the interests of safety and consistency and in recognition of the wide use of *Lecture Notes in Clinical Pharmacology* around the world. For the present, we have kept the names adrenaline and noradrenaline on account of their wide clinical acceptance in Britain, Europe and beyond.

Recent developments in medical education have emphasized self-learning using a problem-based approach. There has been a tendency to reduce the influence of didactic teaching and the perception of the need to require and retain factual information. Whether learning is problem-based or more traditional, it must be underpinned by clear understanding of the principles of the pathophysiology of disease, the molecular mechanisms of drug action in humans, and an appreciation of drug therapy in the context of overall health care.

For those who use it, we hope this book will provide a clear understanding not only of *how* but also *when* to use drugs.

John Reid
Peter Rubin
Brian Whiting

Acknowledgements

We acknowledge the help and assistance freely given by many colleagues, commenting, reviewing and updating chapters related to their specialist interest and expertise. We particularly acknowledge the input and contribution of Roch Cantwell, Stuart Cobbe, John Connell, David Davies, Curtis Gemmell, Ian Hall, Elizabeth Horn, Chris Hawkey, David Lawson, Kennedy Lees, Gordon Lowe, Helen Lyall, Alistair McLellan, Paul O'Donnell, Colin Runcie, David Stott, Roger Sturrock, Alison Thomson and Glyn Volans.

We are grateful to Ann Harold, Louise Sabir and Rhona Little for their role in collecting, collating and coordinating the text and revisions.

SECTION I

Principles of Clinical Pharmacology

CHAPTER 1

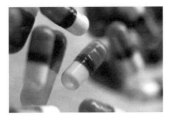

Principles of
Clinical Pharmacology

Prior to the twentieth century, medical practice depended largely on the administration of mixtures of natural plant or animal substances. These preparations contained a number of pharmacologically active agents in variable amounts. Their actions and indications were empirical and based on historical or traditional experience. Their use was rarely based on an understanding of the mechanism of disease or careful measurement of effect.

During the last 90 years an increased understanding has developed of biochemical and pathophysiological factors that influence disease. The chemical synthesis of agents with well characterized, specific actions on cellular mechanisms has led to the introduction of many powerful and effective drugs. Additionally, advances in the detection of these compounds in body fluids have facilitated investigation into the relationships between the dosage regimen, the profile of drug concentration against time in body fluids, notably the plasma, and corresponding profiles of clinical effect. Knowledge of this concentration–effect relationship and the factors that influence drug concentrations are used to determine how much drug an individual patient will require, and how often it should be given.

1.1 Principles of drug action (pharmacodynamics)

Pharmacological agents are used in therapeutics to:

1 Cure disease:
  (a) Chemotherapy in cancer or leukaemia.
  (b) Antibiotics in specific bacterial infections.
2 Alleviate symptoms:
  (a) Antacids in dyspepsia.
  (b) Non-steroidal anti-inflammatory drugs in rheumatoid arthritis.
3 Replace deficiencies:
  (a) Thyroxine in hypothyroidism.
  (b) Insulin in diabetes mellitus.

A drug is a single chemical entity that may be one of the constituents of a medicine.

A medicine may contain one or more active constituents (drugs) together with additives to facilitate administration.

Mechanism of drug action

Action on a receptor
A receptor is a specific macromolecule, usually a protein, to which a specific group of drugs or naturally occurring substances (such as neurotransmitters or hormones) can bind.

An agonist is a substance that stimulates or activates the receptor to produce an effect.

An antagonist prevents the action of an agonist but does not have any effect itself.

A partial agonist is usually an antagonist but under certain circumstances (e.g. high concentrations) can demonstrate agonist activity.

The biochemical events that result from an agonist–receptor interaction and which produce an effect, are still to be determined.

RECEPTORS FOR COMMONLY USED DRUGS

Receptor	Subtype	Main actions of natural agonist	Drug agonist	Drug antagonist
Adrenoceptor	alpha$_1$	Vasoconstriction		Prazosin
	alpha$_2$	Hypotension, sedation		Clonidine
	beta$_1$	Heart rate	Dopamine	Atenolol
			Dobutamine	Metoprolol
	beta$_2$	Bronchodilation	Salbutamol	
		Vasodilation	Terbutaline	
		Uterine relaxation	Ritodrine	
Cholinergic	Muscarinic	Heart rate		Atropine
		Secretion		Benzatropine (benztropine)
		Gut motility		Orphenadrine
		Bronchoconstriction		Ipratropium
	Nicotinic	Contraction of striated muscle	Suxamethonium Tubocurarine	
Histamine	H$_1$	Bronchoconstriction,		Chlorphenamine (chlorpheniramine)
		Capillary dilation		Terfenadine
	H$_2$	↑ Gastric acid		Cimetidine
				Ranitidine
				Famotidine
5-Hydroxy-tryptamine			Fluoxetine	Ondansetron
			Fluvoxamine	Granisetron
	Dopamine	CNS neurotransmitter	Bromocriptine	Chlorpromazine
				Haloperidol
				Thioridazine
Opioid		CNS neurotransmitter	Morphine, pethidine, etc.	Naloxone

Table 1.1 Some receptors involved in the action of commonly used drugs.

There are many types of receptors and in several cases subtypes have been identified which are also of therapeutic importance (Table 1.1).

Action on an enzyme

Enzymes, like receptors, are protein macromolecules with which substrates interact to produce activation or inhibition. Drugs in common clinical use which exert their effect through enzyme action, generally do so by inhibition.

1 Digoxin inhibits the membrane bound Na$^+$/K$^+$ ATPase.

2 Aspirin inhibits platelet cyclo-oxygenase.
3 Captopril inhibits angiotensin converting enzyme.
4 Selegiline inhibits monoamine oxidase B.
5 Carbidopa inhibits decarboxylase.
6 Allopurinol inhibits xanthine oxidase.

Drug receptor antagonists and enzyme inhibitors can act as competitive, reversible, antagonists or as non-competitive irreversible antagonists. The duration of the effect of drugs of the latter type is much longer than that of the former. Effects of competitive antagonists can be overcome by increasing the dose of endogenous or exogenous agonist, while effects of irreversible antagonists cannot usually be overcome.

Atenolol is a competitive beta adrenoceptor antagonist used in hypertension and angina. Its effects last for hours and can be overcome by administering an appropriate dose of a beta-receptor agonist like isoprenaline.

Vigabatrin is an irreversible inhibitor of gamma aminobutyric acid (GABA) amino-transferase and is used in epilepsy. Its action and adverse effects may persist for days as a result of irreversible binding to the target enzyme.

Action on membrane ionic channels

The conduction of impulses in nerve tissues and electromechanical coupling in muscle depends on the movement of ions, particularly sodium, calcium and potassium, through membrane channels. Several groups of drugs interfere with these processes:

1 Antiarrhythmic drugs (Chapter 6).
2 Calcium slow channel antagonists (Chapters 6–8).
3 General and local anaesthetics (Chapter 18).
4 Anticonvulsants (Chapter 20).

Cytotoxic actions

Drugs used in cancer or in the treatment of infections may kill malignant cells or micro-organisms. Often the mechanisms have been defined in terms of effects on specific receptors or enzymes. In other cases chemical action (alkylation) damages DNA or other macromolecules and results in cell death or failure of cell division (Chapter 13).

Dose–response relationship

In clinical practice dose–response relationships rarely follow the classical sigmoid pattern of experimental studies. It is uncommon for the upper plateau or maximum effect to be reached in man or to be relevant therapeutically. Additionally, variability in the relationship between dose and concentration means that it is often difficult to detect a dose–response relationship. Consequently, concentration–response relationships are often more clinically relevant.

Dose– (or concentration–) response relationships may be steep or flat. A steep relationship implies that small changes in dose will produce large changes in clinical response or

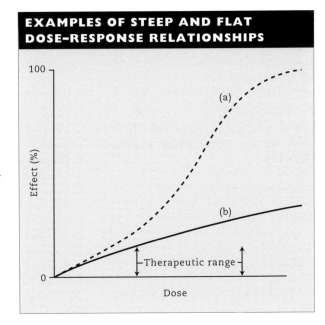

EXAMPLES OF STEEP AND FLAT DOSE-RESPONSE RELATIONSHIPS

Fig. 1.1 Schematic examples of a drug: (a) with a steep dose– (or concentration–)response relationship in the therapeutic range, e.g. warfarin as an oral anticoagulant; and (b) a flat dose– (or concentration–) response relationship within the therapeutic range, e.g. thiazide diuretics in hypertension.

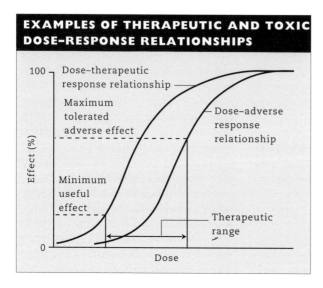

EXAMPLES OF THERAPEUTIC AND TOXIC DOSE–RESPONSE RELATIONSHIPS

Fig. 1.2 Schematic diagram of the dose–response relationship for the desired effect (dose–therapeutic response) and for an undesired adverse effect. The therapeutic index is the extent of displacement of the two curves within the normal dose range.

adverse effects, while flat relationships imply that increasing the dose will offer little clinical advantage (Fig. 1.1).

The potency of a drug is relatively unimportant; what matters is its efficacy or the maximum effect that can be obtained. In clinical practice the maximum therapeutic effect may often be unobtainable because of the appearance of adverse or unwanted effects: few, if any, drugs cause a single pharmacological response. The concentration–adverse response relationship is often different in shape and position to that of the concentration–therapeutic response relationship. The difference between the concentration that produces the desired effect and the concentration that causes adverse effects is called the therapeutic index and is a measure of the selectivity of a drug (Fig. 1.2).

The shape and position of dose–response curves in a group of patients is variable because of genetic, environmental and disease factors. However, this variability is not solely an expression of differences in response to drugs. It has two important components: the dose–plasma concentration relationship and the plasma concentration–effect relationship.

Dose → Concentration → Effect

With the development of specific and sensitive chemical assays for drugs in body fluids, it has been possible to characterize dose–plasma concentration relationships so that this component of the variability in response can be taken into account when drugs are prescribed for patients with various disease states. For drugs with a narrow therapeutic index it may be necessary to measure serum concentrations to assess the relationship between dose and concentration in individual patients. The description of a drug concentration profile against time is known as pharmacokinetics (see pp. 7–15) and its application in clinical practice is clinical pharmacokinetics (Chapter 2).

The residual variability in the relationship between dose and response is the concentration–effect component—a true expression of drug response, and a measure of the sensitivity of a patient to a drug. This is known as pharmacodynamics. Clinical pharmacology seeks to explore the factors that underlie variability in pharmacokinetics and pharmacodynamics and to use this information to optimize drug therapy for individual patients.

1.2 Principles of pharmacokinetics

Absorption

Drug absorption after oral administration has two major components: absorption rate and bioavailability. Absorption rate is controlled partially by the physicochemical characteristics of the drug but in many cases is modified by the formulation. A reduction in absorption rate can lead to a smoother concentration–time profile with a lower potential for concentration-dependent adverse effects and may allow less frequent dosing.

Bioavailability is the term used to describe the fraction of the dose that is absorbed into the systemic circulation and is usually designated *F*. It can range from 0 to 1 (0–100%) and depends on a number of physicochemical and clinical factors. Low bioavailability may occur if the drug has low solubility or is destroyed by the acid in the stomach. Changing the formulation can affect the bioavailability of a drug and it can also be altered by food or the co-administration of other drugs. For example, antacids can reduce the absorption of quinolone antibiotics by binding them in the gut. Other factors influencing bioavailability include metabolism by gut flora, the intestinal wall or the liver.

First-pass metabolism refers to metabolism of a drug that occurs en route from the gut lumen to the systemic circulation. For the majority of drugs given orally, absorption occurs across the portion of gastrointestinal epithelium that is drained by veins forming part of the hepatoportal system. Consequently, even if they are well absorbed, drugs must pass through the liver before reaching the systemic circulation. For drugs that are susceptible to extensive hepatic metabolism, a substantial proportion of an orally administered dose can be metabolized before it ever reaches its site of pharmacological action. Drugs with a high first-pass metabolism are listed in Table 1.2.

The importance of first-pass metabolism is two fold:

1 It is one of the reasons for apparent differences in drug absorption between individuals. Even healthy people show considerable variation in liver metabolizing capacity.

DRUGS UNDERGOING FIRST-PASS METABOLISM	
Analgesics	*Drugs acting on CNS*
Aspirin	Clomethiazole (chlormethiazole)
Morphine	Chlorpromazine
Paracetamol	Imipramine
Pentazocine	Levodopa
Pethidine	Nortriptyline
Cardiovascular drugs	*Respiratory drugs*
Glyceryl trinitrate	Salbutamol
Isoprenaline	Terbutaline
Isosorbide dinitrate	
Labetalol	*Oral contraceptives*
Lidocaine (lignocaine)	
Metoprolol	
Nifedipine	
Prazosin	
Propranolol	
Verapamil	

Table 1.2 Several drugs that undergo extensive first-pass metabolism.

2 In patients with severe liver disease first-pass metabolism may be dramatically reduced, leading to the absorption of greater amounts of parent drug.

Distribution

Once a drug has gained access to the bloodstream it begins to distribute to the tissues. The extent of this distribution depends on a number of factors including plasma protein binding, the pKa of the drug, its partition coefficient into fatty tissue and regional blood flow. The volume of distribution, V, is the *apparent volume* of fluid into which a drug distributes based on the *amount* of drug in the body and the *measured concentration* in the plasma or serum. If a drug was wholly confined to the plasma, V would equal the plasma volume—approximately 3 l in an adult. If, on the other hand, the drug was distributed throughout all body water, V would be approximately 42 l. In reality, drugs are rarely distributed into physiologically relevant volumes. If most of the drug is bound to tissues, the plasma concentration will be low and the apparent V will be high, while high plasma protein binding will tend to maintain high concentrations in the blood and a low V will result. For the majority of drugs V depends on the balance between plasma binding and sequestration or binding by various body tissues, for example, muscle and fat. Volume of distribution can vary therefore from relatively small values (e.g. an average of 0.14 l/kg body weight for aspirin) to large values (e.g. an average of 200 l/kg body weight for chloroquine (Table 1.3).

Plasma protein binding

In the blood, a proportion of the drug is bound to plasma proteins—mainly albumin (acidic drugs) and alpha$_1$-acid glycoprotein (basic drugs). Only the unbound, or free, fraction distributes because the protein bound complex is too large to pass through membranes. Movement of the drug between the blood and other tissues proceeds until equilibrium is established between the unbound drug in plasma and the drug in tissues. It is the unbound portion that is generally responsible for clinical effects—both the target response

VOLUMES OF DISTRIBUTION

Drug	Volume of distribution (l/kg)
Chloroquine	200
Nortriptyline	20
Digoxin	7
Propranolol	4
Phenytoin	0.65
Theophylline	0.50
Gentamicin	0.25
Aspirin	0.14
Warfarin	0.10

In general, a small V occurs when:

1 Lipid solubility is low.
2 There is a high degree of plasma protein binding.
3 There is a low level of tissue binding.

A high V occurs when:

1 Lipid solubility is high.
2 There is a low degree of plasma protein binding.
3 There is a high level of tissue binding.

Table 1.3 Average volumes of distribution of some commonly used drugs.

and unwanted, adverse effects. Changes in protein binding (e.g. resulting from displacement interactions) generally lead to a transient increase in free concentration and are rarely clinically relevant because the equilibrium becomes re-established with the same unbound concentration. However, a lower total concentration will be present and the measurement might be misinterpreted if the higher free fraction is not taken into account. This is a common problem with the interpretation of phenytoin concentrations, where free fraction can range from 10% in a normal patient to 40% in a patient with hypoalbuminaemia and renal impairment.

Clinical relevance of V

Knowledge of volume of distribution can be used to determine the size of a *loading dose* if an immediate response to treatment is required. This assumes that therapeutic success is closely related to the plasma concentration and that there are no adverse effects if a relatively large dose is suddenly administered. It is sometimes employed when drug response would take many hours or days to develop if the regular maintenance dose was given from the outset, e.g. digoxin.

A loading dose can be calculated as follows:

Loading dose = V × desired concentration

$$\text{(Eqn. 1.1)}$$

In practice, because most values for V are related to weight, this calculation is often simplified to a mg/kg dose.

Clearance

Clearance is the sum of all drug eliminating processes, principally determined by hepatic metabolism and renal excretion. It can be defined as the theoretical volume of fluid from which a drug is completely removed in a given period of time.

When a drug is administered continuously by intravenous infusion or repetitively by mouth, a balance is eventually achieved between its input (dosing rate) and its output (the amount eliminated over a given period of time). This balance gives rise to a constant amount of drug in the body which depends on the dosing rate and clearance. This amount is reflected in the plasma or serum as a steady-state concentration (Css). A constant rate intravenous infusion will clearly yield a constant Css, while a drug administered orally at regular intervals will result in fluctuation between peak and trough concentrations (Fig. 1.3).

The average Css in any dosage interval may be *approximated* by the concentration one-third of the way between the trough and the peak.

The relationship between the average Css, drug input and drug output for a constant infusion can be written

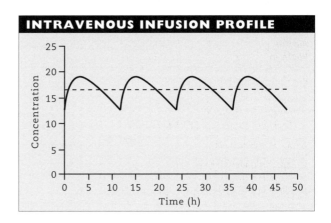

Fig. 1.3 Steady-state concentration–time profile for an oral dose (——) and a constant rate intravenous infusion (- - - - -).

PLOTS OF CONCENTRATION VS. TIME

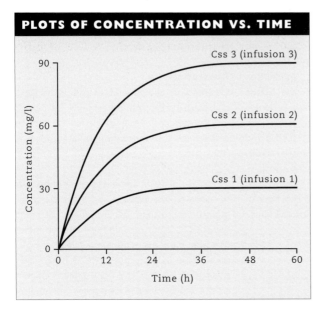

Fig. 1.4 Plots of concentration vs. time for three infusions allowed to reach steady state. Infusion 2 is at a rate twice that of infusion 1; infusion 3 is at a rate three times that of infusion 1. The three steady-state concentrations (Css 1, 2 and 3) are directly proportional to the corresponding infusion rates.

$$Css_{average} = \frac{Input\ rate}{Output\ rate} = \frac{Infusion\ rate}{Clearance}$$

$$(Eqn. 1.2)$$

or for oral therapy

$$Css_{average} = \frac{F \times Dose}{Clearance \times dosage\ interval}$$

$$(Eqn. 1.3)$$

Equations 1.2 and 1.3 highlight the important fact that if an estimate of clearance is available, it can be used to determine the *maintenance dose* for any desired Css, thus:

Infusion rate = Clearance × desired $Css_{average}$

$$(Eqn. 1.4)$$

or for oral therapy,

Maintenance dose = Clearance

× desired $Css_{average}$

× dosage interval/F

$$(Eqn. 1.4a)$$

Clearance depends critically on the efficiency with which the liver and/or kidneys can eliminate a drug; it will vary in disease states that affect these organs *per se*, or that affect the blood flow to these organs. In stable clinical conditions, clearance remains constant and Eqns. 1.2 and 1.3 show that the $Css_{average}$ is directly proportional to dose rate. The important implication is that if the dose rate is doubled, the $Css_{average}$ doubles: if the dose rate is halved, the $Css_{average}$ is halved. This is illustrated in Fig. 1.4. If each $Css_{average}$ is plotted against its corresponding dose rate, the direct proportionality becomes obvious (Fig. 1.5). In pharmacokinetic terms this is referred to as a first-order or linear process, and results from the fact that the rate of elimination is proportional to the amount of drug present in the body.

Single intravenous bolus dose

A number of other important pharmacokinetic principles can be appreciated by considering the concentrations that result following a single intravenous bolus dose (see Fig. 1.6a). If we assume that the drug distributes instantaneously into its volume of distribution, V, then its initial concentration C_0, depends only on the dose (D) and V, thus

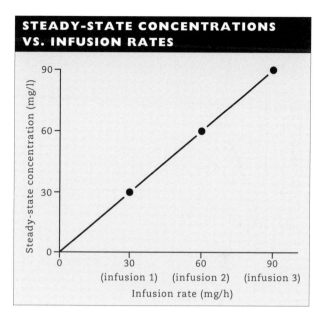

STEADY-STATE CONCENTRATIONS VS. INFUSION RATES

Fig. 1.5 Three steady-state concentrations plotted against corresponding infusion rates showing the linear relationship between dose and $Css_{average}$.

$$C_0 = \frac{D}{V} \tag{Eqn.1.5}$$

This is based on the concept that the body can be depicted as a single homogeneous compartment of volume, V, as shown in Fig. 1.7. The concentration will then decline by a constant proportion per unit time, giving rise to an exponential decline. The concentration at any time, t, after the dose can therefore be determined from the exponential expression

$$C(t) = \frac{D}{V}e^{-kt} \tag{Eqn.1.6}$$

where k is the elimination rate constant of the drug, t is any time after drug administration and e^{-kt} is the fraction of drug remaining at time t. If the concentrations are plotted on a logarithmic scale, a linear decline will be obtained with slope $-k$ and intercept $\ln D/V$; thus

$$\ln C(t) = \ln \frac{D}{V} - kt \tag{Eqn.1.7}$$

Semi-logarithmic graph paper allows $C_0(D/V)$ to be determined directly (Fig.

1.6b). k represents the constant fraction of the volume of distribution from which drug is eliminated in a given period of time and therefore depends on both clearance and volume of distribution; thus

$$k = \frac{\text{clearance}}{\text{volume of distribution}} \tag{Eqn.1.8}$$

k can also be expressed in terms of the half-life of a drug. The half-life, $t_{1/2}$, is the time required for the plasma concentration to fall to half of its original value and can be derived either graphically (Fig. 1.6) or from the expression

$$t_{1/2} = \frac{\ln 2}{k} \tag{Eqn.1.9}$$

where $\ln 2$ is the natural logarithm of 2, or 0.693. It can be used to predict the time at which steady state will be achieved after starting a regular treatment schedule or after any change in dose. As a rule, in the absence of a loading dose, steady state is attained after four to five half-lives (Fig. 1.8). Furthermore, when toxic drug levels have been inadvertently produced, it is very useful to estimate how long it

BOLUS INTRAVENOUS INJECTION

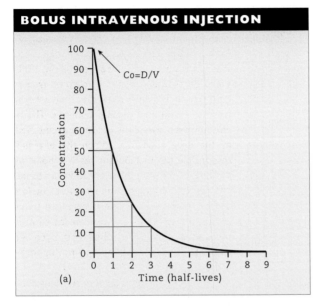

(a)

THE BODY AS A VOLUME

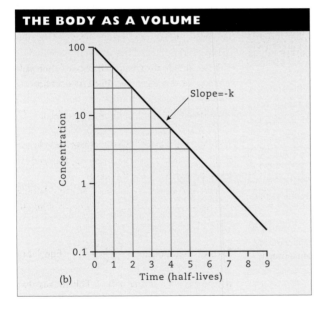

(b)

Fig. 1.6 (a) Plot of concentration vs. time after a bolus intravenous injection. The intercept on the y (concentration) axis, C_0, is the concentration resulting from the instantaneous injection of the bolus dose. (b) Semi- logarithmic plot of concentration vs. time after a bolus intravenous injection. The slope of this line is $-k$, the elimination rate constant (Eqns 1.6 and 1.7) and the elimination half-life of the drug can be easily determined from such a plot by noting the time at which the concentration has fallen to half its original value.

will take for such levels to reach the therapeutic range, or how long it will take for all the drug to be eliminated once the drug has been stopped. Usually, elimination is effectively complete after four to five half-lives (Fig. 1.6).

The elimination half-life can also be used to determine dosage intervals to achieve a target concentration–time profile. For example, in order to obtain a gentamicin peak of 8 mg/l and a trough of 0.5 mg/l in a patient with an elimination half-life of 3 h, the dosage interval should be 12 h. (The concentration will fall from 8 mg/l to 4 mg/l in 3 h, to 2 mg/l in 6 h, to 1 mg/l in 9 h and to 0.5 mg/l in 12 h.)

THE BODY AS A SINGLE COMPARTMENT

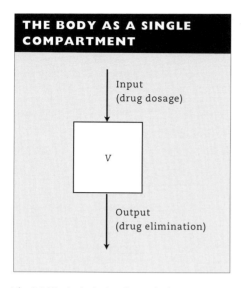

Fig. 1.7 The body depicted as a single compartment of volume V.

ORAL DOSE DRUG ADMINISTRATION

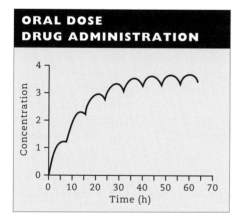

Fig. 1.8 Plot of concentration vs. time illustrating the accumulation to steady state when a drug is administered by regular oral doses.

However, for many drugs, dosage regimens should be designed to maintain concentrations within a range that avoids high (potentially toxic) peaks or low, ineffective troughs. Excessive fluctuations in the concentration-time profile can be prevented by giving the drug at intervals of less than one half-life or by using a slow-release formulation.

Linear vs. non-linear kinetics

In the discussion on clearance, it was pointed out that the hallmark of linear pharmacokinetics is the proportionality between dose rate and steady-state concentration. This arises because the rate of elimination is proportional to the amount of drug in the body, while the clearance remains constant. This is not, however, always the case as is exemplified by the drug phenytoin. When the enzymes responsible for metabolism reach a point of saturation, the rate of elimination, in terms of amount of drug eliminated in a given period of time, does not increase in response to an increase in concentration (or an increase in the amount of drug in the body) but becomes constant. This gives rise to non-linear or zero-order kinetics.

The general relationship between drug concentration (C) and rate of metabolism is shown in Fig. 1.9. The maximum rate at which the enzymes can function, V_{max}, corresponds to the plateau attained by the curve.

The equation relating the rate of metabolism to C is the Michaelis–Menten equation

$$\text{Rate of metabolism} = \frac{V_{max} \times C}{K_m + C} \qquad (Eqn.1.10)$$

and the fundamental difference between linear and non-linear kinetics can be appreciated by considering two extreme cases.

1 The serum concentration is considerably less than K_m. In this case, the Michaelis–Menten equation can be approximated to

$$\text{Rate of metabolism} = \frac{V_{max} \times C}{K_m} \qquad (Eqn.1.11)$$

where V_{max}/K_m is a constant. This means that the rate of change of concentration is then proportional to the concentration (linear kinetics).

2 The serum concentration is considerably greater than K_m.

In this case, the Michaelis–Menten equation can be approximated to

$$\text{Rate of metabolism} = V_{max} \qquad (Eqn.1.12)$$

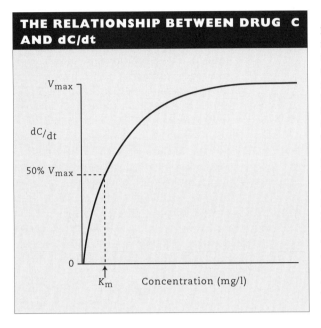

THE RELATIONSHIP BETWEEN DRUG C AND dC/dt

Fig. 1.9 Diagrammatic representation of the general relationship between drug concentration, C, and the rate of metabolism. V_{max} is the maximum velocity at which the drug metabolizing enzyme can function and is a constant (with units of mass/time). K_m is the concentration at which V_{max} is 50%. The K_m is usually much higher than therapeutic concentrations and the rate of metabolism vs. C is essentially linear (Eqn. 1.11). With a few drugs, notably phenytoin, therapeutic plasma concentrations are in the region of K_m so that rate of metabolism vs. C is non-linear and governed by the relationship shown in Eqn. 1.10.

which indicates that the rate of elimination is a constant.

At steady state, dose rate can be substituted for rate of metabolism, i.e.

$$\text{Steady-state dose rate} = \frac{V_{max} \times Css}{K_m + Css}$$

$$(\text{Eqn.1.13})$$

For phenytoin, V_{max} has a typical value of 7.2 mg/kg per day and K_m has a typical value of 4.4 mg/l (17.6 µmol/l). In the case of phenytoin, the range of concentrations used clinically encompasses and exceeds K_m. Consequently, the relationship between the steady-state concentration and dose rate will alter as the concentration changes. At low concentrations, the increase in concentration will be proportional to the dose rate (linear pharmacokinetics). At higher concentrations, the increase will be much greater than would have been anticipated (non-linear pharmacokinetics). Steady state will not be achieved if the dose rate exceeds V_{max}. This can be seen in Fig. 1.10.

Comment. The clinical relevance of non-linear kinetics is that a small increase in dose can lead to a large increase in concentration. This is particularly important when toxic side-effects are closely related to concentration, as with phenytoin.

1.3 Principles of drug elimination

Drug metabolism

Drugs are eliminated from the body by two principal mechanisms: (i) liver metabolism and (ii) renal excretion. Drugs that are already water-soluble are generally excreted unchanged by the kidney. Lipid-soluble drugs are not easily excreted by the kidney because, following glomerular filtration, they are largely reabsorbed from the proximal tubule. The first step in the elimination of such lipid-soluble drugs is metabolism to more polar (water-soluble) compounds. This is achieved mainly in the liver, but can also occur in the gut

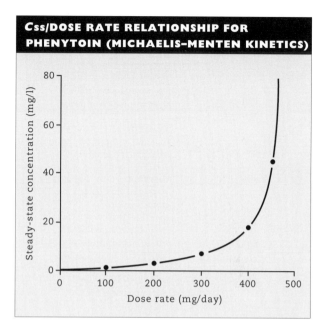

Fig. 1.10 The Css vs. dose rate relationship for phenytoin is governed by Michaelis–Menten kinetics (Eqn. 1.13).

and may contribute to first-pass elimination. Metabolism generally occurs in two phases:

Phase 1 Mainly oxidation (sometimes reduction or hydrolysis) to a more polar compound.

Phase 2 Conjugation, usually with glucuronic acid or sulphate, to make the compound substantially more polar.

Phase 1 metabolism

Oxidation can occur in various ways, including aromatic or aliphatic hydroxylation, oxygenation at carbon, nitrogen or sulphur atoms and N- and O-dealkylation. These reactions are catalysed by the cytochrome P-450-dependent system of the endoplasmic reticulum. Knowledge of P-450, which exists as a superfamily of similar enzymes (isoforms), has increased greatly over the past decade. The P-450 superfamily is divided into a number of families and subfamilies, where genes encoding for proteins within a family have at least 40% nucleotide sequence homology and subfamilies have over 65% homology. Although numerous P-450 isoforms are present in human tissue, only a few of these have a major role in the metabolism of drugs. These

enzymes, which display a distinct but overlapping substrate specificity, are listed in Table 1.4.

Phase 1 metabolites usually have only minor structural differences from the parent drug, but may exhibit totally different pharmacological actions. For example, the aromatic hydroxylation of phenobarbital (phenobarbitone) abolishes its hypnotic activity, while metabolism of azathioprine produces the powerful antimetabolite 6-mercaptopurine.

Phase 2 reactions

These involve the addition of small endogenous molecules to the parent drug, or to its phase 1 metabolite, and almost always lead to abolition of pharmacological activity. Multiple forms of conjugating enzymes are also known to exist, although these have not been investigated to the same extent as the P-450 system.

Metabolic drug interactions

The wide range of drugs metabolized by the P-450 system provides the opportunity for interactions of two types, namely enzyme induction and inhibition.

TYPICAL SUBSTRATES

Major human P-450s	Typical substrates
CYP1A2	Theophylline, caffeine, tacrine, fluvoxamine, oestradiol, phenacetin (R)-warfarin
CYP2C9	(S)-Warfarin, tolbutamide, glipizide, losartan, ibuprofen, diclofenac, phenytoin
CYP2C19	(S)-Mephenytoin, omeprazole, diazepam, citalopram, proguanil, moclobemide
CYP2D6	(S)-Metoprolol, bufuralol, dextromethorphan, fluoxetine, desipramine, nortryptiline
CYP2E1	Enflurane, halothane, chlorzoxazone, ethanol
CYP3A4	Astemizole, terfenadine, cisapride, pimozide, nisoldipine, midazolam, indinavir, lovastatin

Table 1.4 Major human P-450 enzymes involved in drug metabolism.

LIVER ENZYME INDUCERS

Carbamazepine
Phenobarbital (phenobarbitone)
Phenytoin
Rifampicin

Table 1.5 Some of the most potent enzyme inducers in humans.

Induction

Enzyme induction, which may be defined as the increase in amount and activity of drug metabolizing enzymes, is a consequence of new protein synthesis resulting from prolonged exposure to the inducing drug. While a drug may induce its own metabolism, it can also accelerate the metabolism and clearance of unrelated compounds. Many compounds are known to act as enzyme inducers in animals at toxicological dose levels, but relatively few drugs produce clinically significant induction in man when used at therapeutic doses.

The compounds shown in Table 1.5 are the most potent enzyme inducers in clinical use and have produced numerous clinically significant drug interactions, related primarily to increases in the metabolism of CYP2C9, CYP2C19 and CYP3A4 substrates. For example, the anticonvulsants phenytoin, carbamazepine and phenobarbital all induce the enzymes that metabolize the constituents of oral contraceptives. If a woman receiving an oral contraceptive starts taking one of these anticonvulsants, the metabolism of the oestrogen and progestogen in the oral contraceptive increases, with the risk of contraceptive failure. Enzyme induction is not, however, limited to drug administration. Cigarette smoking, for example, results in enzyme induction with

TYPICAL INHIBITORS

Major human P-450s	Typical inhibitors
CYP1A2	Furafylline, fluvoxamine, ciprofloxacin
CYP2C9	Fluconazole, ketoconazole, sulfaphenazole
CYP2C19	Omeprazole, ketoconazole, cimetidine
CYP2D6	Quinidine, fluoxetine, ritonavir
CYP2E1	Disulfiram
CYP3A4	Ketoconazole, itraconazole, ritonavir, erythromycin, diltiazem

Table 1.6 P-450 inhibitors involved in drug interactions.

increased metabolism of CYP1A2 substrates, such as theophylline, and ethanol is an inducer of CYP2E1.

Inhibition

Concurrently administered drugs can also lead to inhibition of enzyme activity, with many P-450 inhibitors showing considerable isoform selectivity. Some of the most clinically relevant inhibitors are listed in Table 1.6, together with the isoform inhibited. For example, ketoconazole decreases the metabolism of the CYP3A4 substrate, terfenadine, leading to potentially dangerous adverse effects, e.g. QT interval prolongation and torsades de pointes.

As with induction, P-450 inhibition is not limited to drug administration. Grapefruit juice is a fairly potent inhibitor of CYP3A4 activity and produces clinically significant interactions with a number of drugs, including midazolam, lovastatin and terfenadine. This type of information, together with some knowledge of the enzymes involved in a particular drug's clearance, makes it much easier to understand and predict drug interactions.

Comment. Enzyme induction produces clinical changes over days or weeks, but the effects of enzyme inhibition are usually observed immediately. In most circumstances, these changes are manifest as decreases in efficacy resulting from induction, or as increases in adverse effects resulting from inhibition. Clinical relevance occurs when drug therapy needs to be

altered to avoid the consequences of the drug interaction and this is most common and most serious in compounds which have a narrow therapeutic index. Clearly, pronounced enzyme inhibition, which may result in plasma concentrations of the inhibited drug being many times higher than intended, can be a major safety issue. For example, co-administration of ketoconazole or ritonavir with the hypnotic dug, midazolam, increases the midazolam plasma AUC by 15–20 times, a situation which should be avoided.

Genetic factors in metabolism

The rate at which healthy people metabolize drugs is variable. Although part of this variability is a consequence of environmental factors, including the influence of inducers and inhibitors, the main factor contributing to interindividual variability in metabolism is the underlying genetic basis of the drug metabolizing enzymes. Although there is probably a genetic component in the control of most P-450 enzymes, some enzymes (e.g. CYP2C19 and CYP2D6) actually show genetic polymorphism. This results in distinct subpopulations of poor and extensive metabolizers, where the poor metabolizers are deficient in that particular enzyme. There are a number of enzymes under polymorphic control and some clinically important examples are shown in Table 1.7. As with enzyme inhibition, genetic polymorphism is primarily a concern for drugs which have a narrow therapeutic index and

ENZYMES DISPLAYING GENETIC POLYMORPHISM

Enzyme	Typical substrates	Characteristics
CYP2C19	(S)-Mephenytoin, diazepam, omeprazole	About 2-5% of white people are poor metabolizers, but 18-23% of Japanese people have this phenotype
CYP2D6	Propafenone, flecainamide, desipramine	About 7% of white people are poor metabolizers, but this frequency is only about 2% in black Americans and <1% in Japanese/Chinese
N-Acetyl-transferase	Hydralazine, sulphonamides, isoniazid, procainamide	About 50% of white people are slow acetylators

Table 1.7 Major enzymes displaying genetic polymorphism.

which are metabolized largely by a single polymorphic enzyme. In such cases, the phenotype of the patient should be determined and lower doses of the drug used, or alternative therapy should be considered.

Renal excretion

Three processes are implicated in renal excretion of drugs:

1 *Glomerular filtration.* This is the most common route of renal elimination. The free drug is cleared by filtration and the protein bound drug remains in the circulation where some dissociates to restore equilibrium.

2 *Active secretion in the proximal tubule.* Both weak acids and weak bases have specific secretory sites in proximal tubular cells. Penicillins are eliminated by this route, as is about 60% of procainamide.

3 *Passive reabsorption in the distal tubule.* This occurs only with un-ionized, i.e. lipid-soluble, drugs. Urine pH determines whether or not weak acids and bases are reabsorbed, which in turn determines the degree of ionization.

If renal function is impaired, for example by disease or old age, then the clearance of drugs that normally undergo renal excretion is decreased (Chapter 3).

CHAPTER 2

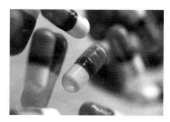

Clinical Pharmacokinetics: Dosage Individualization

2.1 Dosage individualization

If a dose of a drug is prescribed for a number of patients, the blood concentrations achieved can be quite variable. There are several reasons for this:

1 Individual differences in absorption, first-pass metabolism, volume of distribution and clearance.

2 Altered pharmacokinetics because of gastrointestinal, hepatic, renal or cardiac disease.

3 Drug interactions.

4 Poor compliance with drug therapy.

For most drugs there is an accepted 'target' range, i.e. a range of concentrations below which the drug is usually ineffective and above which it is usually toxic. In order to maintain drug concentrations within this range, knowledge about factors that influence the relationships between drug dose and blood concentration is used to design dosage regimens. Dosage adjustments based on age, renal function, hepatic function or other drug therapies are often recommended, especially for drugs with a narrow therapeutic index. For example, the initial dose of gentamicin, a renally cleared antibiotic, is based on the patient's renal function. As a consequence of an interaction that increases digoxin concentrations, the dose of digoxin is usually halved when amiodarone is added to a patient's therapy.

2.2 Therapeutic drug monitoring

In many cases it is relatively easy to evaluate the pharmacological effects of a drug by clinical observation and initial dosage regimens can be modified to increase the therapeutic effect or to eliminate unwanted effects. Measurement of drug concentrations in blood can be performed to help with diagnosis or to optimize therapy for those drugs where response (therapeutic or toxic effects) cannot be readily evaluated from clinical observation alone. Examples of drugs where monitoring has been used as an aid to clinical judgement are shown in Table 2.1.

Because of pharmacokinetic and pharmacodynamic variability, the following factors should be considered when interpreting drug concentration measurements:

1 Is the patient responding to therapy or showing symptoms of toxicity?

2 Was the sample taken at steady state?

3 Was the sampling time appropriate for the drug?

4 Where is the concentration relative to the 'target' range (Table 2.2)?

5 If the patient is not responding or has toxicity, how should the dose be modified? Unexpectedly low concentrations may indicate poor compliance or an absorption problem (e.g. vomiting).

DRUGS FOR WHICH TDM MAY BE USEFUL

Antiarrhythmics (Chapter 6)
Amiodarone
Digoxin
Lignocaine (lidocaine)
Mexiletine
Quinidine

Antimicrobials (Chapter 10)
Aciclovir
Amikacin
Flucytosine
Gentamicin
Netilmicin
Teicoplanin
Tobramycin
Vancomycin

Immunosuppressants (Chapter 13)
Ciclosporin (cyclosporin)
Mycophenolate
Tacrolimus

Anticancer drugs (Chapter 13)
Carboplatin
Methotrexate

Anticonvulsants (Chapter 20)
Carbamazepine
Ethosuximide
Lamotrigine
Phenobarbital
Phenytoin
Sodium valproate

Miscellaneous
Lithium (Chapter 19)
Theophylline (Chapter 11)
Antidepressants (Chapter 19)
Antipsychotics (Chapter 19)
Protease inhibitors

Table 2.1 Drugs for which serum level measurements have been used to guide dosage.

TARGET RANGES

Drug	Target range Mass units	Molar units
Digoxin	0.8–2 μg/l	1–2.6 nmol/l
Carbamazepine	4–12 mg/l	20–50 μmol/l
Phenobarbital	10–30 mg/l	50–150 μmol/l
Phenytoin	10–20 mg/l	40–80 μmol/l
Amikacin*	15–25 mg/l (1h post-dose)	
	<5 mg/l (trough)	
Gentamicin, netilmicin, tobramycin*	5–12 mg/l (1h post-dose)	
	<2 mg/l (trough)	
Vancomycin	5–10 mg/l (trough)	
Lithium		0.4–1.0 mmol/l
Theophylline	5–20 mg/l	28–110 μmol/l

* In some hospitals, high aminoglycoside doses (e.g. gentamicin doses of 5–7 mg/kg) are given at intervals of 24–48 h and the normal target peak and trough ranges do not apply. Samples are usually taken 6–14 h after the dose and the dose is adjusted (if necessary) according to a nomogram.

Table 2.2 Examples of target ranges.

2.3 Clearance estimates

The clinical significance of clearance is that it determines an individual patient's maintenance dose requirements. It is important to note that clearance varies between individuals and within an individual in response to changes in his or her clinical condition.

The physiological and pathological factors that affect the clearance of a drug depend mainly on which organ is primarily responsible for its elimination. For example, clearance of the bronchodilator theophylline, a drug that is eliminated by hepatic metabolism, is influenced by age, weight, alcohol consumption, cigarette smoking, other drugs, congestive cardiac failure, hepatic cirrhosis, acute pulmonary oedema and severe chronic obstructive airways disease.

Clearance in any individual is most accurately determined from concentration measurements. However, in many cases, relationships between clearance and clinical factors have previously been established. For example, the average value for theophylline clearance is 0.04 l/h per kg and this is modified according to the patient's clinical characteristics by multiplying by the factors shown in Table 2.3. This means that on average, smokers require 1.6 times the theophylline dose of non-smokers and patients with cirrhosis require half the dose of patients without cirrhosis. For drugs primarily excreted by the kidney, e.g. digoxin and gentamicin, creatinine clearance closely reflects drug clearance. Thus, digoxin clearance can be estimated from the equation:

$$\text{Digoxin clearance} = \text{Creatinine clearance} + 0.33$$
$$(\text{ml/min/kg}) \qquad (\text{ml/min/kg}) \qquad (\text{Eqn.2.1})$$

The 0.33 in this equation represents the elimination by routes other than the kidney, such as metabolism and clearance by the hepatobiliary system.

An estimate of clearance can then be used to calculate the required dose to achieve a target concentration, as shown in Chapter 1, i.e.

$$\text{Maintenance dose rate} = \text{Clearance} \times \text{Target } Css_{average}$$
$$(\text{Eqn.2.2})$$

$$\text{Maintenance dose} = \text{Clearance} \times \text{Target } Css_{average} \times \text{Dosage interval}/F$$
$$(\text{Eqn.2.3})$$

where F represents oral bioavailability. Factors that influence clearance are now routinely investigated for all new drugs so that dosage adjustments can be made for patients with a low clearance, who might be at risk from toxicity.

2.4 Interpretation of serum concentrations

Serum concentrations can be measured for a number of reasons and it is important to interpret the measured concentration in the light of the clinical situation. If the aim is to assess the patient's maintenance dose requirements, samples should ideally be taken at steady state. However, confirmation of steady state is not

THEOPHYLLINE CLEARANCE AND DOSE REQUIREMENTS	
Factor	Adjustments required
Smoking	×1.6
Congestive cardiac failure	×0.4
Hepatic cirrhosis	×0.5
Acute pulmonary oedema	×0.5
Severe chronic obstructive airways disease	×0.8

Table 2.3 Factors influencing theophylline clearance and therefore dose requirements.

necessary if the aim is to confirm toxicity or to assess the need for a loading dose in a patient who is acutely unwell.

Steady state normally requires that four to five half-lives have elapsed since treatment started or since any change in dose. Doses should be given at regular intervals and it is important to confirm that no doses have been omitted. If these conditions can be satisfied and the pharmacokinetics of the drug are linear, clearance depends on the ratio of the dosing rate to the average steady-state concentration as can be seen by rearranging Eqn. 2.2,

$$\text{Clearance} = \frac{\text{Maintenance dose rate}}{Css_{\text{average}}}$$

(Eqn.2.4)

This means that doses can be adjusted by simple proportion (see Chapter 1) i.e.

New maintenance dose

$$= \frac{\text{Desired } Css_{\text{average}}}{\text{Measured } Css_{\text{average}}} \times \text{Current dose}$$

(Eqn.2.5)

Concentrations that are not at steady state cannot be used in this way, although if accurate details of dosage history and sampling time are available, clearance may be estimated with the help of a pharmacokinetic computer package.

It is important to remember that drugs with non-linear kinetics (such as phenytoin) require special consideration and different techniques are applied to the interpretation of their concentrations.

Successful interpretation of a concentration measurement depends on accurate information. The minimum usually required is:

1 Time of sample collection with respect to the previous dose. Samples taken at inappropriate times may be misinterpreted. Usually, the simplest approach is to measure a trough concentration (i.e. at the end of the dosage interval). However, for some drugs (e.g. the aminoglycoside antibiotics), peaks may also be measured.

2 An accurate and detailed dosage history—drug dose, times of administration and route(s) of administration. This information can be used to assess if the sample represents steady state. Samples taken without knowledge of dosage history can result in an inappropriate clinical action or dosage adjustment.
3 Patient details such as age, sex, weight, serum creatinine (or creatinine clearance) and assessments of cardiac and hepatic function. This information helps to determine expected dose requirements and is necessary for all computerized interpretation methods. Knowledge about the stability of the patient can help to determine the frequency of monitoring, especially if the drug is renally cleared and renal function is changing.
4 Changes in other drug therapy that might influence the pharmacokinetics of the drug being measured.
5 The reason for requesting a drug analysis should be considered carefully. 'On admission' or 'routine' requests are usually of little value and are a waste of valuable resources.

2.5 Examples of therapeutic drug monitoring

Digoxin

Mr AR, a 78-year-old man weighing 72 kg and with a creatinine clearance of 24 ml/min, has been taking 250 μg digoxin daily to control atrial fibrillation. He presents to his general practitioner with anorexia and nausea a month after starting therapy. A digoxin concentration of 3.6 mg/l (4.6 nmol/l) is measured.

(i) Is this concentration expected?

His expected digoxin clearance can be calculated from Eqn. 2.1, i.e.

$$\begin{aligned}
\text{Digoxin clearance} \atop (\text{ml/min/kg}) &= \frac{24}{72} + 0.33 \\
&= 0.663 \text{ ml/min/kg} \\
&= 2.9 \text{ l/h}
\end{aligned}$$

His average steady-state concentration can be estimated from Eqn. 1.3, i.e.

$$\text{Predicted } Css_{average} = \frac{0.6 \times 250 \,\mu g}{2.9 \times 24 \,h}$$

$$= 2.2 \,\mu g/l \; (2.8 \,nmol/l)$$

where 0.6 represents the bioavailability of digoxin tablets.

The reason the measured concentration is higher than expected should be investigated. In this case, it was found that the sample had been withdrawn 2.5 h after the dose. Digoxin is absorbed quickly but distributes slowly to the tissues. Samples taken before distribution is complete (i.e. less than 6 h after the dose) cannot be interpreted. As concentrations only fall by about 20 % from 6 to 24 h after the dose, samples can be taken at any time during this period.

A further (trough) sample withdrawn 24 h after the last dose measured 2.4 μg/l (3.1 nmol/l). This result is more consistent with the expected concentration but suggests that the dose is too high and may be contributing to his symptoms.

(ii) What dose adjustment should be made?

Because digoxin has linear pharmacokinetics, the new dose can be determined by simple proportion. Table 2.4 shows that there are three dosage options for Mr AR. A reduction to 125 μg daily is the most obvious first choice but further adjustment (up or down) could be made if necessary on clinical grounds (e.g. poor control of atrial fibrillation or persistence of adverse effects).

Comment. This case illustrates the importance of sampling time for the correct interpretation of digoxin concentrations Although digoxin is traditionally prescribed to be taken in the morning, changing to a night-time dose can reduce the chances of samples being withdrawn during the distribution phase. Digoxin has a long elimination half-life (50–100 h) and elimination is slow beyond 6 h after the dose. If samples are taken at steady state, dosage adjustment can be performed by simple proportion.

Gentamicin

Mr JL, a 64-year-old man who weighs 80 kg and has an estimated creatinine clearance of 35 ml/min, requires gentamicin therapy for a suspected gram-negative infection. The aim is to achieve a peak concentration around 8 mg/l and a trough around 1 mg/l.

(i) What dosage regimen should be prescribed?

Gentamicin is cleared by excretion through the kidneys and its clearance can be approximated by creatinine clearance. The volume of distribution of gentamicin is around 0.25 l/kg (Table 1.3). A dosage interval of about 3 half-lives will allow the concentration to fall from 8 mg/l to 1 mg/l ($8 \rightarrow 4 \rightarrow 2 \rightarrow 1$). The elimination half-life can be calculated from Eqn. 1.9, i.e.

$$t_{1/2} = \frac{\ln 2}{k}$$

$$t_{1/2} = \frac{0.693 \times V}{Cl}$$

$$t_{1/2} = \frac{0.693 \times 0.25 \,l/kg \times 80 \,kg}{35 \,ml/min \times (60/1000)}$$

$$= \frac{0.693 \times 20 \,l}{2.1 \,l/h}$$

$$= 6.6 \,h$$

STEADY-STATE DIGOXIN		
Dose (μg)	$Css_{average}$ (μg/l)	Css_{trough} (mg/l)
250	3.0	2.4
187.5	2.2	1.8
125	1.5	1.2
62.5	0.75	0.6

Table 2.4 Predicted steady-state digoxin concentrations for Mr AR.

It will therefore take $3 \times 6.6 = 20\,h$ for the concentration to fall from 8 mg/l to 1 mg/l. Because the 'peak' is measured 1 h after the dose, the dosage interval should be 21 h. A 'practical' dosage interval is therefore 24 h. The dose administered should increase the concentration by 7 mg/l (i.e. from 1 to 8 mg/l). It can be calculated from the volume of distribution, i.e.

Dose (mg) $= 7\,mg/l \times 0.25\,l/kg \times 80\,kg$

$\qquad = 140\,mg$

Mr JL was started on a daily dose of 140 mg and after two days of therapy his peak concentration (1 h post dose) was 6 mg/l and his trough (24 h post dose) was 0.5 mg/l.

(ii) Has steady state been reached?

Mr JL's estimated elimination half-life is 6.6 h; therefore, steady state should be reached in $5 \times 6.6 = 33\,h$. He will be at steady state after two days of therapy.

(iii) How should the dose be adjusted?

The peak is slightly lower than the target and the trough is satisfactory. As these represent steady-state concentrations and gentamicin has linear pharmacokinetics, the dose can be adjusted by proportion. Increasing the dose to 200 mg daily should achieve a peak of $(200/140) \times 6 = 8.6\,mg/l$ and a trough of $(200/140) \times 0.5 = 0.7\,mg/l$.

Comment. Elimination half-life is a useful guide to dosage interval and is particularly important when the target concentration–time profile includes both peak and trough concentrations. In this case, because the peaks and troughs were both low, the dose can be adjusted by direct proportion. If the trough had been high, an increase in the dosage interval would also have been necessary.

Phenytoin

Mrs DL, a 38-year-old woman who weighs 55 kg, was prescribed phenytoin at a dose of 300 mg daily (5.5 mg/kg per day) after carbama-zepine failed to control her epilepsy. She attended the outpatient clinic 3 weeks later and her 24 h post dose trough phenytoin concentration was 6 mg/l (24 μmol/l). As her seizures were not well controlled, her dose was increased to 350 mg daily (6.4 mg/kg per day). She presented to her general practitioner 2 weeks later complaining of fatigue and difficulty in walking properly. Her trough phenytoin concentration was 28 mg/l (112 mol/l).

(i) Why was the first concentration so low?

There are two possibilities: the dose was too low; or she was not complying with her prescribed dose. As patients generally require phenytoin maintenance doses in the range 4.5–5 mg/kg per day, both doses were higher than average. Phenytoin has non-linear pharmacokinetics at concentrations normally seen clinically and standard pharmacokinetic equations cannot be used. The relationship between dose rate and average steady-state concentration is controlled by V_{max} (the maximum amount of drug that can be metabolized by the enzymes per day) and K_m (the concentration at half V_{max}). Using average values of V_{max} (7.2 mg/kg per day) and K_m (4.4 mg/l), Mrs DL's expected concentration can be calculated from the Michaelis–Menten equation (Eqn. 1.13), i.e.

$$\text{Dose rate} = \frac{V_{max} \times Css}{K_m + Css}$$

$$Css = \frac{\text{Dose rate} \times K_m}{V_{max} - \text{Dose rate}}$$

$$Css = \frac{300\,mg/day \times 4.4\,mg/l}{(7.2 \times 55)\,mg/day - 300\,mg/day}$$

$$= \frac{1320}{96}$$

$$= 14\,mg/l\ (55\,\mu mol/l)$$

The measured concentration of 6 mg/l is much lower than expected and suggests poor compliance with therapy.

STEADY-STATE PHENYTOIN		
	Steady-state concentration	
Dose (mg/day)	(mg/l)	(μmol/l)
225	6	24
250	7	28
275	9	36
300	13	52
325	18	72
350	28	112
375	55	220

Table 2.5 Predicted steady-state phenytoin concentrations for Mrs DL.

(ii) Why was the second concentration so high?

The predicted concentration on her increased dose can be calculated as before, i.e.

$$Css = \frac{350\,\text{mg/day} \times 4.4\,\text{mg/l}}{(7.2 \times 55)\,\text{mg/day} - 350\,\text{mg/day}}$$

$$= \frac{1540}{46}$$

$$= 33\,\text{mg/l}\ (147\,\mu\text{mol/l})$$

In this case, the measured concentration was reasonably consistent with the predicted value and her actual V_{max} can therefore be estimated from the measured concentration, i.e.

$$V_{max}(\text{mg/day}) = \frac{\text{Dose rate} \times (K_m + Css)}{Css}$$

$$V_{max}(\text{mg/day}) = \frac{350\,(\text{mg/day}) \times (4.4 + 28)\,\text{mg/l}}{28\,\text{mg/l}}$$

$$= 405\,\text{mg/day}$$

Using her actual V_{max} and a K_m of 4.4 mg/l, average steady-state concentrations can be predicted for various doses (Table 2.5). Note that a small change in the dose produces a disproportionately large increase in concentration, especially at higher concentrations.

(N.B. A number of nomograms and graphical approaches are available to estimate V_{max} and K_m but they are beyond the scope of this text.)

It is known that a concentration of 6 mg/l does not control her seizures and she experiences toxicity with 28 mg/l. Her ideal dose is therefore likely to lie in the range 275–325 mg daily. It would be sensible to start with 300 mg daily and adjust the dose (if necessary) according to her response. It would also be useful to emphasize to the patient that she must comply with her prescribed dose in order to obtain the maximum benefit from her therapy.

Comment. This case illustrates the non-linearity of phenytoin dose-concentration relationships and the difficulty of interpreting phenytoin concentrations when dosage history is uncertain (as frequently occurs with outpatients). It also demonstrates the value of using serial measurements (the two results were clearly inconsistent with each other) and average dose requirements to assess compliance.

CHAPTER 3

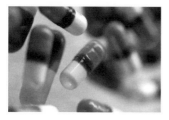

Influence of Disease on Pharmacokinetics and Pharmacodynamics

Drugs are usually considered in terms of their effect on disease processes. However, several diseases can influence the pharmacokinetics of a drug or its pharmacological effect on target organs. This is of considerable clinical importance when diseases of the liver or kidney modify drug elimination, or drug distribution and elimination are altered in congestive cardiac failure.

3.1 Influence of gastrointestinal disease

Oesophageal dysmotility

In our increasingly aged population non-specific disorders of oesophageal motility are more common. Although relatively rare, oesophageal spasm in presenting elderly patients may be associated with neurodegenerative diseases such as Parkinson's disease. In such patients there is an increased risk of drug-induced oesophageal injury. Tablet or pill size makes a considerable difference to the ease of swallowing; large round objects are more difficult to swallow and show significantly higher incidence of impaction in the oesophagus (when wetted) when muco-adhesive coats rather than film coats are used. The precise nature of the drug is not always relevant because any tablet which impacts and releases its contents locally will cause irritation, owing to hypertonicity. The chemical nature of the substance may in some cases be relevant, e.g. iron tablets that are directly toxic.

Achlorhydria

Achlorhydria occurs in around 10% of the elderly population, usually as a result of Helicobacter-induced atrophic gastritis. Iatrogenic achlorhydria is becoming increasingly commonly mainly in patients taking proton pump inhibitors for reflux oesophagitis. This will inhibit the absorption rate of drugs such as doxycycline monohydrate, ketaconazole, whose dissolution and absorption is optimum with an acid gastric pH. Theophylline absorption appears to be increased because of slower small intestinal transit. The absorption rate of solid formulations of aspirin is increased because the higher pH increases its rate of dissolution.

Achlorhydria is induced deliberately by proton pump inhibitors (PPIs) in order to enhance the bioavailability of acid labile drugs, and in particular macrolides such as clarithromycin. This is important in the treatment of Helicobacter pylori; the amount of clarithromycin that remains after 1 h at pH 1 is about 10% but the use of PPIs to raise the pH to 6 can increase this to 90%. Proton pump inhibitors also increase the bioavailability of acid labile penicillins such as benzylpenicillin.

Coeliac disease

There are several pathophysiological factors that can influence drug absorption. Loss of absorptive surface area decreases absorption along with impairment of fat absorption. However first pass metabolism by enterocytes is also decreased and this increases the bioavailability of drugs such as oestrogens, which are usually inactivated by enterocyte sulphatases. Other changes are an increased surface mucosal pH related to the loss of villi and increase in crypt/villous ratio. This enhances the absorption of some drugs, e.g. propranolol, but decreases that of folic acid, a weak acid whose ionization will increase at the higher pH and, hence, reduce the amount of the most readily absorbed, un-ionized form of the drug.

As a result of these varying influences, the outcome is hard to predict with some drugs showing decreased absorption, e.g. amoxicillin (amoxycillin) and pivampicillin, but with others showing increased absorption, e.g. cefalexin (cephalexin). Decreased absorption of dietary folate contributes to the frequent low red cell folate and may increase the risk of bone marrow toxicity from cotrimoxazole.

Dapsone, which may be given to treat coeliac-associated dermatitis herpetiformis, has an impaired absorption in untreated coeliac patients who may need to go on a gluten free diet to get the full benefit of dapsone.

Drugs that are lipid soluble or are absorbed after dissolution in micelles such as vitamin D are usually malabsorbed and may best be given by injection.

Crohn's disease

The characteristic features are focal inflammation with fibrosis and fistulation affecting either the small or large intestine or both. There are subtle defects with villous atrophy reducing the upper small intestinal absorptive area, although this effect is probably small. The biggest effect is diarrhoea, possibly through cytokine-mediated mechanisms and the presence of anaerobic bacteria within the small bowel when colo-intestinal fistulae develop. This bacterial contamination induces fat malabsorption and will impair the absorption of fat-soluble drugs. Rapid transits through the colon and lower small intestine will induce a degree of impairment of the enterohepatic recirculation. This may make certain drugs less effective, e.g. enterohepatic recirculation

of oestrogen is important in maintaining efficacy of the oral contraceptive pill.

The greatest effect is seen after bowel resection which, if repeated, may end up with a short bowel syndrome with malabsorption of many substances including drugs and nutrients and water. Terminal ileal resections may impair vitamin B_{12} absorption.

Comment. Many factors can influence drug absorption when the gastrointestinal tract is abnormal. The presence of a malabsorption syndrome does not imply that drugs are necessarily malabsorbed: the absorption of some can actually increase. Currently there is insufficient information to comment on the clinical importance of these changes, but, theoretically, treatment failure may occur because of malabsorption and drug toxicity may be a consequence of increased absorption. Clinically relevant changes in drug absorption are most likely to result from fat malabsorption and diarrhoea.

3.2 Influence of impaired renal function

Impaired renal function can influence drug therapy for the following reasons:
1 Pharmacokinetics may be altered as a result of:
    (a) Decreased elimination of drugs that are normally excreted entirely or mainly by the kidneys.
    (b) Decreased protein binding.
    (c) Decreased hepatic metabolism.
2 Drug effect may be altered.
3 Existing clinical condition may be worsened.
4 Adverse effects may be enhanced.

Each of these factors is now considered in more detail.

Altered pharmacokinetics

Elimination

Because the kidney represents one of the major routes of drug elimination, a decline in renal function can influence the clearance of many drugs. If a drug normally cleared by the kidney is given to someone with decreased renal function without altering the dose, the steady-state blood concentrations of that drug will be increased. This is of considerable importance in the case of drugs showing concentration-related effects, particularly those that have a narrow therapeutic range.

When such drugs are given to patients with renal dysfunction, the general aim is to achieve similar concentrations to those seen in patients with normal kidneys.

Therapeutic concentrations can be maintained by:

1 Determining renal function, usually by estimating creatinine clearance.

2 Modifying the dose using a nomogram, either increasing the dosage interval, giving a lower dose at the same interval or by altering both the dose and the interval. The extent and precision of dose modification depend very much on the toxicity of the drug concerned. In the case of the aminoglycosides, even minor impairment of renal function requires some dosage alteration, while the dose of penicillins need only be reduced in severe renal failure (creatinine clearance <10 ml/min). Guidance on dosage modification is readily available for most commonly used drugs.

It should be noted that the loading dose is usually not changed by renal impairment because this depends more on the volume of distribution of the drug than its rate of elimination.

3 Monitoring drug concentrations. This is useful for drugs with concentration-related adverse effects, such as the aminoglycosides, digoxin, aminophylline, phenytoin and carbamazepine, and mandatory for lithium, ciclosporin (cyclosporin) and methotrexate. Nomograms are useful guides to the doses likely to be appropriate, but every patient is different. Concentrations of drugs in the blood can be used to assess clearance and to determine the most appropriate dose for individual patients.

Decreased protein binding

The following changes occur in patients with impaired renal function:

1 Acidic drugs are less bound to serum albumin and the decrease in binding correlates with the severity of renal impairment. The binding of basic drugs (to α_1 acid glycoprotein) undergoes little or no change.

2 The structure of albumin is changed in renal failure and endogenous compounds may compete with drugs for binding.

3 Haemodialysis does not return binding to normal but renal transplantation does.

In most cases changes in protein binding have limited clinical relevance and do not require alterations in dose. However, protein binding is important for the interpretation of serum phenytoin concentrations.

Hepatic metabolism

The hepatic metabolism of some drugs (e.g. nicardipine, propranolol) may be decreased in patients with renal failure. The reasons for this are not clear, but may indicate the presence of a metabolic inhibitor in uraemic plasma because regular haemodialysis appears to normalize the clearance of these compounds.

Altered drug effect

There are several examples of increased drug sensitivity in patients with renal failure. Opiates, barbiturates, phenothiazines and benzodiazepines all show greater effects on the nervous system in patients with renal failure than in those with normal renal function. The reasons are not known, but increased meningeal permeability is one possible explanation.

Various antihypertensive drugs have a greater postural effect in renal failure. Again the reasons are not clear, but changes in serum balance and autonomic dysfunction may be partly responsible.

Worsening of the existing clinical condition

Drug therapy can result in deterioration of the clinical condition in the following ways:

1 By further impairing renal function. In patients with renal failure it is clearly advisable to avoid drugs that are known to be nephrotoxic and for which alternatives are available. Examples include aminoglycosides, amphotericin, cisplatin, gold, mesalazine, non-steroidal anti-inflammatories, penicillamine and vancomycin.

2 By causing fluid retention. Fluid balance is a major problem in the more severe forms of renal failure. Drugs that cause fluid retention should therefore be avoided, e.g. carbenoxolone and non-steroidal anti-inflammatory drugs (NSAIDs) such as indometacin (indomethacin).

3 By increasing the degree of uraemia. Tetracyclines, except doxycycline, have an anti-anabolic effect and should be avoided.

Enhancement of adverse drug effects

In addition to decreased elimination, digoxin is more likely to cause adverse effects in patients with severe renal failure if there are substantial electrolyte abnormalities, particularly hypercalcaemia and/or hypokalaemia.

Because potassium elimination is impaired in renal failure, diuretics that also conserve potassium (amiloride, spironolactone) are more likely to cause hyperkalaemia.

3.3   Influence of liver disease

Impaired liver function can influence the response to treatment in several ways.

1 Altered pharmacokinetics:
(a) Increased bioavailability resulting from reduced first-pass metabolism or, potentially, decreased first-pass activation of pro-drugs.
(b) Decreased protein binding.
(c) Decreased elimination.

2 Altered drug effect.

3 Worsening of metabolic state.

Altered pharmacokinetics

The liver is the largest organ in the body, has a substantial blood supply (around 1.5 l/min) and is interposed between the gastrointestinal tract and the systemic circulation. For these reasons it is uniquely suited for the purpose of influencing drug pharmacokinetics.

Decreased first-pass metabolism

A decrease in hepatocellular function decreases the capacity of the liver to perform metabolic processes, while portosystemic shunting directs drugs away from sites of metabolism. Both factors are usually present in patients with severe cirrhosis.

Knowledge of the drugs that undergo first-pass metabolism is important in situations where it is decreased as a result of disease. Considerably greater quantities of active drug then reach the site of action and any given dose of drug has unexpectedly intense effects.

Examples of changes in bioavailability found in some patients with severe cirrhosis are:
• Clomethiazole (chlormethiazole) (100% increase)
• Labetalol (91% increase)
• Metoprolol (65% increase)
• Nicardipine (500% increase)
• Paracetamol (50% increase)
• Propranolol (42% increase)
• Verapamil (140% increase).

Conversely, first-pass activation of pro-drugs such as many ACE inhibitors (e.g. enalapril, perindopril, quinapril) may potentially be slowed or reduced.

Decreased elimination by liver metabolism and decreased protein binding

High extraction drugs

These are drugs that the liver metabolizes at a very high rate. Their bioavailability is low and their clearance is dependent mainly upon the rate of drug delivery to the enzyme systems. The clearance of these drugs is therefore relatively sensitive to factors which can influence hepatic blood flow, such as congestive cardiac failure, and relatively insensitive to small changes in enzyme activity or protein binding. Examples include labetalol, lidocaine, metoprolol, morphine, propranolol, pethidine, nortriptyline and verapamil.

Low extraction drugs
In low extraction drugs the rate of metabolism is sufficiently low that hepatic clearance is relatively insensitive to changes in hepatic blood flow, and dependent mainly on the capacity of the liver enzymes. Examples include chloramphenicol, paracetamol and theophylline. The hepatic clearance of drugs in this group that are also highly protein bound, such as diazepan, tolbutamide, phenytoin and valproic acid, depends on both the capacity of the enzymes and the free fraction; it is thus difficult to predict the consequences of hepatic disease on total drug concentration. However, as with renal disease, care must be taken in the interpretation of concentrations of highly protein bound drugs such as phenytoin.

The influence of liver disease on drug elimination is complex: the type of liver disease is critical. In acute viral hepatitis the major change is in hepatocellular function, but drug-metabolizing ability usually remains intact and hepatic blood flow can increase. Mild to moderate cirrhosis tends to result in decreased hepatic blood flow and portosystemic shunting, while severe cirrhosis usually shows reduction both in cellular function and blood flow. Cholestasis leads to impaired fat absorption with deficiencies of fat-soluble vitamins and impairment of absorption of lipophillic drugs. Alcoholic liver disease is common and chronic ethanol abuse is associated with increased activity of the microsomal ethanol-oxidizing system. This effect is a result primarily of induction by ethanol of a specific cytochrome P-450 (CYP2E1) responsible for enhanced oxidation of ethanol and other P-450 substrates and, consequently, for metabolic tolerance to these substances. This may lead to enhanced clearance and, hence, decreased response to certain drugs such as benzodiazepine sedatives, anticonvulsants (phenytoin) and warfarin. By contrast, simultaneous alcohol ingestion may decrease clearance of drugs metabolized via the P-450 (CYP2E1) enzyme system.

Comment. Unlike the measurement of creatinine clearance in renal disease, there is no simple test that can predict the extent to which drug metabolism is decreased in liver disease. A low serum albumin, raised bilirubin and prolonged prothrombin time give a rough guide.

The fact that a drug is metabolized by the liver does not necessarily mean that its pharmacokinetics are altered by liver disease. It is not easy, therefore, to extrapolate the findings from one drug to another. This is because superficially similar metabolic pathways are mediated by different forms of cytochrome P-450.

The documentation of modestly altered pharmacokinetics does not necessarily imply clinical importance. Even normal subjects show quite wide variations in pharmacokinetic indices and therefore pharmacokinetics should not be viewed in isolation from alterations in drug effect, which are much more difficult to assess. However, if a drug is known to be subject to substantial pharmacokinetic changes, clinical significance is much more likely.

If it is clinically desirable to give a drug that is eliminated by liver metabolism to a patient with cirrhosis, it should be started at a low dose and the drug levels or effect monitored very closely.

Altered drug effect

Deranged brain function
The more severe forms of liver disease are accompanied by poorly understood derangements of brain function that ultimately result in the syndrome of hepatic encephalopathy. However, even before encephalopathy develops, the brain is extremely sensitive to the effects of centrally acting drugs and a state of coma can result from administering normal doses of opiates or benzodiazepines to such patients.

Decreased clotting factors

Patients with liver disease show increased sensitivity to oral anticoagulants. These drugs exert their effect by decreasing the vitamin K dependent synthesis of clotting factors II, VII, IX and X. When the production of these factors is already reduced by liver disease, a given dose of oral anticoagulant has a greater effect than in subjects with normal liver function.

Worsening of metabolic state

Drug-induced alkalosis

Excessive use of diuretics can precipitate encephalopathy. The mechanism involves hypokalaemic alkalosis, which results in conversion of NH_4^+ to NH_3, the un-ionized ammonia crossing easily into the central nervous system (CNS) to worsen or precipitate encephalopathy.

Fluid overload

Patients with advanced liver disease often have oedema and ascites secondary to hypoalbuminaemia and portal hypertension. This problem can be worsened by drugs that cause fluid retention, e.g. NSAIDs, and antacids that contain large amounts of sodium. NSAIDs should be avoided anyway, because of the increased risk of gastrointestinal bleeding.

Hepatotoxic drugs (Table 3.1)

Where an acceptable alternative exists, it is wise to avoid drugs that can cause liver damage, e.g. sulphonamides, rifampicin, and repeated exposure to halothane anaesthesia.

3.4   Influence of congestive heart failure

Congestive heart failure can influence drug kinetics in the following ways:
- Decreased rate or extent of gastrointestinal absorption, e.g. hydrochlorothiazide and metolazone.
- Altered volume of distribution, e.g. lidocaine and aminoglycosides.

- Decreased elimination, e.g. lidocaine, theophylline.

Altered pharmacokinetics

Decreased gastrointestinal absorption

The main factors involved are:
1 Mucosal oedema.
2 Reduced epithelial blood supply.
3 Splanchnic vasoconstriction.
4 Reduced secretion of bile salts leading to fat malabsorption.

The most important effect is impaired absorption of fat-soluble vitamins A, D, E and K, which is common in childhood cholestatic disease. This leads to osteomalacia, prolonged clotting and neurological defects. Oral vitamin supplements may need to be replaced in the more advanced stages by the better absorbed alphacalcidol (vitamin D analogue) and D-alpha-tocopheryl polyethylene glycol 1000 succinate (vitamin K analogue). This latter preparation is a water-soluble form of vitamin K that forms micelles, and when given with vitamin D actually enhances its absorption.

Altered volume of distribution

Decreased volume is thought to result from decreased tissue perfusion and is clearly documented for lidocaine. Therefore, for any given dose, higher blood concentrations are achieved. The practical importance of this is that initial loading doses should be correspondingly reduced. Conversely, increased volumes can be observed for water-soluble drugs (such as the aminoglycosides) in the presence of oedema. In this case higher doses would be required to achieve target peak concentrations.

Decreased elimination

The main factors involved for the liver are:
1 Decreased perfusion.
2 Decreased oxidizing capacity due to hypoxia.
3 Decreased metabolizing capacity due to congestion.

For the kidney they are:

DRUGS CAUSING LIVER DAMAGE

Hepatitis
Halothane (repeated exposure)
Isoniazid
Rifampicin
Methyldopa
Phenelzine
Trimipramine
Desipramine
Carbimazepine
Trasidone
Propylthiouracil
Augmentin
Erythromycin
Nitrofurantoin
Chloroguanidee
Tienilic acid
Dihydralazine
Azothiaprine
Sulfasalazine (sulphasalazine)
Naproxen
Amiodarone

Cholestasis with mild hepatic component
Phenothiazines
Carbamazepine
Tricyclic antidepressants
Non-steroidal anti-inflammatory drugs (especially phenylbutazone)
Rifampicin, ethambutol, pyrazinamide
Sulphonylureas, trimethoprin
Sulphonamides, ampicillin, nitrofurantoin, erythromycin estolate
Oral contraceptives (stasis without hepatitis)

Cirrhosis
Methotrexate

Table 3.1 Drugs that can cause liver damage.

1 Decreased glomerular filtration rate.
2 Increased tubular reabsorption.

The clearance of lidocaine is dependent upon liver blood flow and in heart failure it can be reduced by up to 50%. For theophylline the metabolic capacity of the liver is important and again clearance is reduced in heart failure (Chapter 2, Table 2.3). As these drugs have concentration-related toxicity, the rate of administration must be reduced in heart failure and therapeutic drug monitoring may be used to adjust therapy.

3.5 Influence of thyroid disease

Thyroid disease alters a patient's response to digoxin. Hyperthyroid patients are relatively resistant to the drug while hypothyroid patients are extremely sensitive to it. The reasons are in part kinetic and in part dynamic. The volume of distribution of digoxin is lower in hypothyroidism and higher in hyperthyroidism and its clearance is roughly proportional to thyroid function. Consequently, for any given dose lower concentrations are achieved in hyperthyroid patients and higher concentrations are achieved in hypothyroid patients compared to normal patients. In addition, hypothyroid patients may experience adverse effects at relatively low concentrations while hyperthyroid patients often require higher concentrations, and possibly additional drugs, to control atrial fibrillation.

Lithium can cause hypothyroidism by inhibiting the release of thyroid hormone from the gland. It is important to recognize this complication in order to avoid mistaking hypothyroidism for a relapse in the depressive illness. Thyroxin can be prescribed concurrently with lithium.

CHAPTER 4

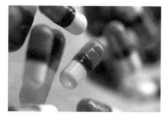

Drugs and the Elderly

The elderly (65 years and over) constitute approximately 16% of the population yet they consume 40% of the drug prescriptions in the UK. Two-thirds of those over the age of 65 receive regular medication. This high consumption of drugs is related to an increasing prevalence of acute and chronic disease, resulting in increasing numbers of prescriptions (see p. 36). Multiple drug prescribing can lead to problems with compliance and carries increased risk of side effects. The overall incidence of drug side effects in the elderly is up to three times that seen in the young. Adverse drug reactions in the elderly tend to be dose related rather than idiosyncratic and are related to changes in pharmacokinetics and pharmacodynamics. The drugs that have the highest incidence of side effects in the elderly are those that are most commonly prescribed (sedatives, diuretics and non-steroidal anti-inflammatory drugs). However, in one study, insulin and nitrofurantoin had the highest incidence of adverse effects when related to the total number of doses administered.

Drug absorption, distribution, metabolism, excretion and activity can all change as a result of ageing. However, the presence of multiple pathology in the old frequently has a greater effect than ageing alone.

4.1 Drug absorption

Ageing is associated with increased gastric pH, delayed gastric emptying, decreased intestinal motility and reduced splanchnic blood flow.

PRESCRIBING FOR THE ELDERLY

1 Make an accurate diagnosis. The presentation of disease in the elderly is often non-specific (e.g. confusion, dizziness and incontinence). It is important to make an accurate diagnosis to allow appropriate therapy.
2 Treat only important disorders. Elderly patients frequently have multiple pathology. This can lead to polypharmacy with a resultant increase in side effects and poor compliance.
3 Avoid ineffective drugs. Prescriptions for marginally effective or ineffective drugs can only lead to side effects and poor compliance. It should be remembered that there is no drug treatment for dementia and those advertised for the treatment of atherosclerosis or urinary incontinence have little, if any, measurable effect.
4 Review drugs regularly. It is important to review the need for each prescription. If a drug is considered necessary, make sure the minimum dose required is used.
5 Understand the changes in pharmacology with age for each drug used, remembering that relative renal insufficiency is very common in the elderly.

Despite these changes, there is little evidence to suggest that intestinal drug absorption changes with age. For example, the rate of absorption of digoxin is slower in the elderly but the overall bioavailability remains the same.

4.2 Drug distribution

Age-related changes in body composition, in protein binding and in organ blood flow can all affect drug disposition.

Ageing is associated with a relative increase in body fat and corresponding reduction in body water. The volume of distribution of water-soluble drugs is smaller and this tends to cause an increase in initial drug concentration (e.g. digoxin and cimetidine). Lipid-soluble drugs tend to have an increased volume of distribution (e.g. nitrazepam and diazepam) which prolongs the elimination half-life and may prolong effect.

The extent of plasma protein-drug binding changes little with age but the plasma albumin may fall considerably with the onset of disease. There is no strong evidence that protein binding interactions are more common in the elderly than in the young.

4.3 Drug metabolism and age

There is evidence for age-related changes in the rates of metabolism of some drugs. In general, drugs that undergo microsomal oxidation (e.g. chlordiazepoxide) are likely to be metabolized more slowly in the elderly. Despite this, there is no evidence that the concentration or activity of hepatic microsomal oxidizing enzymes is reduced in the elderly. The age-related reduction in oxidizing capacity may be related to the reduction in hepatic volume and blood flow that occurs in the elderly. Conjugation pathways do not appear to be affected by age. Overall, the changes in metabolism with age alone are not of great clinical significance.

First-pass metabolism may be reduced considerably in the elderly (see below). This is probably the consequence of the age-associated reduction in liver mass and blood flow. As a result, drugs that undergo extensive first-pass metabolism (e.g. labetolol and propranolol) may show considerably increased bioavailability in the elderly.

This effect is amplified by the presence of chronic liver disease.

4.4 Renal excretion

In old age there is a fall in both renal blood flow and renal function. Glomerular filtration falls by approximately 30% by the age of 65 years, compared with young adults. Digoxin and the aminoglycoside antibiotics are excreted mainly by glomerular filtration and these will tend to accumulate in the elderly if the dose is not reduced. Renal tubular function also declines and drugs such as penicillin and procainamide, which undergo active tubular secretion, have a marked reduction in clearance. In addition, the elderly are more likely to suffer a further reduction in renal function as a result of renal tract disease such as infection. Illness in the elderly is frequently accompanied by dehydration and this reduces renal function even further. The overall effect of physiological ageing and disease considerably diminishes the elderly kidney's capacity to excrete drugs.

4.5 Receptor sensitivity

In practice, it is very difficult to assess accurately drug receptor numbers or sensitivity. In most cases information is derived from drug effect related to drug plasma concentration. Using this approach it can be shown that the elderly are more sensitive to the effect of benzodiazepine drugs such as nitrazepam, temazepam and diazepam. Warfarin is more potent in the elderly because of a greater effect on coagulation factor synthesis

PHARMACOKINETICS/PHARMACODYNAMICS IN THE ELDERLY

Reduced first-pass metabolism
- propranolol (in sick elderly)

Reduced protein binding (in sick elderly)
- phenytoin
- diazepam

Increased volume of distribution (relative increased body fat)
- diazepam

Decreased hepatic oxidation
- chloridiazepoxide

Decreased renal excretion
- digoxin
- gentamicin
- cimetidine

Decreased drug-receptor sensitivity
- cardiac $beta_1$–adrenoceptor drugs

Increased drug-receptor sensitivity
- warfarin
- benzodiazepines

and this is a reflection of the increased receptor affinity to warfarin that occurs in the elderly.

Perhaps most is known about the effects of ageing on the autonomic receptors. On the one hand there is a modest decline in the tachycardia produced by stimulation of $beta_1$–adrenoceptors; on the other, there appears to be no age-related change in $beta_2$–adrenoceptor-mediated vascular or bronchial relaxation. The effect of the vasconstrictor $alpha_1$–adrenoceptor is also unchanged with age.

4.6 Impairment of homeostasis

The effect of drugs in the elderly may be affected by a loss of homeostatic control that is often seen in the elderly patient.

Cardiovascular postural reflexes are commonly less effective in the aged. Elderly patients tend to fall more easily than the young and this is made worse by the use of drugs that cause postural hypotension. There are many such drugs, including diuretics, antihypertensive agents and sedatives.

The elderly have impaired thermoregulation. Many of the major tranquillizers may precipitate hypothermia. This is the result not only of a direct hypothermic effect, but also of a reduction in physical activity.

4.7 Compliance

There is no evidence that an elderly patient whose mental function is normal is more likely to make mistakes with their medication than a younger patient. However, one of the main contributory factors to poor drug compliance at all ages is polypharmacy—the rate of errors when three drugs are prescribed is approximately 20% but it is close to 100% when 10 drugs are prescribed—and the high consumption of drugs in the elderly results in a greater opportunity to make errors. This is often made worse by the prevalence of mental impairment, which is as high as 25% in those over the age of 85 years. Physical handicap can also contribute to poor compliance. Arthritic hands have great difficulty in opening 'child-proof' containers or 'bubble-packed' drugs.

CHAPTER 5

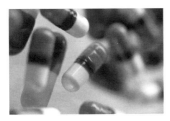

Drugs in Pregnant and Breast Feeding Women

Nearly 40% of women in the UK take at least one drug during pregnancy, excluding iron, vitamins and drugs used during delivery. Once in the maternal circulation, drugs are separated from the fetus by a lipid placental membrane, which any given drug crosses to a greater or lesser extent depending on the physicochemical properties of the molecule.

Drugs in pregnancy can be viewed from two standpoints:
1 Effect of drugs on the fetus.
2 Effect of pregnancy on the drug.

5.1 Effect of drugs on the fetus

Drugs can influence fetal development at three separate stages:
1 Fertilization and implantation period: conception to about 17 days gestation.
2 Organogenesis: 18–55 days.
3 Growth and development: 56 days onward.

The possible consequences of drug exposure are quite different at each stage. In addition, drugs given at the end of pregnancy can influence structure or function in the neonate.

Fertilization and implantation period

Interference by a drug with either of these processes leads to failure of the pregnancy at a very early and probably subclinical stage. Therefore, very little is known about drugs that influence this process in the human.

Organogenesis

It is during this period that the developing embryo shows great sensitivity to the teratogenic effects of drugs. A teratogen is any substance (virus, environmental toxin or drug) that produces deformity. Before discussing the teratogenic properties of certain drugs, the following points must be appreciated:
1 Teratogenesis in the human is very difficult to predict from animal studies because of considerable species variation. Thalidomide, the most notorious drug teratogen of recent times, showed no teratogenicity in mice and rats.
2 Serious congenital deformities are present in 1–2% of all babies; therefore, a drug is only readily identified as teratogenic if its effects are frequent, unusual and/or serious. A low-grade teratogen that infrequently causes minor deformities is likely to pass unnoticed.

Table 5.1 lists some drugs that are known to be teratogenic. It is important to realize that, even for known teratogens, first trimester use often results in a normal baby, e.g. phenytoin is teratogenic in about 5% of exposures and warfarin in up to 25%. Also, there will be occasions, such as the use of warfarin in women with prosthetic heart valves, where the risks to the mother of not using the drug outweigh the risks of exposure in the fetus.

Comment. The greatest risk of teratogenesis occurs at a time when a woman might not even be aware that she is pregnant. Only a

KNOWN TERATOGENS

Drug	Deformity
Danazol	Virilization of female fetus
Lithium	Cardiac (Ebstein's complex)
Phenytoin	Craniofacial; limb
Carbamazepine	Craniofacial; limb
Primidone	Facial clefting; cardiac
Retinoids	Central nervous system
Sodium valproate	Neural tube
Diethylstilbestrol (stilboestrol)	Adenocarcinoma of vagina in teenage years
Warfarin	Multiple defects; chondrodysplasia punctata

Table 5.1 Drugs which are known to be teratogenic.

few drugs are known definitely to be teratogenic, but many more could be under certain circumstances. When prescribing for a woman of childbearing age, remember that she might be pregnant and ask yourself if the benefits of drug use outweigh the risks, however small, of teratogenesis.

Growth and development
During this stage major body structures have been formed, and it is their subsequent development and function that can be affected:

1 Antithyroid drugs cross the placenta and can cause fetal and neonatal hypothyroidism.
2 Tetracyclines inhibit bone growth and discolour teeth.
3 Angiotensin converting enzyme inhibitors can seriously damage fetal kidney function.
4 Warfarin can cause bleeding into the fetal brain.
5 Drugs with dependence potential, e.g. benzodiazepines, opiates and dextropropoxyphene, which are taken regularly during pregnancy can result in withdrawal symptoms in the neonate.

Drugs given at the end of pregnancy
1 Aspirin in analgesic doses can cause haemorrhage in the neonate.

2 Indometacin (and possibly high doses of aspirin) causes premature closure of the ductus arteriosus with resulting pulmonary hypertension.
3 Central nervous system (CNS) depressant drugs (e.g. opiates, benzodiazepines) can cause hypotension, respiratory depression and hypothermia in the neonate.

5.2 Effect of pregnancy on drug absorption, distribution and elimination

The substantial physiological changes that occur in pregnancy can influence drug disposition, while pathological conditions in pregnancy can accentuate these changes.

Drug distribution
Maternal plasma volume and extracellular fluid volume increase by about 50% by the last trimester, and this should decrease the steady-state concentration of drugs with a small volume of distribution. Considerable changes in protein concentration occur during the last trimester, with serum albumin falling by about 20% while alpha$_1$–acid glycoprotein increases in concentration by about 40% in normal pregnancies. These changes are accentuated in pre-eclampsia, with albumin concen-

tration falling by about 35% and glycoprotein rising by as much as 100%. This means that the free fraction of acidic drugs can increase substantially, while that of basic drugs can be decreased greatly, in the last trimester. Diazepam, phenytoin and sodium valproate have been shown to have significantly elevated free fractions in the last trimester.

Drug elimination

Effective renal plasma flow doubles by the end of pregnancy but this has been shown to be important in only a few cases; for example, the clearance of ampicillin doubles and the dose must also be doubled for systemic (but of course not for renal tract) infections. The hepatic microsomal mixed function oxidase system undergoes induction in pregnancy, probably as the result of high circulating levels of progesterone. This leads to an increased clearance of drugs that undergo metabolism by this pathway, and there is evidence that the steady-state concentrations of the anticonvulsants sodium valproate, phenytoin, carbamazepine and phenobarbital are decreased to a clinically significant extent during the

second and third trimesters. Therefore, higher doses are required as the pregnancy progresses, with careful monitoring of drug concentrations.

5.3 Drug treatment of common medical problems during pregnancy

Infection

Urinary tract infections are common during pregnancy. Penicillins are the preferred treatment (subject to appropriate sensitivity testing), because these drugs have never been implicated in teratogenesis and are generally well tolerated. Nitrofurantoin is not harmful to the fetus but frequently causes nausea. Tetracyclines are contraindicated (Table 5.2). Co-trimoxazole should be avoided. In early pregnancy, the trimethoprim component can possibly cause limb reduction and cleft palate, while at the end of pregnancy the sulphonamide component can cross the placenta and displace bilirubin from protein-binding sites in the neonate.

DRUGS TO AVOID IN BREAST FEEDING	
Drug	Effect of drug
Amiodarone	Iodine content may cause neonatal hypothyroidism
Aspirin	Theoretical risk of Reye's syndrome
Barbiturates	Drowsiness
Benzodiazepines	Lethargy
Carbimazole	Use lowest effective dose to avoid hypothyroidism
Contraceptives (combined oral)	May diminish milk supply and reduce nitrogen and protein content
Cytotoxic drugs	Potential problems include immune suppression and neutropenia
Ephedrine	Irritability
Tetracyclines	Theoretical risk of tooth discoloration

Table 5.2 Commonly used drugs which should be avoided in women who are breast feeding.

Fortunately, severe infections in pregnancy are rare. Aminoglycosides cause fetal eighth nerve damage, and the benefits of their use must be seen in this context. At present there is no evidence to suggest fetal damage from cephalosporins, metronidazole or chloramphenicol. However, chloramphenicol can cause cardiovascular collapse in neonates and should not be used at the end of pregnancy unless absolutely necessary.

In the case of tuberculosis, both isoniazid and ethambutol have been used extensively during pregnancy, including the first trimester, with no fetal defects. The incidence of fetal deformity following rifampicin is three times greater than with isoniazid or ethambutol, and this drug should be avoided in the first trimester if possible. Streptomycin definitely causes auditory deficit and should not be used.

Diabetes mellitus

Diabetic pregnancies are associated with a twofold increase in perinatal mortality. Liveborn neonates are prone to respiratory distress syndrome, hypoglycaemia, hypocalcaemia and jaundice. The aim of therapy is obsessionally to maintain preprandial blood glucose concentrations between 3 and 6 mmol/l (55–110 mg/100 ml). The adequacy of therapy in the short term is monitored by daily preprandial glucose estimation.

Gestational diabetes, i.e. the development of mild glucose intolerance during pregnancy, can sometimes be managed adequately by carbohydrate restriction. If this fails, insulin is used.

Insulin is usually given as twice daily injections of a highly purified preparation containing a mixture of short- and intermediate-acting types. Insulin-dependent diabetics who are on different regimens should be changed when they become pregnant or, preferably, before conception. Insulin requirements often increase from around the 15th to the 30th week of pregnancy, remain constant until delivery and then fall rapidly to prepregnancy levels. Therefore, daily monitoring of blood glucose is mandatory to maintain normoglycaemia.

Asthma

Poorly controlled asthma is associated with increased perinatal mortality. Maternal hypoxia and respiratory alkalosis are the major determinants of fetal distress in asthmatic pregnancies. Theophylline, salbutamol by metered aerosol, and steroids have good safety records at all stages of pregnancy. There has been little experience with newer bronchodilators.

Pregnancy should not alter the general approach to asthma as described in Chapter 11. It is important to control bronchospasm and avoid prolonged abnormalities of blood gases or acid–base balance.

Epilepsy

The main issues are possible teratogenicity associated with anticonvulsants and the need for therapeutic drug level monitoring to control fits.

The incidence of congenital malformations in children of epileptic mothers is about 5% (see Table 5.1, p. 38), which is three times higher than in the general population. In part, this could reflect a genetic predisposition, but anticonvulsants seem largely to be responsible. Cleft palate and congenital heart disease are the most common findings. Troxidone, phenytoin and phenobarbital are almost certainly teratogenic. Sodium valproate probably increases the likelihood of neural tube defects. Coadministration of anticonvulsants produces a greater risk than when either drug is used alone.

At the present time the guidelines shown below seem appropriate to the management of pregnant epileptics.

The pharmacokinetic changes associated with pregnancy are clinically important in the treatment of epilepsy. Anticonvulsant concentrations tend to fall during pregnancy (see above) and, although partially offset by a decrease in protein binding, this change in drug level can be accompanied by increased

MANAGEMENT OF PREGNANT EPILEPTICS

1 Management should begin before conception:
  (a) If a woman has been seizure-free for 2–3 years, consider slowly stopping treatment.
  (b) There is no justification for changing from, for example, phenytoin to a drug about which even less is known. However, control should be optimized on monotherapy if possible.
2 Discuss the possibility of a birth defect in the context of around a 95% likelihood of a normal child compared to 98% in the general population.
3 There is no point in changing treatment if a woman presents after the first 8–9 weeks of pregnancy as any damage will already have occurred.
4 A scan around 20 weeks is likely to detect major structural defects.

seizure frequency. Therefore, concentration monitoring is required at regular intervals during pregnancy. In women whose epilepsy has been well controlled, the aim should be to maintain early or prepregnancy concentrations with doses being increased as necessary to achieve this. Following delivery, there is a return to normal kinetics over 5–10 days and monitoring is again required to aid dosage adjustment. A further issue concerns drug-induced suppression of vitamin K-dependent clotting factors. Mothers receiving anticonvulsants should be given 20 mg/day vitamin K for the last 2 weeks of pregnancy and vitamin K should also be given to the newborn baby.

Hypertension

Methyldopa is widely used in the management of essential hypertension during pregnancy. This drug is now rarely used outside of pregnancy because of a wide range of side effects, notably sedation. However, it has an unrivalled safety record in pregnancy.

Beta-blockers successfully lower blood pressure in pregnancy, but have not been shown conclusively to improve fetal outcome. They are not teratogenic. When given throughout pregnancy, beta-blockers can cause growth retardation of the fetus.

Hyperthyroidism

Propylthiouracil tends to be used more often than carbimazole during pregnancy. Propylthiouracil is less lipid soluble and more protein bound and crosses less well into the fetus and breast milk. The dose should be titrated against maternal thyroid function.

5.4 Breast feeding

The factors that determine the transfer of drugs into breast milk are the same as those influencing drug distribution in general (Chapter 1, Section 1.2).

Most drugs enter breast milk to a greater or lesser extent but, because the concentration has been greatly reduced by distribution throughout the mother's body, the amount of drug actually received by the breast-fed baby is usually clinically insignificant.

Drugs that can safely be given to breast feeding mothers are listed below.

DRUGS SAFE FOR BREAST FEEDING MOTHERS

- Penicillins, cephalosporins.
- Theophylline, salbutamol by inhaler, prednisolone.
- Valproate, carbamazepine, phenytoin.
- Beta-blockers, methyldopa, hydralazine.
- Warfarin, heparin.
- Haloperidol, chlorpromazine.
- Tricyclic antidepressants.

Certain drugs achieve sufficient concentration in breast milk, and they are sufficiently potent that their use in breast feeding mothers should be avoided (Table 5.2).

Comment. Most commonly used drugs can be safely used in women who are breast feeding. If in doubt, seek further information.

SECTION 2

Aspects of Therapeutics

CHAPTER 6

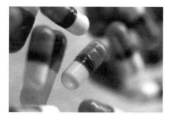

Cardiac Arrhythmias

Not all electrocardiographically documented arrhythmias require treatment. In each instance, the physician must consider the balance between the symptomatic or prognostic significance of the arrhythmia and the potential side effects of therapy. The indications for active treatment in certain circumstances are clear, such as in the termination or prophylaxis of arrhythmias that are life threatening, producing major haemodynamic sequelae, or troublesome symptoms. Treatment of arrhythmias may involve either pharmacological or non-pharmacological therapy. Where pharmacological therapy is indicated, the choice of the most appropriate antiarrhythmic drug depends on several factors:

1 Patient-related:
   (a) Electrocardiographic diagnosis.
   (b) Possible mechanism of the arrhythmia.
   (c) Nature of underlying cardiac disease (if any), especially coronary artery disease and/or left ventricular dysfunction.
   (d) Requirement for acute or long-term therapy.
2 Drug-related:
   (a) Mechanism of drug action—primary and secondary.
   (b) Pharmacokinetics.
   (c) Haemodynamic effects of the drug.
   (d) Non-cardiac effects of the drug.

Under different circumstances, the aim of the therapy may be termination of a tachycardia with restoration of sinus rhythm (e.g. supraventricular tachycardia), control of ventricular rate without restoration of sinus rhythm (e.g. atrial fibrillation) or prevention of recurrent episodes of tachycardia.

6.1 Relevant pathophysiology

Normal electrophysiology

Cardiac muscle may be divided into three electrophysiologically distinct types:

1 Tissue with spontaneous pacemaker activity, i.e. the sinoatrial (SA) and atrioventricular (AV) nodes.
2 Specialized high velocity conducting tissue—the His–Purkinje system.
3 'Working' atrial and ventricular myocardium.

The action potentials of SA and AV nodal cells undergo diastolic depolarization, which results in the generation of spontaneous action potentials. The upstroke of the cardiac action potential in these cells is dependent on the 'slow' inward calcium current. Conduction velocity in nodal tissue, e.g. AV node, is slow, accounting for the delay between atrial and ventricular systole, and for the limitation of the rate at which atrial impulses are transmitted to the ventricles.

Depolarization in His–Purkinje tissue and atrial and ventricular myocardium depends on the rapid inward sodium current. The action potential upstroke and conduction velocity are much faster than those in nodal tissue, allowing electrical activation of the atria or ventricles in a short period of time, permitting coordinated contraction. Under normal circumstances, atrial and ventricular myocardium has no intrinsic automaticity, while that of the His–Purkinje network is slow (30 beats/min).

Mechanisms of arrhythmias

Arrhythmias may arise either from abnormal automaticity or from disorders of impulse conduction. Most clinically important arrhythmias depend on the latter mechanism, and are examples of the 're-entry' phenomenon. Re-entry occurs when an advancing wave of depolarization finds one pathway temporarily inexcitable (refractory) as a result of prematurity, resulting in conduction block. Depolarization may proceed by another route and reach the distal part of the refractory area after a long enough period to allow partial excitability to have recovered. The impulse can then travel slowly in a retrograde direction through the area of previous conduction block. If the time taken for the impulse to pass around such a circuit exceeds the refractory period of the normal tissue at the site proximal to the area of conduction block, this tissue will be re-excited, and the potential for a continuous 'circus' movement will exist. Atrial flutter and fibrillation, supraventricular tachycardias, recurrent ventricular tachycardia secondary to previous myocardial infarction, and ventricular fibrillation are all examples of re-entry.

Abnormal automaticity is the likely basis for the arrhythmias of digitalis toxicity.

Classification of antiarrhythmic drugs

The most commonly used classification of antiarrhythmic drug action was proposed by Singh and Vaughan Williams, following observations on the electrophysiological effects of drugs on isolated tissues. Four principal modes of action have been identified (Table 6.1). However, individual drugs may have actions in more than one category, and their effects in abnormal myocardium (e.g. during ischaemia) differ from those under normal physiological conditions. The antiarrhythmic actions of digitalis and adenine nucleotides are not included in the Vaughan Williams classification, and are considered separately in Sections 6.6 and 6.7.

Class I action

Agents with class I activity interfere with the rapid sodium current, resulting in slowing of conduction, an increase in refractory period, or both. This action is sometimes termed 'local anaesthetic' or 'membrane stabilizing'. Class I drugs are subdivided according to their subsidiary properties. Class Ia agents

ANTIARRHYTHMIC DRUG ACTIONS

Class	Drugs
I: Fast sodium channel inhibitors	Ia: Quinidine, procainamide, disopyramide Ib: Lidocaine, phenytoin, mexiletine, tocainide Ic: Flecainide
II: Antisympathetic agents	Beta-blockers
III: Prolongation of action potential duration	Amiodarone, bretylium, sotalol
IV: Slow calcium channel antagonists	Verapamil, diltiazem
Not classified	Digoxin, adenine nucleotides

Table 6.1 Classification of antiarrhythmic drug actions.

lengthen action potential duration moderately and cause minor slowing of intracardiac conduction and widening of the QRS complex in therapeutic concentrations. Class Ib drugs shorten action potential duration and have no effect on intracardiac conduction or the QRS complex in sinus rhythm. Class Ic drugs have no net effect on action potential duration, but slow intracardiac conduction, and widen the QRS complex.

Class II action

Drugs with class II action decrease the arrhythmogenic effects of catecholamines. This may occur by competitive antagonism at beta-adrenoceptors (e.g. beta-blockers), by non-competitive adrenoceptor antagonism (e.g. amiodarone) or by inhibition of noradrenaline release at sympathetic nerve terminals (e.g. bretylium).

Class III action

Class III activity involves inhibition of outward (repolarizing) currents, resulting in lengthening of action potential duration and effective refractory period without interference with the inward sodium current. The basis of this action in clinically available drugs in this category is inhibition of the rapid component of the delayed rectifier current I_{kr}. The action of class Ia drugs in lengthening action potential duration is also mediated by I_{kr} inhibition. Currently available drugs in this category possess additional class II (e.g. bretylium, sotalol) or both class I, II and IV activity (e.g. amiodarone), but drugs with 'pure' class III activity are under development and are likely to be licensed shortly.

Class IV action

Inhibition of the slow inward Ca^{2+} current by this class of drugs results in slowed conduction and increased refractoriness in the atrioventricular node. This action is of value in blocking supraventricular tachycardia involving the AV node as one limb of a re-entry circuit, or in slowing the ventricular response to atrial fibrillation.

Pharmacological vs. non-pharmacological therapy

Antiarrhythmic drugs exert powerful electrophysiological effects on the heart. While these may be beneficial, it is increasingly recognized that potentially lethal arrhythmias may be provoked by drug action. This phenomenon, termed proarrhythmia, has been identified increasingly in recent years as a result of randomized clinical trials that demonstrated an increased mortality in patients receiving certain antiarrhythmic drugs compared with placebo. As a result of this problem, and the limited efficacy of drug therapy in many instances, there has been an impetus towards the development of non-pharmacological approaches to the management of arrhythmias. In many instances, a non-pharmacological approach is now used for the definitive treatment of arrhythmias. However, drug treatment, by virtue of its ease of administration and widespread availability, is still the commonest initial therapeutic approach. Full discussion of the indications for drug vs. non-pharmacological treatment is beyond the scope of this chapter, but an indication of the arrhythmias in which non-pharmacological approaches are used is given in Table 6.2.

6.2 Class I agents

General

Although class I drugs have been the mainstay of antiarrhythmic drug therapy for many years, results from several recent clinical trials have shown them to be inferior to other (class III) agents in terms of efficacy and safety in the prophylaxis of symptomatic arrhythmias. Class I drugs increase the risk of death in patients with asymptomatic ventricular premature beats after myocardial infarction. Overall, the benefit/risk margin for class I agents is narrow, the risks of producing conduction block or exacerbating arrhythmias are considerable and use of these drugs is declining. They should only be used under expert supervision. All class I agents interfere with sodium channel

NON-PHARMACOLOGICAL THERAPY OF ARRHYTHMIAS

Arrhythmia	Indication	Technique
Atrial fibrillation	Termination	DC cardioversion
	Rate control	AV nodal ablation/ pacemaker
Atrial flutter	Termination	DC cardioversion
	Prophylaxis	Radiofrequency ablation
AV nodal re-entry	Termination	Valsalva manoeuvre
Atrioventricular re-entry	Prophylaxis	Radiofrequency ablation
Ventricular tachycardia	Termination	DC cardioversion, overdrive pacing
	Prophylaxis	Implantable cardioverter-defibrillator radio-frequency ablation, surgery
Ventricular fibrillation	Termination	DC cardioversion Implantable cardioverter-defibrillator

Table 6.2 Non-pharmacological therapy of arrhythmias.

activity, and reduce Na^+ influx. This may reduce intracellular Na^+ concentrations and, by Na^+/Ca^{2+} exchange, result in a reduced intracellular Ca^{2+} concentration. Thus all class I agents have a potentially negative inotropic effect and need to be used with great caution in patients with overt or incipient heart failure. In some instances (e.g. quinidine) the negative inotropic effect may be balanced by peripheral vasodilation. Of the subgroups, group Ib agents have the least negative inotropic action, and group Ia the most.

Class Ia agents

Quinidine

Mechanism
Quinidine reduces the maximal rate of depolarization, depresses spontaneous phase 4 diastolic depolarization in automatic cells, slows conduction and also prolongs the effective refractory period of atrial, ventricular and Purkinje fibres.

Pharmacokinetics
Seventy per cent of the drug is absorbed from the gut. With conventional preparations measurable levels are obtained within 15 min and the peak effect occurs between 1 and 3 h. However, because the average half-life is of the order of 6 h, slow-release preparations are more commonly used. It is 80–90% bound to plasma proteins and is metabolized by hydroxylation; the inactive metabolites are excreted in the urine. Antiarrhythmic effects are seen with drug levels of 2.3–5 mg/l. In cirrhosis the clearance of quinidine is reduced. There is also less binding to plasma proteins and hence lower plasma levels are effective.

Adverse effects
Quinidine has a vagolytic action, which increases AV conduction. This may lead to acceleration in ventricular rate in patients with atrial flutter or fibrillation. Progressive QRS and QT prolongation may occur, the latter leading to atypical ventricular tachycardia (torsades de pointes). Higher concentra-

tions are associated with decreased myocardial contractility, hypotension, or electrophysiological effects with possible sinus arrest, sinoatrial or AV block. Other adverse effects include: gastrointestinal symptoms with nausea, vomiting, and diarrhoea; cinchonism; hypersensitivity reactions with fever, purpura, thrombocytopaenia and hepatic dysfunction.

Drug interactions
Quinidine increases digoxin plasma levels and may precipitate digoxin toxicity if the dose of digoxin is not reduced to compensate.

Clinical use and dose
Quinidine now has limited use. The dose is 200–600 mg orally 6-hourly after an initial test dose.

Procainamide

Mechanism
Procainamide has similar electrophysiological properties to quinidine.

Pharmacokinetics
Procainamide can be administered orally, being 75% bioavailable. However, because it has a relatively short half-life of the order of 3.5 h, it is usually given as a slow-release preparation. The compound is metabolized to N-acetyl procainamide (NAPA), which has class III antiarrhythmic activity in its own right. Antiarrhythmic activity of procainamide occurs at blood levels of 4–10 mg/l and toxic effects are likely with blood levels of 16 mg/l. Relatively high plasma levels of both parent drug and NAPA occur in renal impairment and cardiac failure.

The drug is metabolized by acetylation in the liver by an enzyme that also metabolizes isoniazid and hydralazine. The enzyme is bimodally distributed in the population; slow acetylators theoretically require smaller doses for antiarrhythmic activity than fast acetylators.

Adverse effects
Rapid intravenous administration may cause hypotension with vasodilatation and reduced cardiac output. ECG changes include QRS and QT prolongation. In toxic doses PR prolongation may occur, leading ultimately to AV block. On chronic oral therapy at high dosage many patients develop a drug-induced lupus erythematosus syndrome with a positive antinuclear factor.

Drug interactions
Procainamide reduces the antimicrobial effect of sulphonamides. The mechanism appears to be formation of p-aminobenzoic acid from procaine.

Clinical use and dose
Procainamide is used predominantly in the termination or prophylaxis of ventricular tachycardias, including lidocaine-resistant arrhythmias. It is administered intravenously, 50–100 mg every 5 min to a total dose of 1000 mg or until hypotension or QRS widening occurs. It is rarely used in chronic oral form.

Disopyramide

Mechanism
Disopyramide has electrophysiological properties similar to quinidine.

Pharmacokinetics
Disopyramide is 70–80% bioavailable. The half-life in normal subjects is 6–8 h. Fifty per cent is excreted unchanged in the urine; a further 25% is excreted in the form of the main metabolite—the N-dealkylated form of disopyramide. The dose should be reduced in severe renal failure when creatinine clearance levels are less than 25 ml/min. The therapeutic range is 2–5 mg/l.

Adverse effects
Disopyramide has marked negative inotropic actions and should be avoided in patients with left ventricular dysfunction. Other adverse

effects are related primarily to anticholinergic activity, with urinary retention, glaucoma and blurred vision. QT prolongation occurs with increasing plasma concentrations, and may predispose to torsades de pointes. Contraindications to therapy include sick sinus syndrome and prostatic hypertrophy.

Clinical use and dose
Disopyramide is occasionally used for atrial and ventricular arrhythmias, including those resistant to lidocaine. The dose is 100–200 mg 6-hourly orally or by slow-release preparation. It is also available for slow intravenous injection 2 mg/kg over 20 min.

Class Ib agents

Lidocaine (formerly lignocaine)

Mechanism
Lidocaine causes only marginal slowing of conduction velocity in Purkinje fibres and in ventricular muscle, but is selectively active in suppressing ventricular premature beats and ventricular tachycardia. Like other class Ib agents, it has no useful action against supraventricular tachycardias.

Pharmacokinetics
Lidocaine is not given orally because it is hydrolysed in the gastrointestinal tract and is subjected to extensive first-pass metabolism in the liver so that adequate blood levels are not achieved. Following intravenous administration, the elimination half-life is about 100 min. The clearance of lidocaine is reduced in cardiac failure and lower rates of infusion are required.

Adverse effects
Although therapeutic concentrations have little haemodynamic effect, high levels of lidocaine cause bradycardia, hypotension and even asystole. Nausea and vomiting may also occur. At levels $\geq$5 mg/l, central nervous system (CNS) adverse effects may occur with paraesthesiae, twitching and even grand mal seizures.

Clinical use and dose
Lidocaine has no action on atrial arrhythmias, but it is used in the termination of haemodynamically stable ventricular tachycardia and the short-term prevention of recurrent ventricular tachycardia or fibrillation after myocardial infarction. Lidocaine is given by the intravenous route, with a loading dose of 1–2 mg/kg body weight by rapid injection followed by an infusion of 1–2 mg/min to maintain arrhythmia suppression. The dose requires reduction in the presence of cardiac failure or liver disease. Therapeutic blood levels are 1.5–5 mg/l.

Mexiletine

Mechanism
This primary amine has similar electrophysiological action to lidocaine.

Pharmacokinetics
Mexiletine is active after both oral and intravenous administration. It is extensively metabolized to p-hydroxy- and hydroxymethylmexiletine and to their corresponding deaminated alcohols by hepatic metabolism. The half-life in normal subjects is 9–12 h. However, this may be increased, particularly following acute myocardial infarction. Oral absorption is reduced when given with morphine or diamorphine.

Adverse effects
Toxic effects include nausea, dizziness, drowsiness, tremor and hypotension, common at plasma levels above 2.0 mg/l.

Clinical use and dose
Mexiletine is occasionally used in the treatment of ventricular arrhythmias but therapy is commonly limited by patient intolerance. Mexiletine is given initially as a 1–3 mg/kg i.v. bolus injection, then 20–45 μg/kg per min by intravenous infusion, followed by 0.6–1.2 g orally in 24 h. Effective plasma levels are 0.75–2.0 mg/l; the therapeutic range is narrow.

Phenytoin

Phenytoin has class Ib activity similar to lidocaine. Haemodynamic adverse effects include dose-related impairment of myocardial contractility following intravenous use. Adverse effects are reviewed in the chapter on anticonvulsants. It finds occasional use as an alternative to lidocaine or in digoxin-induced arrhythmias, given in 50–100 mg rapid intravenous doses over 5 min, up to 1000 mg.

Class Ic agents

Flecainide

Mechanism

Flecainide slows conduction in the atria, His–Purkinje system, accessory pathways and ventricles. In therapeutic concentration it causes lengthening of the PR and QRS intervals. Flecainide is effective against atrial arrhythmias and tachycardias involving accessory pathways (Wolff–Parkinson–White syndrome).

Pharmacokinetics

Flecainide is well absorbed orally, and about 27% is excreted unchanged in the urine. The remainder undergoes biotransformation to active metabolites, but the plasma concentrations of the unconjugated, pharmacologically active forms are considerably less than those of the parent drug. Flecainide is not extensively protein bound. The average elimination half-life in normal subjects is 14 h, permitting twice daily administration. The half-life is increased in cardiac and renal failure.

Adverse effects

Flecainide may exacerbate pre-existing conduction disorders and should be used with great care in patients with sinoatrial disease, AV nodal disease or bundle branch block. It may cause an acute increase in the ventricular stimulation threshold, with a risk of asystole in pacemaker-dependent patients. Exacerbation of ventricular arrhythmias may occur. These are not normally of the torsades de pointes type, but rather a sustained (often incessant) monomorphic ventricular tachycardia with gross widening of the QRS complex and a relatively slow rate (120–140/min). Neurological disturbances such as ataxia and taste disturbance may occur at higher doses.

Clinical use and dose

Flecainide is effective in the chemical cardioversion of recent-onset atrial fibrillation, and in the maintenance of sinus rhythm after cardioversion or in paroxysmal atrial fibrillation. The drug is also used in the prophylaxis of atrioventricular re-entry tachycardia in the Wolff–Parkinson–White syndrome. Flecainide should not be used in patients with prior myocardial infarction or left ventricular dysfunction. It is a potentially hazardous drug, and its use should be restricted to arrhythmia specialists.

Chronic oral doses range from 50 to 150 mg twice daily with target therapeutic plasma concentrations of 0.2–1.0 mg/l. Intravenous flecainide (up to 2 mg/kg) may be given by slow infusion over 30 min.

Propafenone

This class Ic agent has additional minor beta blocking and calcium antagonist properties.

Pharmacokinetics

Propafenone undergoes variable metabolism. Fast acetylators metabolize the drug rapidly to an active metabolite, in contrast to slow acetylators. There is therefore a marked variability in the plasma half-life of the native drug, but the overall pharmacodynamic properties of the active drug and metabolite are similar. Propafenone exhibits non-linear kinetics as a result of saturation of hepatic metabolism. For this reason, an increase in the daily dose from 300 mg to 600 mg daily results in doubling of the plasma concentration, while a further doubling in plasma concentration occurs when the dose is increased from 600 mg per day to 900 mg per day.

Adverse effects

The cardiac and non-cardiac adverse effects of propafenone are similar to those of flecainide. In addition, the weak beta-blocking action may be of significance in patients with asthma in whom the drug is contraindicated. The calcium antagonist properties also render the drug unsuitable for patients with myasthenia gravis.

Clinical use and dose

Propafenone is indicated for the prophylaxis of paroxysmal atrial fibrillation or supraventricular tachycardia. As with flecainide, its use should be avoided in patients with prior myocardial infarction or impaired left ventricular function The dosage ranges from 450 to 900 mg daily in two or three divided doses.

6.3 Class II agents

Beta-adrenoceptor antagonists

The pharmacokinetics, adverse effects and mechanisms of action are discussed in Chapter 8.

Clinical use

These compounds are useful in antiarrhythmic therapy in view of their freedom from significant proarrhythmic effects. They may be used for the control of inappropriate sinus tachycardia, or the prophylaxis of paroxysmal atrial fibrillation or supraventricular tachycardia. Beta-blockers are ineffective in restoring sinus rhythm in atrial fibrillation. However, they are used either singly or in conjunction with digoxin to control the ventricular rate in permanent atrial fibrillation by virtue of their slowing effect on atrioventricular nodal conduction. Beta-adrenoceptor antagonists reduce the risk of sudden death in long-term therapy after myocardial infarction and in congestive heart failure. Other clinical situations in which the beta-blockers have useful antiarrhythmic action include mitral valve prolapse, and the congenital long QT syndromes.

Bretylium

This agent has adrenergic neurone blocking activity and suppresses noradrenaline release. It is eliminated by the kidney with a half-life of 7–12 h. Bretylium also has class III action on Purkinje fibres and is effective in ventricular arrhythmias, particularly ventricular fibrillation refractory to lidocaine or procainamide, and repeated electrical defibrillation.

Adverse effects include hypotension.

It is administered by the intravenous route, 5–10 mg/kg or by the intramuscular route, 5 mg/kg.

6.4 Class III agents

Amiodarone

Mechanism

Amiodarone prolongs the action potential duration and effective refractory period in all cardiac tissues. It is a non-competitive alpha- and beta-adrenoceptor antagonist, and also has class I, class II and class IV activity.

Pharmacokinetics

After oral administration, considerable accumulation occurs in muscle and fat, and the therapeutic action may take several weeks to develop fully. Amiodarone is metabolized in the liver to desethylamiodarone, which is also electrophysiologically active. The steady-state therapeutic plasma concentrations of amiodarone and desethylamiodarone are 1–2 mg/l. Elimination of amiodarone is complex, with an initial relatively rapid (1–2 days) and extremely slow terminal half-life (more than 30 days).

Adverse effects

Amiodarone has little negative inotropic effect, and is the best tolerated of all the antiarrhythmic agents in heart failure. Amiodarone depresses sinus node automaticity and intracardiac conduction; therefore, it should be used with caution in the presence of SA or

AV nodal disease. In common with all drugs that prolong ventricular repolarization, amiodarone may provoke torsades de pointes ventricular tachycardia, but this occurs less frequently than with other class III agents. The use of amiodarone is limited principally by its non-cardiac side effects, of which the most important are pulmonary (alveolitis), hepatic (hepatitis), neurological (tremor, ataxia), thyroid (hyper- or hypothyroidism), testicular (orchitis) and cutaneous (photosensitivity). The last effect occurs in a high percentage of patients, of whom a small minority develop a slate-grey discoloration of light-exposed areas, especially the nose and cheeks. Corneal microdeposits occur in almost all patients, but do not interfere with vision.

Clinical use and dose

Amiodarone is effective in a wide variety of supraventricular and ventricular arrhythmias, including those associated with the Wolff–Parkinson–White syndrome. In view of its adverse effects, chronic amiodarone therapy should be used only in life-threatening or severely disabling arrhythmias, when other antiarrhythmic agents have failed or are contraindicated, and non-pharmacological therapy is not appropriate. An oral loading dose of 600–1200 mg daily is given for 2 weeks, then reduced to 100–400 mg daily. Intravenous amiodarone may be effective in the acute conversion or control of troublesome supraventricular and ventricular arrhythmias, including recent-onset atrial flutter and fibrillation. It has a relatively slow onset of action, which makes its use suitable only for haemodynamically stable arrhythmias. The initial dose is 300 mg i.v. given over 30 min to avoid hypotension, followed by up to 1200 mg/24 h. The intravenous preparation is irritant, and should be given via a central vein.

Drug interactions

Amiodarone potentiates the effect of warfarin and increases plasma digoxin levels. Dose reduction is required in both cases.

Sotalol

Mechanism

Sotalol is a non-selective beta-blocker, which also possesses class III activity and thus prolongs atrial and ventricular action potential duration and refractory period. It has no class I activity at therapeutic concentrations.

Clinical use

Sotalol appears to be more effective than other beta-blockers, particularly in supraventricular tachycardias involving accessory pathways and in ventricular arrhythmias. It may be used in the prophylaxis of recurrent ventricular tachycardia. The side effects are those of other beta-blockers (see Chapter 8) with the additional predisposition to torsades de pointes. The principal risk factors for this are female gender, bradycardia, left ventricular hypertrophy or dysfunction, high plasma concentrations, coexisting potassium depletion and coadministration of other drugs which lengthen QT interval. The dosage of sotalol in antiarrhythmic therapy ranges from 80 to 320 mg twice daily.

6.5 Class IV agents

Verapamil

Mechanism

Verapamil inhibits the slow inward Ca^{2+} current. Its antiarrhythmic actions stem from decreasing AV conduction.

Pharmacokinetics

Bioavailability is only 10–20% owing to extensive first-pass metabolism. It is eliminated by the kidneys.

Adverse effects

In view of its depressant effects on the SA and AV nodes, verapamil is contraindicated in heart block or sinoatrial disease. Verapamil has significant negative inotropic action, and is contraindicated in heart failure. Additional effects include nausea, dizziness, facial flushing and constipation.

Drug interactions

Verapamil potentiates the negative effects of digoxin and beta-blockers on AV nodal conduction. Verapamil and beta-blockers in combination may cause high grade AV block or asystole, particularly if either is administered intravenously. Beta-blockers also enhance the negative inotropic action of verapamil.

Clinical use and dose

Verapamil is ineffective in restoring sinus rhythm in atrial flutter and atrial fibrillation, but its effect on increasing AV block allows control of the ventricular rate. Verapamil is useful in terminating re-entry supraventricular arrhythmias by transient block of AV nodal conduction. Verapamil should not be used in the termination of undiagnosed wide-complex tachycardias where ventricular tachycardia cannot be excluded. Verapamil can be used by both oral and intravenous routes. Intravenous verapamil is administered by infusion or rapid injections of 5–10 mg, with infusion rates of 0.005 mg/kg per min. Oral dosage is 80–120 mg three times daily, or an equivalent daily dose of a slow-release preparation.

Diltiazem

This calcium channel blocker has similar antiarrhythmic properties to verapamil. Dosage is 60–120 mg thrice daily of conventional release diltiazem. Sustained-release preparations may be taken once or twice daily.

Comment. Calcium channel blockers of the dihydropyridine class (e.g. nifedipine) do not interfere with AV nodal conduction and have no antiarrhythmic action.

6.6 Digitalis glycosides

The term digitalis or digitalis glycoside refers to any of the cardioactive steroids which share an aglycone ring structure and have positive inotropic and electrophysiological effects. In the UK, the vast majority of clinicians use the cardiac glycoside, digoxin.

Mechanism

A major effect is to decrease sodium transport out of the cardiac cell by inhibiting Na^+/K^+ ATPase (the sodium pump). The resulting accumulation of sodium results in an increase of intracellular calcium ions by Na^+/Ca^{2+} exchange, which is responsible for the positive inotropic effects of digitalis glycosides. These drugs exert their antiarrhythmic effect by virtue of enhancing vagal inhibition of sinus node automaticity and atrioventricular nodal conduction. At high concentrations, digitalis glycosides increase myocardial automaticity as a result of intracellular calcium overload.

The three major effects of digitalis glycosides on the heart are:

1 Positive inotropy.

2 Decreased ventricular rate in atrial fibrillation or flutter, by decreasing AV conduction. This effect is diminished on exercise as a result of withdrawal of underlying vagal tone.

3 Increased myocardial automaticity in high (toxic) concentrations, or at 'therapeutic' concentrations if other factors such as hypokalaemia are present.

Digoxin

Pharmacokinetics

Digoxin can be given orally or intravenously. The average volume of distribution is approximately 7.3 l/kg; this is decreased in patients with renal disease, hypothyroidism and in patients taking quinidine. It is increased in thyrotoxicosis. Clearance varies from individual to individual and is the result of both renal and metabolic elimination mechanisms. In healthy adults, the metabolic component is of the order of 40–60 ml/min per 70 kg, and the renal component approximates creatinine clearance. Metabolic clearance is reduced in congestive cardiac failure. Clearance in any individual can be calculated by the equations discussed in Chapters 1 and 2.

In patients with normal renal function, the elimination half-life is approximately 2 days. This is increased to approximately 4–6 days in severe renal disease.

Adverse effects

Adverse effects are determined in part by plasma concentration (>2.5 μg/l for digoxin) and in part by electrolyte balance. Digoxin and potassium compete for cardiac receptor sites and hypokalaemia can precipitate digitalis adverse effects. Hypercalcaemia also potentiates toxicity.

The common extracardiac adverse effects are anorexia, nausea, diarrhoea, vomiting, fatigue or weakness.

Less commonly, neurological symptoms occur, including difficulty in reading, confusion or even psychosis. Abdominal pain is another less common manifestation.

The cardiac adverse effects may include depression of automaticity or conduction resulting in sinus bradycardia, sinus arrest, junctional rhythm, or various degrees of AV block, including complete heart block. Additionally, digoxin may produce excitatory effects, resulting in ventricular ectopic beats, atrial or ventricular tachycardia, or ventricular fibrillation. The typical effects of digitalis glycosides on the electrocardiogram (ECG), i.e. prolonged PR interval and ST segment depression, does not indicate toxicity. Cardiac signs precede extracardiac signs in about 50% of cases of toxicity.

Drug interactions

Digoxin absorption is decreased by drugs that increase intestinal motility (e.g. metoclopramide), and increased by drugs that decrease motility (e.g. propantheline). Many antacids, particularly magnesium trisilicate, reduce digoxin absorption. Digoxin levels increase if quinidine or amiodarone is coadministered and toxicity can occur. The potential for toxicity is enhanced for all cardiac glycosides when diuretics are coadministered because of hypokalaemia.

Digitoxin and ouabain

Digitoxin is more lipid soluble than digoxin and is practically 100% absorbed from the gastrointestinal tract. It is given orally and intravenously. It is extensively metabolized by the liver, and the elimination half-life is 5–7 days. Renal impairment does not appreciably alter digitoxin kinetics but binding to plasma proteins, normally of the order of 90–97%, may be slightly decreased in uraemia.

It seems likely that digitoxin is excreted in the bile and is then reabsorbed to some extent, i.e. it has an enterohepatic circulation. Colestyramine (cholestyramine), which can bind cardiac glycosides in the gut, can interrupt the enterohepatic circulation; whether it can shorten the duration of digitoxin toxicity is still a matter for speculation.

Ouabain is poorly absorbed from the gut and is administered exclusively by the intravenous route. Its onset of action is rapid, and it has a somewhat shorter half-life than digoxin, approximately 1 day. Elimination is mainly renal.

Clinical use and doses

The principal use of cardiac glycosides is in the control of ventricular rate in atrial fibrillation, particularly when a return to sinus rhythm is not expected (e.g. chronic mitral valve disease). Combination therapy with verapamil or beta-blockers provides better control of exercise heart rate with a lower risk of toxicity than high-dose glycosides. The onset of action even after intravenous administration is delayed for several hours. Thus if clinical circumstances require urgent control of ventricular rate, other approaches such as cardioversion or intravenous amiodarone may be more appropriate. Acute digitalization has been superseded by the use of intravenous adenosine or verapamil in the termination of supraventricular tachycardias. The use of digoxin in patients with heart failure in sinus rhythm is discussed elsewhere (Chapter 7).

The dosing schedules used with the cardiac glycosides depend not only on the pharmacokinetic properties of the drug, but also on factors that determine individual susceptibility. The loading dose is determined by the volume of distribution and the desired plasma concentration; the maintenance dose by clearance (Chapters 1 and 2). Nomograms and simple equations are available for dose calculation. However, these must remain approximations and the patient's clinical response must influence long-term management. If a maintenance dose is employed without a loading dose, drug accumulation and activity develop slowly because steady state is not reached for four to five half-lives. The major determinant of digoxin clearance is renal function and the maintenance dose for this glycoside must be reduced if renal function is impaired. The average loading dose of digoxin is 1.0–1.5 mg orally, or 0.3–1.0 mg intravenously. The usual oral maintenance dose in the presence of normal renal function is 0.125–0.25 mg daily.

The use of drug monitoring of the glycoside plasma levels has been useful, particularly in renal impairment and toxicity. The normal therapeutic range of digoxin is 1–2 μg/l. Venous sampling should be performed 3–4 h after an i.v. dose or 6–8 h after an oral dose. If blood levels are low then compliance should be checked, and possible causes of malabsorption considered.

Treatment of digitalis-induced toxicity

Treatment of digitalis-induced arrhythmias is often difficult. The glycoside should be withdrawn, and if hypokalaemia is present, potassium chloride should be administered by infusion at a rate of 20 mmol/h (not exceeding 100 mmol total) with electrocardiographic and biochemical monitoring. Severe digitalis intoxication is treated with specific Fab anti-digoxin antibodies, which bind and inactivate digoxin.

Ventricular arrhythmias may require lidocaine or phenytoin administration. Supraventricular arrhythmias may respond to beta blockade or phenytoin. Care must be observed when using verapamil and procainamide, as increased degrees of heart block may occur. Temporary pacing may be required for heart block with haemodynamic effects or in the rare instance of SA node arrest. Intravenous amiodarone infusion has shown promise in digitoxic arrhythmias.

6.7 Adenine nucleotides

Mechanism

The adenine nucleotides adenosine and adenosine triphosphate (ATP) act via purinergic receptors situated in the SA and AV nodes. Stimulation of these receptors causes hyperpolarization of the cells resulting in suppression of automaticity and conduction. This results in transient sinus bradycardia and AV block. Adenine nucleotides transiently interrupt the re-entrant circuit in AV nodal tachycardia or in atrioventricular tachycardia involving an accessory pathway, while increasing the degree of AV block in atrial flutter or fibrillation.

Pharmacokinetics

ATP is rapidly metabolized to adenosine in the plasma and probably exerts its antiarrhythmic effects as adenosine. Adenosine is metabolized to the inactive inosine. The plasma half-life of adenosine is approximately 10 s. Both nucleotides are inactive orally.

Adverse effects

Adenine nucleotides are vasodilators, and produce marked flushing. Bolus injection causes a transient increase followed by a small fall in blood pressure, but the duration of action of a bolus dose is normally insufficient to cause clinically significant hypotension. A feeling of chest tightness or sometimes chest pain is experienced, which may be very unpleasant but is transient. Transient complete heart block lasting a few seconds may occur. This usually responds to coughing. Adenine nucleotides may precipitate bronchoconstriction in asthmatics.

Clinical use and dose

Adenine nucleotides are the drugs of choice for the termination of regular supraventricular tachycardias. Tachycardias involving the AV node as an integral part of the re-entry circuit will be terminated, while atrial tachycardias will demonstrate transient slowing of the ventricular rate which allows identification of the underlying rhythm, e.g. atrial flutter. Dosing of adenosine is by rapid intravenous bolus injection, starting with a bolus of 3 mg, followed by a saline flush. The antiarrhythmic effect occurs shortly after the onset of flushing, usually 20–30 s after injection. If the initial dose is ineffective, repeat boluses of 6 or 12 mg are given at 2- to 3-min intervals until success is achieved or the dose is limited by patient intolerance.

Drug interactions

The effects of adenine nucleotides are inhibited by purinoceptor antagonists (methylxanthines, e.g. theophylline and its derivatives) and accentuated by dipyridamole. Adenine nucleotides may be given safely to patients already receiving beta-adrenoceptor antagonists or calcium channel blockers.

CHAPTER 7

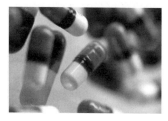

Heart Failure and Angina Pectoris

7.1 Heart failure

Definition

Physiological: an inability of the heart to maintain a cardiac output sufficient to meet the requirements of the metabolizing tissues despite a normal filling pressure.

Clinical: symptoms suggestive of heart failure (e.g. exertional breathlessness, ankle swelling, etc.) accompanied by objective evidence (usually by echocardiography) of cardiac dysfunction of sufficient severity to account for these. Most patients with heart failure have left ventricular systolic dysfunction and it is these patients for which there is evidence-based treatment. The treatment of other causes of heart failure is less clearcut and empirical (e.g. valve repair or replacement, diuretics for patients with left ventricular hypertrophy and preserved systolic function). In patients who do not respond to appropriate therapy the diagnosis should be reviewed.

There is a poor relationship between haemodynamic abnormalities (the physiological definition of heart failure; see above and symptoms and signs of heart failure (the clinical definition of heart failure).

Relevant pathophysiology

There is a poor relationship between symptoms and cardiac performance in chronic heart failure. Treatment that improves cardiac function does not necessarily improve symptoms or prognosis and many treatments that have only modest beneficial effects on cardiac function may have clearly beneficial effects on symptoms and prognosis.

In contrast, there does appear to be a relationship between haemodynamics, symptoms and prognosis in patients with acute pulmonary oedema or cardiogenic shock. Treatments directed at haemodynamic abnormalities in this setting do appear to relieve symptoms and probably improve prognosis.

Cardiac performance is influenced by:

1 *Preload*: which determines ventricular end-diastolic pressure and volume. In normal hearts an increased preload leads to increased end-diastolic fibre length, which, in turn, causes increased force of contraction. In heart failure this response is reduced or even reversed.

2 *Force of cardiac contraction*: determined largely by the intrinsic strength and integrity of the muscle cells. Force of contraction is decreased by:

  (a) Ischaemic heart disease (myocardial infarction or chronic severe ischaemia).

  (b) Specific disorders affecting heart muscle, such as hypertension, myocarditis.

  (c) Disorders of heart muscle of unknown cause, e.g. idiopathic dilated cardiomyopathy.

3 *Myocardial compliance*: an important determinant of ventricular filling and therefore of cardiac output. Compliance is decreased by:

  (a) Fibrosis.

  (b) Hypertrophy.

AETIOLOGY/MANAGEMENT OF HEART FAILURE

Principal aims:
Improve quality of life by:
- improving symptoms,
- avoiding side-effects,
- preventing major morbid events such as myocardial infarction or stroke, and
- delaying death.

Secondary aims:
- improve cardiac performance,
- improve exercise capacity,
- reduce arrhythmias (ventricular and supraventricular),
- maintain renal function, and
- prevent electrolyte disturbance.

Aetiology:
In westernized countries heart failure is usually caused by one of the following:
- ischaemic heart disease,
- hypertension (Chapter 8),
- heart muscle disorders, and
- valvular heart disease.

DRUGS USED TO TREAT HEART FAILURE

1 Diuretics: thiazides, loop diuretics.
  (a) Decrease peripheral and pulmonary oedema.
  (b) Decrease preload by reduction in circulatory volume.
2 Neuroendocrine antagonists.
  (a) ACE inhibitors.
  (b) Aldosterone antagonists.
  (c) Alpha-adrenoceptor antagonists.
  (d) Beta-receptor antagonists.
3 Drugs with a positive inotropic effect.

Cardiac glycosides (mainly chronic heart failure). Beta-adrenoceptor agonists (acute heart failure only).
4 Vasodilator agents.
  (a) Mainly decrease preload: nitrates (glyceryl trinitrate, isosorbide dinitrate and isosorbide mononitrate).
  (b) Mainly decrease afterload: hydralazine.
  (c) Decrease preload and afterload: sodium nitroprusside.

(c) Ischaemia.

4 *Afterload*: is the ventricular wall tension developed during ejection. Afterload is increased by:
  (a) Systemic arterial vasoconstriction
  (b) Increased arterial pressure.
  (c) Obstruction to outflow, e.g. aortic stenosis.

5 *Neuroendocrine activation*: after an acute cardiac insult plasma concentrations of renin, angiotensin II, aldosterone, noradrenaline, endothelin, antidiuretic hormone and the natriuretic peptides are increased. If the patient survives and does not require treatment then activity of the renin–angiotensin–aldosterone system (RAAS) returns to normal, probably a consequence of compensatory salt and water retention, but plasma concentrations of other neuroendocrine systems remain elevated. Once diuretics have been administered RAAS activity increases, as do the concentrations of other neuro-hormones with the exception of the natriuretic peptides, which may decline. However, as heart failure progresses all the above neuroendocrine systems become markedly activated. Increased sympathetic activation via arterial baroreflexes (and possibly a down-regulation of inhibitory activity of baroreceptors) leads to sympathetically mediated increases in renal renin secretion and further increases in angiotensin II and aldosterone. Local haemodynamic factors probably play an important role in activation of other systems.

Neuroendocrine activation may be responsible for many of the characteristic features of heart failure. Examples include:

Angiotensin II: vasoconstriction (especially renal), sodium retention, continuing cardiac myocyte damage causing progressive ventricular dilatation (remodelling), stimulates aldosterone secretion.

Aldosterone: sodium retention; potassium loss and myocardial fibrosis (both may lead to arrhythmias).

Sympathetic activation: vasoconstriction, arrhythmias, hypokalaemia, sodium retention. May initially increase cardiac contractility but has adverse effects on long-term cardiac function.

Diuretics

These drugs are first-line treatment for patients with heart failure. In mild failure a thiazide (Chapter 8) may suffice. Moderate or severe failure requires a loop diuretic.

Loop diuretics

Furosemide (frusemide), bumetanide.

Mechanism

Inhibition of active chloride reabsorption and also of Na^+/K^+ ATPase in the ascending limb of the loop of Henle with increased salt and water loss. The increased delivery of sodium to the distal tubule encourages Na^+/K^+ exchange with a tendency to hypokalaemic alkalosis.

Pharmacokinetics

Both drugs are well absorbed following oral administration and are also available in intravenous formulations. Elimination is largely by renal excretion with a small contribution by liver metabolism. These drugs have a rapid onset and short duration of action.

Adverse effects

Salt and water depletion can occur. May cause prerenal uraemia (increase in blood urea and creatinine concentrations). Regular monitoring of serum potassium is required. Urate retention can occur as with thiazides. Rapid intravenous injection of large doses can produce deafness.

Drug interactions

These include potentiation of nephrotoxic effects of gentamicin and cephaloridine. Hypokalaemia enhances the risk of digoxin toxicity. Loop diuretics may be combined usefully with thiazide diuretics resulting in an extremely potent diuretic combination. It is not clear if this combination is superior to the use of large doses of loop diuretic alone. Non-steroidal anti-inflammatory drugs (NSAIDs) may impair diuresis and provoke hyperkalaemia and renal failure.

Doses

Furosemide: oral—20 mg each morning up to 1 or 2 g each day in very resistant oedema or cardiac failure. Intravenous—20–40 mg slowly. In resistant cases up to 1 g can be infused over 2–4 h.

Bumetanide: oral—0.5–5 mg each day. Intravenous—0.5–2 mg or infusion up to 5 mg slowly.

Prevention and treatment of hypokalaemia

There is no evidence that potassium supplements (other than intravenous) are effective in preventing or treating hypokalaemia in patients with heart failure. Hypokalaemia is much less of a problem in patients with heart failure treated with angiotensin-converting enzyme (ACE) inhibitors but may still occur in patients taking very large doses of diuretics. There are three occasions where hypokalaemia is likely to be a problem:

1 Administration of high doses of loop diuretics in treating heart failure without an ACE inhibitor.

2 Coadministration of digoxin since hypokalaemia potentiates digoxin toxicity.

3 Administration of a thiazide diuretic to a patient with a low potassium intake, e.g. the older patient.

In general, persistent serum potassium below 3.5 mmol/l is an indication for potassium correction usually by coadministration of a potassium sparing diuretic the most appropriate of which is spironolactone.

Potassium sparing diuretics

Amiloride, triamterene, spironolactone: These drugs are all diuretics themselves, but their effect is weak and they are rarely used alone. They act mainly on the distal tubule inhibiting sodium/potassium exchange. Spironolactone acts by inhibiting the effect of aldosterone on the distal tubule and is discussed further under the heading of neuroendocrine antagonists.

The adverse effect common to all of these drugs is hyperkalaemia and is particularly likely in patients with impaired renal function. Potassium supplements should rarely be required with potassium sparing diuretics. If they are used, close monitoring of serum potassium is necessary. Potassium sparing drugs (with the exception of spironolactone—see below) should generally be avoided in patients taking ACE inhibitors as both agents raise potassium and severe hyperkalaemia may occur especially in the presence of renal failure. Spironolactone should only be used in a low dose and with caution in patients prescribed an ACE inhibitor (see below). When combined with thiazide diuretics hyponatraemia may occur.

Doses
Amiloride: 5–20 mg/day
Triamterene: 100–200 mg/day
Spironolactone: 100–200 mg/day for refractory oedema. (Lower doses are of benefit in severe heart failure—see below).

Comment. Potassium sparing diuretics are available in proprietary formulations combined with a thiazide or furosemide. Combination tablets are more expensive but may improve compliance by reducing the number of tablets to be taken.

Neuroendocrine antagonists

ACE inhibitors

ACE inhibitors not only improve symptoms, but also reduce mortality in all grades of heart failure resulting from left ventricular systolic dysfunction treated with diuretics.

Mechanism. The precise mechanism of action of ACE inhibitors has yet to be elucidated. The ACE not only converts angiotensin I to angiotensin II, but also degrades bradykinin. Angiotensin II is a powerful vasoconstrictor, stimulates aldosterone and antidiuretic hormone release, enhances sympathetic activity, causes renal sodium retention and can cause direct damage to cardiac myocytes, increase myocardial fibrosis and stimulate vascular and myocardial hypertrophy. Bradykinin is a powerful vasodilator and also has antiproliferative effects on smooth muscle and stimulates the production of vasodilator postaglandins and nitric oxide.

ACE inhibitors produce both arterial and venous dilatation. The latter may be mediated through increased bradykinin or reduced sympathetic activation. ACE inhibitors increase serum and total body potassium by reducing aldosterone and should not, generally, be used with potassium sparing drugs. (One exception is spironolactone—see below).

Adverse effects. Profound hypotension may occur after the first dose in patients on diuretics or with hyponatraemia. The magnitude and duration differs between different ACE inhibitors. Other adverse reactions include postural hypotension, renal dysfunction, hyperkalaemia, cough and angioneurotic oedema.

Drug interactions. Include hyperkalaemia when combined with a potassium sparing diuretic and renal failure when combined with an NSAID.

Doses. Captopril was the first orally active ACE inhibitor and has a shorter duration of action than enalapril, which is a pro-drug for the active constituent enalaprilat which is longer acting. Several other ACE inhibitors including lisinopril are licensed for heart failure and their long-term benefits are likely to be a class effect.

Captopril: 6.25–50 mg three times daily.
Enalapril: 2.5–20 mg twice daily.
Lisinopril: 2.5–20 mg once daily.

The large trials showing benefit used high doses of ACE inhibitors (e.g. captopril 25–50 mg three times daily, enalapril 10–20 mg twice daily). Dose ranging studies have not shown a convincing difference between doses on symptoms or prognosis. It would seem advisable to use in practice the same doses shown to be of benefit in large clinical trials.

Angiotensin II antagonists
There is evidence that Angiotensin II receptor antagonists have comparable haemodynamic and neurohumoral effects to those of ACE inhibitors in congestive heart failure (CHF). These drugs may also improve symptoms. Their effect on prognosis in CHF is not yet known. Angiotensin II antagonists have the advantage of not causing troublesome cough and could be used as an alternative to ACE inhibitors if the latter are not tolerated. Results of comparative studies are awaited.

Spironolactone
Spironolactone competitively inhibits the effects of aldosterone. It is useful in treating the resistant oedema of conditions associated with excess aldosterone including nephrotic syndrome and cirrhosis. Recently spironolactone has been shown to reduce mortality in patients with New York Heart Association (NYHA) class III and IV heart failure already treated with a diuretic, digoxin and an ACE inhibitor.

Spironolactone commonly causes nausea, gynaecomastia in men and menstrual irregularities in women. It can decrease the renal secretion of digoxin. There is a risk of hyper-

kalaemia when given with other potassium sparing diuretics or an ACE inhibitor. Careful monitoring of blood chemistry is mandatory, especially when combined with an ACE inhibitor.

Spironolactone: 25–50 mg/day has been reported in a clinical trial to improve outcome in heart failure. This indication and dosing regimen has not yet been approved by drug license authorities.

Beta-adrenoceptor antagonists
For the last 30 years heart failure has generally been regarded as a contraindication to beta-blockade, although a series of small studies in heart failure has consistently suggested benefit. Recent large trials suggest not only that beta-blockers are safe, at least in some patient groups (NYHA class I–III patients), but also that they reduce mortality, progression of heart failure and hospital readmission. The reduction in morbidity and mortality is substantial and incremental to that of ACE inhibitors. Whether they have any striking benefit on symptoms is a matter of some controversy. About 5–10% of patients will deteriorate within the first few days of receiving a beta-blocker and it takes 2–6 months for benefits to become obvious. The mechanism of action of beta-blockers in heart failure remains obscure but may involve retarding or even reversing progressive ventricular dysfunction due to excessive sympathetic activity. Currently, the most promising results have been achieved with bisoprolol, carvedilol, and slow release metoprolol. Beta-blockers must be used with extreme caution in patients with heart failure. They should only be started under the supervision of a hospital specialist. In heart failure, beta-blockers are initiated in a very low dose and the dose is up-titrated slowly over 2–3 months. Carvedilol is the first 'licensed' beta-blocker in heart failure but others (bisoprolol, metoprolol) have shown evidence of improving outcome in controlled trials. Carvedilol: 50 mg once or twice daily orally for heart failure (under hospital specialist supervision).

Drugs with a positive inotropic effect

Digoxin

The pharmacodynamics and pharmacokinetics of digoxin together with clinical uses and doses are discussed in full in Chapter 6. Digoxin improves cardiac performance in patients with atrial fibrillation. In patients with sinus rhythm digoxin has a positive inotropic effect when given acutely. There has been controversy as to whether this effect is maintained during long-term therapy. Digoxin has autonomic actions that may be more important in heart failure. Double blind studies have confirmed the long-term beneficial effect of digoxin on symptoms and morbidity (but not mortality) in sinus rhythm, an effect best seen in patients with severe heart failure. If digoxin is used the dose should be adjusted to take account of renal function.

Monitoring of plasma drug levels is of limited use as there is a poor relationship between therapeutic effect (in terms of symptoms) and plasma level. Toxicity may be best judged by the occurrence of side effects (anorexia, nausea). However, in elderly patients the symptoms of digoxin toxicity are protean and the first evidence may be serious arrhythmia; therefore, monitoring for toxicity may be warranted in this group.

Adrenoceptor agonists: dopamine and dobutamine

These drugs are currently used only in acute severe heart failure accompanied by hypotension and poor tissue perfusion. They have established short-term effects when given intravenously.

Mechanism. Both drugs produce their inotropic effect by beta$_1$-adrenoceptor stimulation of the myocardium. The effects of dopamine are dose dependent and result partly from direct action and partly from indirect effects through increased noradrenaline release. Below 5 μg/kg per min the major effect is to increase renal blood flow by stimulation of dopamine receptors. As the dose is increased in the 5–20 μg/kg per min range both beta$_1$- and alpha-adrenoceptor stimulant effects are seen with increased cardiac output and a modest rise in blood pressure. Above this dose range alpha-receptor effects are more marked, with a further rise in blood pressure. This tends to increase afterload and is undesirable. Dobutamine has no renal vasodilator effect, less vasoconstrictor (alpha) effect and a similar inotropic effect to dopamine.

Pharmacokinetics. These drugs undergo rapid clearance. Dopamine and dobutamine must be given intravenously.

Adverse effects. Mainly tachyarrhythmias from beta$_1$-receptor stimulation when used in excessive doses. Stimulation of beta-receptors in skeletal muscle can cause hypokalaemia.

Dose. Dopamine: 5 μg/kg per min initially, increasing as required by the clinical response. Dobutamine: 2.5 μg/kg per min initially increasing as necessary.

Vasodilator agents

Venodilators reduce the left ventricular end diastolic pressure and volume, thus reducing pulmonary congestion and the symptoms of breathlessness in acute heart failure. Arteriolar vasodilators reduce aortic impedance and enhance cardiac output and are appropriate during episodes of acute heart failure when arterial pressure is maintained adequately, especially if valvular regurgitation is present. Vasodilators should be used with caution in the presence of obstructive or stenotic valvular lesions.

Drugs affecting preload

Glyceryl trinitrate

Sub-lingual nitroglycerin leads to direct relaxation of smooth muscle of the systemic venous system, although such treatment is rarely adequate for acute pulmonary oedema.

Subsequent venous pooling in cardiac failure leads to a reduction in left ventricular end diastolic pressure and volume, reducing pulmonary congestion. There is usually no associated rise in cardiac output. Intravenous glyceryl trinitrate can be used acutely until oral agents can be introduced.

Isosorbide dinitrate and mononitrate

The combination of intravenous isosorbide dinitrate and intravenous diuretic has been shown to be a better treatment for acute heart failure than high dose diuretic alone.

Drugs affecting afterload

Hydralazine

This has a direct vasodilator effect confined to the arterial bed. Reduction in systemic vascular resistance leads to a considerable rise in cardiac output. Changes in arterial blood pressure, as a consequence of the rise in cardiac output and heart rate resulting from blunting of baroreflexes, are smaller than in patients with hypertension. Its use may be of benefit in chronic heart failure when used in combination with oral nitrates. Doses up to 200 mg daily are used in heart failure.

Calcium antagonists

Until recently heart failure was considered a contraindication to calcium antagonist use with evidence that nifedipine, diltiazem and verapamil could have adverse effects on prognosis after myocardial infarction in patients with heart failure. Recent studies with long-acting dihydropyridine calcium antagonists (amlodipine, felodipine) suggest that these agents may be safe in heart failure. Their only use is for the treatment of concomitant angina or hypertension when given in addition to an ACE inhibitor.

Drugs affecting preload and afterload

Alpha-adrenoceptor antagonists (see Chapter 8 on p. 82) and ACE inhibitors: see above.

Sodium nitroprusside

This is a mixed venous and arteriolar dilator also used for acute reduction of blood pressure (Chapter 8). It must be given intravenously by continuous infusion in a dose range 25–125 μg/min. Blood pressure falls rapidly and the effects wear off over 1–2 min after stopping the infusion. This agent is particularly useful in acute valvular insufficiency, such as mitral incompetence following an acute infarct or aortic incompetence in bacterial endocarditis. However, randomized controlled trials show a trend to increased mortality in patients with post-infarction heart failure treated routinely with this agent. It should not be used for more than 24–48 h because of accumulation of thiocyanate.

Comment. Vasodilator agents are generally reserved for patients who are intolerant of, or who have contraindications to, ACE inhibitors. A hydralazine/nitrate combination has been favoured in the past but was attended by a high incidence of side effects, poor tolerability and low compliance. Angiotensin II antagonists may be about to take over this role, although no formal trials have addressed this issue. Currently there is no evidence that adding a vasodilator to an ACE inhibitor routinely is of benefit in heart failure.

General principles of management

Acute left ventricular failure or pulmonary oedema presents with severe breathlessness, orthopnoea or nocturnal dyspnoea.

1 Sit the patient up.
2 100% oxygen.
3 Establish an i.v. line.
4 Give 5 mg diamorphine or 10 mg morphine i.v. (with an antiemetic) because:
   (a) It has a venodilator effect reducing preload.
   (b) It reduces the intense distress of the patient.
5 Give furosemide 40 mg i.v., more if the patient is already receiving a loop diuretic, because:

(a) It has a rapid off-loading effect resulting from venous dilatation.

(b) It has a slower off loading effect resulting from diuresis and natriuresis.

6 If the systolic blood pressure is ≥ 100 mmHg and obstructive valve disease has been excluded start on intravenous glyceryl trinitrate or isosorbide dinitrate infusion:

(a) It has a venodilator effect, reducing preload.

(b) It has a arterial vasodilator effect, reducing afterload.

(c) It reduces myocardial ischaemia which is often a coexistent problem in patients with acute heart failure.

7 In resistant patients invasive haemodynamic monitoring is indicated to help selection of appropriate vasodilator therapy with i.v. sodium nitroprusside or inotropic therapy, e.g. with dobutamine.

Cardiogenic shock consists of hypotension and oliguria with clinical signs of poor tissue perfusion. It is usually caused by recent extensive myocardial infarction.

1 Where possible monitor both arterial and pulmonary wedge pressure.

2 Give 100% oxygen.

3 Improve cardiac performance with dobutamine or a similar inotropic drug.

4 Low dose dopamine intravenously may improve renal function.

5 If this fails, then depending on the haemodynamic features try either reduction of afterload with sodium nitroprusside or glyceryl trinitrate, either instead of or in addition to dobutamine.

Long-term management of chronic heart failure

1 Modify cardiovascular risk factor profile, e.g. cigarette smoking, obesity. Arrange once only pneumococcal vaccination and regular immunization against influenza.

2 Underlying causes should be treated, e.g. anaemia, hypertension, valvular disease.

3 If this proves inadequate or when there is no treatable underlying cause, diuretics should be given. The type of diuretic and dose depends on severity of failure.

4 All patients without contraindication who have heart failure resulting from left ventricular systolic dysfunction should be treated with an ACE inhibitor, to improve symptoms further (if still present), to delay worsening heart failure and to reduce major morbidity and mortality.

5 All patients without contraindication who have heart failure due to left ventricular systolic dysfunction should be treated with a beta-blocker, to delay worsening heart failure and to reduce major morbidity and mortality.

6 In patients with persisting symptoms and/or signs of congestion add spironolactone to improve symptoms (if still present), reduce major morbidity and mortality.

7 Digoxin currently remains the drug of choice for the control of ventricular rate in patients with atrial fibrillation and heart failure.

8 In patients with persisting symptoms several strategies can be adopted:

(a) Add digoxin.

(b) An increase in diuretic dose.

(c) Ensure that the patient is on the maximally tolerated dose of ACE inhibitors.

(d) If arterial pressure is still elevated add a dihydropyridine calcium antagonist (amlodipine, felodipine) or hydralazine.

(e) If angina is present add a nitrate or calcium antagonist (amlodipine, felodipine).

(f) If marked oedema is present increase loop diuretic or add a thiazide diuretic or metolazone (careful monitoring of blood chemistry required).

(g) In resistant cases patients may be admitted for intravenous diuretic therapy. If this fails haemodynamic monitoring may be considered. Although empirical vasodilator therapy is not of proven benefit, observational experience suggests that vasodilator therapy tailored to optimize haemodynamics may be beneficial. Haemodynamic investigation often reveals overzealous diuretic therapy with too low a filling pressure to be the cause of the patient's symptoms.

9 Patients with atrial fibrillation should be considered for warfarin therapy.

7.2 Angina pectoris

Aims
Relief of symptoms, prevention of worsening angina and myocardial infarction and improved survival.

Relevant pathophysiology
Angina is the symptom experienced when myocardial oxygen delivery is insufficient to meet myocardial energy requirements. The major determinants of myocardial oxygen consumption are heart rate and the force of myocardial contraction. Angina occurs in two forms.

Stable angina
Attacks are predictably provoked by exertion or excitement and recede when the increased energy demand is withdrawn. The underlying pathology is usually chronic coronary artery disease, with moderate to severe fixed stenosis of the coronary arteries with super-added variation in coronary tone. Anaemia and thyrotoxicosis can precipitate or aggravate angina by reducing oxygen delivery and increasing energy requirements, respectively. Treatment can be directed at increasing myocardial oxygen supply (coronary vasodilatation) or reducing myocardial oxygen consumption (reduce heart rate, contractility, preload and afterload). Drugs that reduce heart rate also increase the duration of diastole, the time when most myocardial blood flow occurs.

Unstable angina
Attacks occur with increasing frequency and severity and on lesser exertion or at rest and are unpredictable. The underlying pathology is usually rupture or dissection of an atheromatous plaque with thrombus formation or extension in the coronary arteries. Spasm may be an additional mechanism. Acute changes in coronary artery pathology are pre-sumed and therapeutic attention directed to halting, reversing or bypassing the coronary arterial occlusive process in the hope of avoiding myocardial infarction. Given the nature of the pathophysiological process, antithrombotic therapy is the key. At the same time, treatment is aimed at reducing myocardial energy requirements. Severe unstable angina can progress to myocardial infarction or death.

Where medical measures have failed to stabilize or reverse the progress of severe unstable angina, coronary angiography and bypass surgery or coronary angioplasty should be considered on an urgent basis. Although there is little evidence that these reduce the risk of infarction or death, they may be effective in reducing or relieving symptoms.

Drugs used in angina

Glyceryl trinitrate

Mechanism
A potent, direct, short-acting, smooth muscle relaxant with widespread vasodilator activity. Whether the predominant effect is a direct action on the coronary arteries to increase flow or a peripheral (systemic) reduction in pre- and afterload is disputed.

Pharmacokinetics
Virtually 100% first-pass metabolism and it is therefore given sublingually, buccally, transdermally as a patch or paste, or intravenously. Very rapid clearance by liver metabolism: half-life about 2 min.

Adverse effects
These are dose related and result from vasodilatation and hypotension: headache, flushing and postural dizziness. These symptoms can be terminated by swallowing the tablet or spitting it out or by removing the patch.

Clinical use and dose
Glyceryl trinitrate tablets are generally kept as a 'rescue' treatment for 'breakthrough' angina.

Ideally, prophylactic therapy should prevent angina. Glyceryl trinitrate can also be taken sublingually by the patient before carrying out a task known to produce angina. The total daily dose may be determined individually as that required to control symptoms. Glyceryl trinitrate is also available in patch form. The shelf-life of sublingual glyceryl trinitate is only 6 months. For patients with infrequent angina chewable isosorbide dinitrate or a sublingual spray have a much longer shelf-life and are more appropriate.

Isosorbide dinitrate and isosorbide mononitrate

The clinical pharmacology of isosorbide dinitrate is similar to glyceryl trinitrate, but it is also effective orally and has a longer half-life of 40 min. Isosorbide mononitrate has an even longer half-life. It is the active metabolite of isosorbide dinitrate and is claimed to have more consistent pharmacokinetics and longer duration of action.

Early trials demonstrated loss of efficacy with long-acting nitrates after several weeks, especially with high doses. This was shown to be a result of tolerance and drug effect could be restored by a short break of treatment. Subsequently it has been shown that a 6- to 8-h nitrate-free interval in each 24 h allows restoration of nitrate efficacy. A long-acting formulation of isosorbide mononitrate can be used once daily while short-acting formulations of isosorbide dinitrate should be prescribed 2–3 times per day but with no doses given between 6 p.m. and 8 a.m. (i.e. an eccentric dosing regimen to give a nitrate-free interval). It must be realized that the patient has no anti-anginal cover over this period and, hence, is most vulnerable to a coronary event. If nocturnal angina is troublesome then the nitrate-free interval can be switched to the day time.

Doses
Isosorbide dinitrate: 30–120 mg daily in 2–3 doses.

Isosorbide mononitrate: 20–120 mg daily in one dose (or 2 doses not more than 8 h apart). Transdermal glyceryl trinitrate: 5–15 mg.

Comment. Nitrate patches should be removed at night to ensure efficacy during the day.

Potassium channel activators

Currently only nicorandil, a compound that has several mechanisms of action including activation of potassium channels and nitrate-like activity, is available for the management of angina in the UK. Nicorandil's pharmacodynamic profile is very similar to that of nitrates although tolerance is thought to be less of a problem.

Beta-receptor blockers

The detailed clinical pharmacology of these drugs is described in Chapter 8. Their value in angina depends mainly on decreasing myocardial oxygen consumption by:

1 Limiting the increased heart rate associated with exercise and anxiety.
2 Limiting the increased force of contraction associated with the same stimuli.
3 Increasing the length of diastole, the period during which coronary blood flow occurs.

Beta-blockers have been shown to reduce sudden death and reinfarction following a myocardial infarct.

Adverse effects (see pp. 75–77)
Rebound worsening of angina, myocardial infarction or tachycardia have been reported when beta-blockers are suddenly withdrawn. Reduce dose over 24–48 h if beta-blockers are being withdrawn in such patients.

Clinical use
There are no reliable data to say whether beta$_1$ selective or non-selective beta-blockers should be preferred in stable and unstable angina. The major post-myocardial infarction trials showing beta-blocker benefit used non-selective agents. The only absolute contra-indication for a beta-blocker is asthma.

Doses

Atenolol: 50–200 mg daily in two divided doses.

Metoprolol: 100–400 mg daily in two or three divided doses.

Bisoprolol: 5–20 mg once daily.

These drugs must all be given in an individually titrated dose to control symptoms and attenuate postural and exercise-induced tachycardia.

Calcium antagonists

There are two major groups:

1 Dihydropyridines including nifedipine, nicardipine, nitrendipine, felodipine and amlodipine.

2 Heart rate limiting ones including verapamil and diltiazem.

Calcium antagonists are further described in Chapter 8. Their principal action is inhibition of the slow calcium-ion channel component of the smooth muscle action potential leading to:

1 Decreased tone in vascular smooth muscle cells including coronary arteries.

2 Decreased contractility in myocardial cells.

3 Verapamil and diltiazem also have depressant effects on sinus node and AV node function (Chapter 6) and therefore slow heart rate. They have additional antiarrhythmic activity.

Pharmacokinetics

All drugs are well absorbed following oral administration. They are cleared by liver metabolism. All undergo extensive first-pass metabolism. Active metabolites may contribute to their effects.

Adverse effects

Headache, nausea, flushing and ankle swelling with nifedipine and other dihydropyridines. The side effects of nifedipine appear to be diminished markedly by combination with a beta-blocker. Constipation occurs with verapamil.

A recent meta-analysis suggested an increase in mortality with the use of nifedipine in patients with ischaemic heart disease. These studies were conducted with the standard formulation that has a rapid onset and offset of effect. Marked increases in sympathetic drive occurred concurrent with vasodilatation and may be responsible for this adverse effect. The most striking adverse effects on mortality were in patients with unstable angina; there is no evidence of an increase in mortality with stable angina. Most authorities suggest avoidance of short-acting formulations of calcium antagonists, particularly dihydropyridines. Slow release formulations of nifedipine have a smoother pharmacodynamic profile, as do long-acting calcium antagonists like amlodipine.

Increases in the risk of developing heart failure after myocardial infarction have been observed with diltiazem.

There is a general perception that beta-blockers may be more effective anti-anginal agents than calcium channel blockers and should be the first choice agent for angina prophylaxis.

Drug interactions

Verapamil or diltiazem should not be given routinely with beta-blockers since the combined negative inotropic and chronotropic effects can cause bradyarrhythmias and rarely precipitate heart failure.

Clinical use

They may be used in stable or unstable angina. Verapamil and diltiazem are alternative first line agents for a beta-blocker in intolerant patients in stable angina. Nifedipine and other dihydropyridines are used to best effect in combination with beta-blockers in severe angina.

Doses

Verapamil: 40 mg two or three times daily up to 360 mg daily in divided doses or as a single dose of a slow-release preparation.

Nifedipine: up to 120 mg daily as a long-acting preparation.

Amlodipine: 5–10 mg once per day.

Diltiazem: 60 mg two or three times daily up to 480 mg daily in divided doses or as a slow-release formulation once or twice daily.

General principles of management

It is important to remember that there are three major components to the treatment of angina:

1 Management of the risk factors for coronary atherosclerosis (e.g. lipid lowering, aspirin, antihypertensive drugs, cessation of smoking).

2 Treatment of symptoms.

3 Preventing or delaying myocardial infarction and death.

There is considerable evidence that treating the first two goals will achieve the third goal by default. There is also evidence that surgical revascularization of patients with angina and severe coronary artery disease improves prognosis.

Where possible, objective evidence of coronary disease should be sought using electrocardiography and exercise testing. This provides diagnostic confirmation and, importantly, objective evidence of the severity of the underlying ischaemia, providing the indication for coronary angiography.

Stable angina

1 Modify cardiovascular risk factors such as cigarette smoking, hypertension and hypercholesterolaemia (this may require drug therapy with a 'statin').

2 Prescribe prophylactic aspirin; clopidogrel is an alternative in aspirin intolerant patients.

3 Recent evidence suggests that ramipril 10 mg once daily may prevent cardiovascular events and death in patients with angina.

4 Treat any underlying precipitating cause such as anaemia, arrhythmias.

5 Prescribe prophylactic therapy with a beta-blocker or a rate-limiting calcium antagonist if a beta-blocker is contraindicated.

6 Prescribe treatment with glyceryl trinitrate for breakthrough attacks of angina or to be taken before undertaking the effort or activity that provokes pain.

7 If prophylaxis with a beta-blocker is unsuccessful use a combination of dihydropyridine calcium antagonist and beta-blocker or long-acting nitrate and calcium antagonist. Calcium antagonists that slow heart rate may be more efficacious than those that do not.

8 Coronary angiography is indicated under three circumstances:

(a) The diagnosis of angina is in doubt.

(b) Symptoms are not controlled with medical therapy, i.e. revascularization by coronary artery bypass graft (CABG) or percutaneous transluminal coronary angioplasty (PTCA) is indicated on symptomatic grounds.

(c) Stress testing suggests the presence of severe coronary artery disease, i.e. surgical revascularization might be indicated on prognostic grounds.

Unstable angina

Patients with suspected unstable angina should be treated with aspirin. There is also recent evidence that the new platelet glycoprotein receptor (GPIIb/IIIa) antagonists improve outcome in patients with severe unstable angina. Once the diagnosis is established (by demonstration of ST segment changes accompanied by symptoms and relieved by nitrates), the patient should receive intravenous nitrates and heparin (either intravenous unfractionated heparin or low molecular weight heparin), a beta-blocker (or verapamil if contraindicated). If symptoms persist a dihydropyridine calcium antagonist or diltiazem (the latter only if heart rate is >65/min) should be added. Symptoms lasting longer than 48 h indicate that angiography should be performed with a view to revascularization for symptom relief. In patients who settle, aspirin should be continued for 12 weeks. The evidence for longer term benefit is doubtful but is probably safe in those with well-preserved ventricular function. Thereafter, patients should be treated as for stable angina.

CHAPTER 8

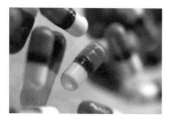

Hypertension and Hyperlipidaemia

Cardiovascular diseases, particularly myocardial infarction and stroke, constitute the commonest causes of death in westernized industrialized countries. Raised blood pressure, lipid disorders and cigarette smoking are major predictors of cardiovascular risk because they accelerate the development of atherosclerosis leading, ultimately, to occlusive thrombotic vascular diseases. Hypertension also predisposes to haemorrhagic stroke, cardiac failure and progressive renal failure.

There is evidence from clinical trials in both hypertension and hyperlipidaemia that preventive treatment can significantly reduce cardiovascular morbidity and mortality. The benefits of antihypertensive treatment are widely accepted and recent studies confirm the benefits of lipid lowering treatments. It is generally accepted that an integrated approach to the management of these two major risk factors is indicated in individuals at increased cardiovascular risk.

8.1 Hypertension

Aim

The aim of treatment is to reduce blood pressure in order to reduce the risk of death or disability from cardiovascular disease, especially stroke, coronary artery disease and cardiac failure. However, because hypertension is an asymptomatic condition, the treatment should control blood pressure without inducing adverse effects or otherwise interfering with the well-being of the patient. A target blood pressure of 140/85 mmHg or less is generally advocated, although this may be modified for particular patients, e.g. those with coexistent diabetes (target BP < 140/80) and patients at the highest risk of cardiovascular disease (Fig. 8.1).

Relevant pathophysiology

Blood pressure is the hydrostatic pressure within the systemic arteries and is determined by total peripheral resistance and cardiac output. Total peripheral resistance is invariably increased in established hypertension, although the causative mechanism is not clearly understood, but increases in heart rate or cardiac output are not consistently found.

Blood pressure values are distributed normally (unimodally) in a given population and there is no clear cut-off between normotensive and hypertensive values. Long-term prospective epidemiological studies indicate that, for both systolic and diastolic blood pressure, the higher the blood pressure the greater the risk of cardiovascular disease. The definition of hypertension is therefore dependent upon the selection of an arbitrary value for normal blood pressure in a given population and the frequency of hypertension varies according to the age, sex and ethnic origin, for example, in the population studied.

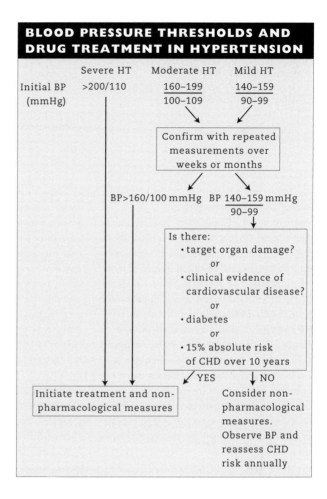

BLOOD PRESSURE THRESHOLDS AND DRUG TREATMENT IN HYPERTENSION

	Severe HT	Moderate HT	Mild HT
Initial BP (mmHg)	>200/110	160–199 / 100–109	140–159 / 90–99

Confirm with repeated measurements over weeks or months

BP>160/100 mmHg   BP 140–159 mmHg / 90–99

Is there:
• target organ damage?
  or
• clinical evidence of cardiovascular disease?
  or
• diabetes
  or
• 15% absolute risk of CHD over 10 years

YES   NO

Initiate treatment and non-pharmacological measures

Consider non-pharmacological measures. Observe BP and reassess CHD risk annually

Fig. 8.1 Treatment decisions based on observed blood pressure.

Primary and secondary hypertension

Hypertension is either primary or secondary. No underlying cause can be identified in about 95% of cases and the terminology of primary or idiopathic or, most commonly, essential is applied. There is a strong polygenic familial trend and environmental factors such as salt and alcohol consumption also contribute. Secondary types of hypertension are relatively rare, even in younger age groups, and usually have an endocrine or renal basis. The following are some potential causes of secondary hypertension.

Risks of hypertension

There is a direct relationship between the severity of hypertension and the increase in morbid and mortal cardiovascular events. Even mild hypertension, which affects the greatest number of individuals, carries an increased risk of cardiovascular disease. Malignant hypertension, i.e. severe hypertension associated with renal damage (proteinuria) and vascular damage (seen on fundoscopy as haemorrhages and exudates and papilloedema), requires urgent treatment otherwise it leads to death in 90% of cases within 1 year, usually from cerebral haemorrhage or renal failure.

CAUSES OF SECONDARY HYPERTENSION

1 Renal diseases
(a) Glomerulonephritis.
(b) Renovascular disease, particularly renal artery stenosis (as a result of fibromuscular hyperplasia in young patients and atheroma in older patients).
2 Endocrine disease
(a) Phaeochromocytoma.
(b) Hyperaldosteronism (Conn's syndrome).
(c) Hypercorticism (Cushing's syndrome).
(c) Acromegaly.
(d) Hypothyroidism.
3 Coarctation of the aorta.
4 Drugs, e.g. oral contraceptives, corticosteroids, NSAIDs, ciclosporin.

Benefits of treatment

Although some clinical trials have produced equivocal results, there is now overall evidence that antihypertensive treatment significantly reduces stroke and the progression of renal and cardiac failure. These benefits have been clearly established in moderate hypertension (systolic 160–199 mmHg and/or diastolic 100–109 mmHg), in severe hypertension (systolic greater than 200 mmHg and/or diastolic greater than 110 mmHg) and in malignant or accelerated phase hypertension. In the treatment of mild hypertension (systolic 140–159 mmHg and/or diastolic blood pressure 90–99 mmHg) there again have been substantial reductions in stroke but only partial benefits in respect of coronary artery disease, and there is not yet a clear explanation for this. The benefits of treatment in mild hypertension are greatest among those patients who have evidence of target organ damage (e.g. left ventricular hypertrophy (LVH), retinopathy or proteinuria), diabetes, pre-existing cardiovascular disease (e.g. prior myocardial infarction (MI)), or a high risk of coronary heart disease (CHD) (>15% over 10 years) by virtue of other risk factors such as raised cholesterol levels.

Principles of antihypertensive treatment

Drugs may be given alone or in rational combinations which do not lead to adverse effects or

ANTIHYPERTENSIVE TREATMENT

1 Hypertension should be confirmed by several measurements of blood pressure over several days, weeks or months.
2 Patients should be counselled about hypertension, and its risk, and the relevance of other risk factors. The reason for long-term treatment should be carefully explained.
3 Hypertension should be treated as part of a management plan for reducing all identifiable cardiovascular risk factors. Mild to moderate hypertension should seldom be treated in isolation and it is important to attempt to modify all of the individual patient's risk factors including cigarette smoking, hyperlipidaemia and diabetes mellitus and to take account of other factors such as a family history of premature cardiovascular disease.
4 Non-pharmacological approaches should always be considered; for example:
(a) for the obese patient, weight reduction of 10 kg may lower blood pressure by about 20/10 mmHg.
(b) if salt intake is very high (more than 200 mEq per day), a modest reduction by the simple avoidance of excessively salty foods and the use of table salt may aid blood pressure control.
(c) consider regular physical exercise.
5 Arrangements should be made for regular and convenient long-term follow-up with blood pressure measurements.
6 As required, a simple and well tolerated antihypertensive drug regimen should be established.

long-term toxicity and the simplest drug regimen is likely to be the most successful. In this respect, compliance with treatment is likely to be maintained best if drugs are administered only once daily. A wide range of suitable first-line antihypertensive drugs is now available and the classes of drug which are currently in widespread use are thiazide diuretics, beta-blockers, calcium antagonists, angiotensin converting enzyme (ACE) inhibitors and angiotensin II (AT$_1$) receptor blockers. Whilst a systematic and rather rigid regimen based upon diuretics and beta-blockers either alone or in combination was previously recommended, there is now a tendency to try to select the most appropriate therapy to meet the particular requirements of the individual patient. The response to treatment can then be evaluated over a period of weeks or months and, if the effect is insufficient and if there are no side effects, the dosage can be increased. If side effects occur or if there is clearly no useful blood pressure response to treatment then it would be appropriate to change to one of the alternative types of therapy. As an alternative, combination treatments may prove particularly suitable, not only for blood pressure control and compliance but also for satisfying the requirements of the individual patient in terms of other CHD risk factors, or concomitant disease states.

Clinical comment. The management of hypertension is a long-term undertaking often in asymptomatic patients. The simplest, safest and most effective treatment should be determined for each individual. Reduction of blood pressure and control of other risk factors is designed to reduce cardiovascular morbidity and mortality without impairing the quality of life. Most patients are started on single drug therapy but more than half of them will require a second or third drug from different classes to achieve treatment targets of 140/85 or less.

Antihypertensive drugs
The following are the most important antihypertensive drug classes (Table 8.1):

1 Thiazide diuretics.
2 Beta-adrenoceptor antagonists.
3 Calcium antagonists.
4 ACE inhibitors.
5 AT$_1$ receptor antagonists.
6 Alternative—alpha$_1$-antagonists; vasodilators; centrally acting agents.

Diuretics

Mechanism of action
These drugs increase sodium excretion and urine volume by interfering with sodium, chloride and water transport across renal tubular cell membranes (Table 8.2). Thus, diuretics are used in states of salt and water overload such as congestive heart failure (Chapter 7, p. 60), nephrotic syndrome and hepatic failure with ascites. The diuretic activity was thought initially to be the mechanism of the antihypertensive effect. However, it is now recognized that the antihypertensive effect is not related directly to the diuretic potency, but instead that the blood pressure lowering action appears to depend upon more subtle alterations to the contractile responses of vascular smooth muscle. Thus, although thiazide diuretics are not powerful diuretics, they are the preferred drugs for the treatment of hypertension. In contrast, loop diuretics, such as furosemide, have greater diuretic potency but their effects on blood pressure are relatively short-acting and liable to provoke reflex stimulation of the renin–angiotensin system to counter any fall in blood pressure. Potassium sparing diuretics are the weakest agents in terms of their diuretic potency but they are not associated with potassium loss, which occurs with both thiazide and loop diuretics. Thus, in refractory oedema they are very useful in combination with the loop diuretics and in some hypertensive patients they can usefully be combined with a thiazide diuretic. The antihypertensive effect of thiazide diuretics manifests at relatively low dosages and there is no additional benefit from high doses in terms of blood pressure reduction. In contrast, it is

MAJOR CLASSES OF ANTIHYPERTENSIVE DRUGS

	Indications		Contraindications	
	Strong	Possible	Possible	Strong
Thiazide diuretics	Elderly patients	–	Dyslipidaemia	Gout
Beta-blockers	Myocardial infarction Angina	Heart failure*	Heart failure*	Asthma or COPD Heart block
Calcium antagonists I (dihydropyridine)	Isolated systolic HT in elderly subjects	Angina Elderly patients	–	–
Calcium antagonists II (rate-limiting drugs)	Angina	Myocardial infarction	Combination with beta-blockers	Heart block Heart failure
ACE inhibitors	Heart failure LV dysfunction Type I diabetic nephropathy	Chronic renal disease†	Renal impairment Peripheral vascular disease	Pregnancy Reno-vascular HT
ANGII antagonists	ACE inhibitor induced cough	Heart failure Intolerance of other antihyper- tensives	Peripheral vascular disease	Pregnancy Reno-vascular HT

ACE, angiotensin converting enzyme; COPD, chronic obstructive pulmonary disease; HT, hypertension; LV, left ventricular; ANGII, angiotensin II.
* Beta blockers may worsen heart failure, but in specialist hands may be used to treat heart failure.
† ACE inhibitors may be beneficial in chronic renal failure but should be used with caution under specialist supervision.

Table 8.1 Indications and contraindications for the major classes of antihypertensive drugs.

possible to increase the diuretic response with higher dosages but this also leads to greater potassium loss, for example, and is therefore unnecessary and unwanted in hypertension.

Clinical pharmacology

Thiazides are well absorbed orally, widely distributed and subject to a variable amount of hepatic metabolism. The effects on the renal tubule depend upon excretion of the drug into the tubule and thiazide diuretics become less effective in renal impairment where loop diuretics retain some efficacy. With thiazides, the onset of the diuretic effect is usually observed within 1 h and may last for about 12 h but, with repeated dosing, the acute diuretic effect tends to diminish in the majority

of hypertensive patients. The antihypertensive effect, however, is more gradual in onset and more long lasting so that, at steady state, the antihypertensive effect persists for more than 24 h and once-daily dosing is therefore appropriate for most agents.

Pharmacologically predictable adverse effects

Hypokalaemia. Because of the increased urinary loss of potassium there may be a reduction in blood potassium to levels below normal. As severe hypokalaemia may precipitate cardiac arrhythmias (especially in patients also receiving digoxin), it may be necessary to provide potassium supplements or to use a combination diuretic treatment with both a thiazide diuretic and a potassium sparing diuretic. In general, to avoid this problem, thiazide diuretics are recommended in low dosage but if severe hypokalaemia persists with low-dose thiazide treatment it should raise the suspicion of an underlying problem such as mineralocorticoid excess (Conn's syndrome).

Hyperuricaemia. Because thiazide diuretics also interfere with the excretion of uric acid, there may be an increased blood level of uric acid and, rarely, the provocation of an acute gouty episode.

Hyperglycaemia. Long-term diuretic therapy is associated with an impairment of glucose tolerance and an increased incidence of non-insulin-dependent diabetes mellitus. The mechanism appears to be mainly related to interference with the action of insulin in peripheral tissues (so-called 'insulin resistance').

Hypercalcaemia. This is a rare adverse effect of thiazide diuretics resulting from reduced renal excretion of calcium.

Other adverse effects
Hyperlipidaemia. By mechanisms that are not entirely clear, long-term use of thiazide diuretics is associated with modest changes in the plasma lipid profile with increases in total and low density lipoprotein (LDL) cholesterol, increases in triglycerides and a reduction in high density lipoprotein (HDL) cholesterol.

ACTION OF DIURETICS

	Site of action	Comment
Thiazides, e.g. Bendroflumethiazide (bendrofluazide) Hydrochlorothiazide Chlortalidone (chlorthalidone)	Proximal part of the distal tubule	All have an antihypertensive effect. Little evidence that newer agents have any advantages over older established agents
Loop diuretics, e.g. Furosemide (frusemide) Bumetanide	Ascending limb of loop of Henle	Potent diuretic and saliuretic but less useful for the treatment of hypertension
Potassium sparing diuretics, e.g. Spironolactone	Distal tubule Aldosterone antagonist	May be used in combination with loop diuretics in refractory oedema
Triamterene	Sodium potassium exchange	May cause hyperkalaemia in renal failure or in the elderly
Amiloride		

Table 8.2 Classification and site of action of diuretics.

Impotence. This is a well-recognized but occasional problem with long-term diuretic treatment. The mechanism is not known and the problem is usually reversible on treatment withdrawal.

Others. Thrombocytopenia and skin rash occur rarely.

Clinical comment. Thiazide diuretics (for example, bendroflumethiazide (bendrofluazide) 2.5 mg daily; hydrochlorothiazide 25 or 50 mg daily; chlortalidone (chlorthalidone) 12.5 or 25 mg daily) are widely used and are effective antihypertensive drugs in mild, moderate and severe hypertension. Where the hypertension is complicated by chronic renal failure, or is proving refractory to treatment, it may be necessary to use a loop diuretic. Because diuretic-induced hypokalaemia has been associated in the past with cardiac rhythm disturbances, it may be necessary to add a potassium sparing drug such as amiloride or triamterene; the combination of a thiazide and a potassium sparing drug is a popular and effective first-line treatment. Serum potassium tends to rise in renal failure, a potassium sparing diuretic should be avoided in this condition. As an alternative a combination of low-dose diuretic with an ACE inhibitor or an angiotensin receptor antagonist is a very effective well-tolerated regimen.

Beta-adrenoceptor antagonists (beta-blockers)

Mechanism of action
Beta-blockers antagonize the effects of sympathetic nerve stimulation or circulating catecholamines. Beta-adrenoceptors are widely distributed throughout the body systems and are subclassified as beta$_1$- and beta$_2$-receptors according to their location. Beta$_1$-receptors are predominant in the heart and beta$_2$-receptors predominate in other organs such as lung, peripheral blood vessels and skeletal muscle. This is a clinically useful subclassification but it is not absolutely accurate: for example, there

are beta$_2$-receptors in the heart and there are beta$_1$-receptors in the kidney.
1 *Heart*: stimulation of beta$_1$-receptors in the sino-atrial node causes an increase in heart rate (a positive chronotropic effect) and stimulation of the beta$_1$-receptors in the myocardium increases the force of cardiac contractility (a positive inotropic effect).
2 *Kidney*: stimulation of beta-receptors in the kidney promotes the release of renin from the juxtaglomerular cells and thereby increases the activity of the renin–angiotensin–aldosterone system.
3 *Central and peripheral nervous system*: stimulation of beta-receptors in the brainstem and stimulation of prejunctional beta-receptors in the periphery promote the release of neurotransmitters and increased sympathetic nervous system activity.

Overall, therefore, stimulation of beta-receptors in the heart, kidney and nervous system leads to an increase in cardiac output, an increase in peripheral vascular resistance and an increase in aldosterone-mediated sodium and water retention. Treatment with beta-blockers is able to antagonize all of these effects to cause a reduction in blood pressure but it remains unclear which is the principal antihypertensive mechanism of these drugs. Acutely, beta blockade leads to a reduction in cardiac output but during long-term treatment the antihypertensive effect is instead associated with a reduction of the elevated peripheral vascular resistance.

Beta-adrenoceptors are also found in the eye. Beta$_2$-receptors control the formation of aqueous humour and beta-blockers applied topically to the eye are used in the treatment of glaucoma. Beta$_2$-receptors are also found in the uterus and stimulation of these receptors relaxes the gravid uterus: beta$_2$-agonists are used to delay premature labour.

Clinical pharmacology
Beta-blockers vary in the extent to which they are eliminated via the kidney or via the liver, usually with extensive first-pass metabolism. The lipid soluble beta-blockers, such as pro-

pranolol, typically depend upon hepatic metabolism for their clearance, whereas the relatively water-soluble beta-blockers, e.g. atenolol are eliminated via the kidney. Propranolol is often quoted as a reference example of a drug which undergoes extensive first pass hepatic metabolism: this is flow limited because it is directly dependent upon hepatic blood flow (see Chapter 1, p. 14). Thus, particularly for the drugs eliminated by the liver, a wide range of doses will be required in clinical practice because of the wide inter-individual variability in bioavailability combined with the inter-individual variability in response. The half-life of most beta-blockers is relatively short: those which depend upon the liver usually require multiple daily dosing, whereas those eliminated via the kidney tend to have longer half-lives and may be suitable for once daily administration, particularly at high doses.

Pharmacologically predictable adverse effects
Bradycardia and impairment of myocardial contractility. An excessive reduction in heart rate and bradycardia are relatively common but seldom symptomatic. Rarely, an excessive reduction in inotropic activity may precipitate or exacerbate cardiac failure in a susceptible individual. Whilst these depressant effects on cardiac function are occasionally deleterious, they also lead to a reduction in cardiac work and a reduction in myocardial oxygen demand which contributes to the antianginal efficacy of these agents (see Chapter 7). Although beta-blockers can worsen left ventricular dysfunction, there is recent evidence that, under specialist supervision, beta-adrenoceptor antagonists may improve symptoms and prolong survival in patients with congestive heart failure.

Peripheral vasoconstriction. The beta$_2$-receptors in the smooth muscle of peripheral blood vessels subserve a vasodilator role, especially in skeletal muscle beds, and blockade of these receptors leads to a relative vasoconstriction which typically gives rise to impairment of the peripheral circulation with cold hands and feet and, possibly, also the development of Raynaud's phenomenon or the worsening of peripheral vascular disease. It must be noted that this peripheral vascular effect does not contribute to the blood pressure lowering effect and, as such, it is distinctly different from the effects mediated via beta-receptors in the peripheral nerves.

CNS effects. Blockade of these beta-receptors is associated with reduced sympathetic outflow, which is the probable cause of a sense of malaise which may occur insidiously during long-term treatment. Additionally, vivid dreams, nightmares and, rarely, hallucinations may occur with highly lipid soluble beta-blockers, and propranolol in particular, because of their greater penetration into the central nervous system (CNS).

Bronchospasm. Beta$_2$-receptors mediate dilatation of the bronchi and obviously blockade of these receptors may precipitate bronchospasm in susceptible individuals.

Tiredness and fatigue. Stimulation of beta$_2$-receptors in skeletal muscle is associated with increased muscle activity and blockade of these receptors leads to a sense of tiredness and ready fatigue during exercise.

Masking of hypoglycaemia. The awareness of hypoglycaemia in the insulin-dependent diabetic depends partly upon sympathetic nervous activation. This response will be blunted by beta-blockers.

Metabolic disturbances. Beta-blockers, especially non-selective agents, tend to cause a small increase in triglycerides and reduced high density lipoprotein (HDL) cholesterol.

Additional pharmacological characteristics (see Table 8.3)
1 Partial agonist activity (sometimes known as intrinsic sympathomimetic activity) manifests

BETA-BLOCKERS

Clinical class	Approved name	Beta$_1$-selectivity	Major route of elimination
Non-selective	Propranolol	–	Liver
Selective	Atenolol	++	Kidney
	Bisoprolol	++	Liver/kidney
	Metoprolol	++	Liver
Additional properties			
Intrinsic sympathomimetic activity (also, partial agonist activity)	Pindolol	–	Liver
Anti-arrhythmic properties	Sotalol	–	Liver
Dual antihypertensive mechanism	Labetalol	–	Liver

Table 8.3 Examples of the pharmacological properties and route of elimination of some beta-blockers in clinical use.

as a beta-stimulant effect when background adrenergic activity is minimal (e.g. during sleep) but the drug's beta-blocker effect manifests when adrenergic activity is increased (e.g. during exercise).

2 Membrane-stabilizing activity: this is a local anaesthetic and antiarrhythmic effect but it is of negligible relevance in humans.

3 Selectivity: the prototype beta-blocker, propranolol, was non-selective insofar as it blocked the responses mediated via both beta$_1$- and beta$_2$-receptors. Because many of the potential adverse effects are mediated through beta$_2$-receptors and many of the desirable effects require blockade of beta$_1$-receptors in the heart, there has been the development of relatively beta$_1$-selective (or cardioselective) blockers. It is important to recognize, however, that this selectivity is not absolute and that all beta-blockers are potentially capable of causing, for example, bronchospasm.

4 Additional pharmacological properties: it is possible to augment the beta-blocker molecule with an ability to also block effects mediated through peripheral alpha-adrenoceptors (e.g. labetalol and carvedilol) or to harness some beta$_2$-agonist or direct vasodilator activity (e.g. celiprolol).

Clinical comment. All beta-blockers, irrespective of their additional characteristics, lower blood pressure to a similar extent. In hypertension those which are beta$_1$-selective ('cardioselective') and which can be administered once daily tend to be preferred, e.g. bisoprolol 10 mg daily, atenolol 25–100 mg once daily. It is important to recognize that, irrespective of their apparent 'cardioselectivity', these drugs are contraindicated in people with asthma and that they should be used with caution in patients at risk of cardiac failure.

In addition to their use in hypertension, beta-blockers are also used to treat the following conditions: supraventricular cardiac arrhythmias, angina pectoris, anxiety neurosis, thyrotoxicosis, migraine and glaucoma. There is also some evidence that prophylactic treatment with propranolol reduces the risk of gastrointestinal bleeding among patients with chronic liver disease and proven oesophageal varices.

Calcium antagonists

Mechanism of action

Increased peripheral vascular resistance depends upon increased constrictor 'tone' in peripheral blood vessels, which, in turn, reflects increased contractility of vascular smooth muscle. This process is calcium dependent and, fundamentally, the calcium antagonist drugs which are also known as calcium entry blockers are able to promote vasodilator activity by reducing calcium influx into the cell by interfering with the voltage operated calcium channels (and to a lesser extent the receptor-operated channels) in the cell membrane of vascular smooth muscle.

Interference with intracellular calcium influx is also important in cardiac muscle, cardiac conducting tissue and the smooth muscle of the gastrointestinal (GI) tract: thus, the potential cardiac effects of calcium antagonism are negative inotropic, chronotropic and dromotropic activities and the GI effects lead to constipation. These effects vary with different agents according to the ability to penetrate cardiac and other tissues and, in particular, because the receptor or recognition site close to the calcium channel is slightly different for each drug class.

Thus, although they are often considered as a single class, there are very clear distinctions to be made between the three principal types of calcium antagonist drug:

1 Dihydropyridine derivatives: prototype drug, nifedipine.

2 Phenylalkalamines: prototype drug, verapamil.

3 Benzothiazipine derivatives: prototype drug, diltiazem.

The dihydropyridine derivatives have pronounced peripheral vasodilator properties, whereas verapamil and diltiazem also have cardiac effects and reduce heart rate.

Clinical pharmacology

The three prototype drugs have low and variable oral bioavailability because all are subject to extensive first-pass metabolism. Numerically the dihydropyridine derivatives are most important and all are similarly susceptible to first-pass metabolism with one exception (amlodipine) which, although it is extensively metabolized, has a substantially longer half-life than any of the other agents (more than 40 h compared to less than 10 h) (see Table 8.4).

Both diltiazem and verapamil have short half-lives because of extensive first-pass metabolism. During chronic treatment they have a tendency to inhibit hepatic drug metabolism

CALCIUM ANTAGONISTS			
Drugs		Half-life (h)	Dosing frequency
Dihydropyridines			
Short-acting	Nifedipine	4–6	Multiple
	Nicardipine	4–6	
Intermediate	Isradipine	8–12	Once or twice daily
Long-acting	Amlodipine	> 40	Once
	Nifedipine	(special formulation)	Once
Verapamil		8–12	Multiple*
Diltiazem		6–10	Multiple*
* Unless special formulation.			

Table 8.4 Clinical classification of calcium antagonist drugs.

and therefore their own half-lives during steady-state treatment are slightly longer than those following the first dose. This enzyme inhibitory effect is a potential source for drug interactions, e.g. with ciclosporin.

Pharmacologically predictable adverse effects

1 Dihydropyridines: particularly with rapid onset and short-acting agents, there is a well-recognized pattern of vasodilator side effects with headache and facial flushing and an associated reflex activation of the sympathetic nervous system which provokes cardioacceleration and palpitations. These symptoms usually decline with time. The longer acting agents and the longer acting formulations, however, are less likely to promote these so-called vasodilator effects. Swelling of the ankles and occasionally of the hands is a well-recognized long-term effect of the dihydropyridine derivatives, including the long-acting agents, but this does not appear to be attributable to a generalized fluid retention and instead reflects a drug-related disturbance of the haemodynamics of the microcirculation in the periphery, plus the effect of gravity.

2 Verapamil: the early onset vasodilator effects are less common with verapamil but the cardiac effects may manifest as bradycardia or atrioventricular (AV) conduction delay. Constipation is a well-recognized symptomatic complaint.

3 Diltiazem: the early vasodilator effects are again less apparent but bradycardia and AV conduction effects are recognized. Skin rash occurs occcasionally.

Clinical comment. All types of calcium-antagonist drugs are effective antihypertensive agents because of their peripheral vasodilator activity. The long-acting dihydropyridine drugs, such as amlodipine or nifedipine in its long-acting once-daily formulation, are generally preferred in the treatment of hypertension because of their lack of negative cardiac effects and because of their suitability

for once-daily dosing. This has additional practical implications when drug combination with a beta-blocker is required (a well-established and effective combination in both hypertension and angina) where there are concerns about the combined cardio-depressant effects of the two drugs. In contrast, the negative cardiac effects of diltiazem and verapamil lead to reduced myocardial oxygen demand such that these drugs tend to be the preferred types of calcium antagonist as monotherapy in angina (see Chapter 7). Dihydropyridine calcium antagonists are particularly suitable for elderly patients with isolated systolic hypertension.

ACE inhibitors

Mechanism of action

ACE inhibitors are drugs which competitively inhibit the activity of angiotensin coverting enzyme (which is also termed kininase II) to prevent the formation of the active octapeptide angiotensin II from its inactive precursor, angiotensin I. This occurs in blood and in tissues including the kidney, heart, blood vessels, adrenal gland and brain. Angiotensin II has a range of activities but most importantly it is a potent vasoconstrictor, it promotes aldosterone release and it facilitates sympathetic activity both centrally and peripherally. Whilst the reduction in blood pressure following ACE inhibition is greatest in patients with a stimulated renin–angiotensin system (such as in sodium depletion, or diuretic treatment, or renal artery stenosis or in malignant phase hypertension) it is now recognized that ACE inhibitors also lower blood pressure in essential hypertensive patients with normal or low activity of the renin–angiotensin system. Although these drugs can functionally be considered to be peripheral vasodilators, it is noteworthy that the response to ACE inhibition does not provoke any reflex cardioacceleration.

The enzyme, kininase II, is also responsible for the breakdown of kinins that have vasodilator and other properties. Inhibition in this system leads to an accumulation of kinins which promotes vasodilator activity and may make a contribution to the overall effectiveness of ACE inhibitor drugs.

Clinical pharmacology
All ACE inhibitor drugs are bound to tissues and plasma proteins and this gives rise to a characteristic concentration–time profile whereby free drug is relatively rapidly eliminated by the kidney, predominantly by glomerular filtration, such that there is little evidence of drug accumulation during chronic dosing. However, because of the binding to tissue sites the plasma drug concentration–time profile shows a long-lasting terminal elimination phase of several days.

There are significant pharmacological differences between the early ACE inhibitors. For example, the prototype drug captopril is absorbed rapidly but has a short duration of action and is usually administered twice or three times daily. Enalapril, like many of the other later ACE inhibitors, is an inactive prodrug that requires hydrolysis in the liver to its active form enalaprilat. Lisinopril is an analogue of enalapril and is itself active (see Table 8.5).

The dose–response relationship for blood pressure reduction is linear initially, but a 'plateau' is quickly reached within the therapeutic dose range; further increases in dosage do not increase the intensity of effect, either on blood pressure reduction or on plasma ACE inhibition, but will prolong the duration of action. The fall in blood pressure following ACE inhibition is not associated with a change in heart rate, in particular there is no reflex tachycardia.

Pharmacologically predictable adverse effects
Profound hypotension. This may complicate the first dose of ACE inhibitor drugs especially in patients with sodium or volume depletion in whom the renin–angiotensin system is activated. This only rarely occurs in uncomplicated essential hypertension but is occasionally seen in patients with cardiac failure.

Impairment of renal function. This is a recognized complication of ACE inhibition, particularly in patients with renovascular disease (bilateral renal artery stenosis). Reversible renal failure may be precipitated in these patients.

Cough. This is the most frequent adverse effect and is probably attributable to the effect on the kinin system rather than upon ACE inhibition. Thus, non-productive, irritant cough is widely reported in the treatment of

RENIN–ANGIOTENSIN SYSTEM

ACE inhibitors	Typical dose regimens
First generation	
Captopril	25 mg two or three times daily
Enalapril	5–20 mg once or twice daily
Lisinopril	5–20 mg once daily
Second generation	
Fosinopril	10–20 mg once daily
Perindopril	2–4 mg once daily
Quinapril	20–40 mg once or twice daily
Ramipril	2.5–5 mg daily
Trandolapril	1–2 mg daily

Table 8.5 Drugs acting on the renin–angiotensin system.

hypertension in up to about 15% of patients. The reported incidence is considerably less in patients with cardiac failure, presumably as a reflection of their much higher background incidence of respiratory symptoms.

Other adverse effects. Angioneurotic oedema is a rare but well-recognized class effect that also has been attributed to the kinin potentiation. Increases in serum potassium and, occasionally, hyperkalaemia occur because ACE inhibitors have potassium saving effects (mediated via the reduction in aldosterone). Taste disturbance and skin rash occur slightly more frequently with captopril, perhaps as a consequence of its chemical structure that contains a sulphydryl group.

Clinical comment. Although many of these agents are recommended for once-daily dosing, it appears that a more consistent response is produced by twice-daily administration. In elderly patients, or in patients with compromised renal function, or in patients with cardiac failure, it is advisable to initiate treatment with lower than usual dosages. In general these drugs are considered to be well tolerated by patients, especially in comparison with 'old-fashioned' competitor agents. ACE inhibitor drugs combine well with thiazide diuretics, and with calcium antagonists, to produce overall antihypertensive effects which are at least additive. However, it is recommended that potassium supplements and potassium sparing diuretics should not be used in combination because hyperkalaemia may result, especially if

there is pre-existing renal impairment. The effectiveness of ACE inhibitors in both hypertension and cardiac failure may be compromised by non-steroidal anti-inflammatory drugs (NSAIDs) and, if possible, NSAIDs should be avoided in these patients.

A new generation of ACE inhibitors with additional endopeptidase inhibitory properties and potential natiuretic peptides are under evaluation. Further experience will confirm whether the enhanced efficacy observed is associated with acceptable tolerability and long-term benefits.

Angiotensin (AT_1) receptor antagonists

Angiotensin II receptors are classified into two subtypes, AT_1 and AT_2. The AT_1 receptor mediates all of the classical pharmacological effects of angiotensin II, e.g. vasoconstriction and aldosterone release, whereas the functional role of the AT_2 receptor remains unclear. Because many tissues contain enzymatic pathways capable of converting angiotensin I to angiotensin II, independently of ACE, there are theoretical advantages in blocking the renin–angiotensin system via AT_1 receptor antagonism. Losartan was the first AT_1 receptor antagonist; irbesartan, valsartan and candesartan have followed (Table 8.6). All four drugs are well absorbed after oral administration but differ slightly in their pharmacokinetic and pharmacodynamic properties. Losartan is converted to an active metabolite, EXP 3174; candesartan is the active metabolite of the compound adminis-

ANGIOTENSIN II (AT_1) RECEPTOR ANTAGONISTS			
Drug	Prodrug	Route of elimination	Half-life (h)
Losartan	Yes	Hepatic	6–9
Valsartan	No	Unchanged in urine	6
Irbesartan	No	Hepatic	15–17
Candesartan cilexetil	Yes	Hepatic	6–12

Table 8.6 Angiotensin II antagonists used in hypertension.

tered as candesartan cilexetil. Irbesartan, valsartan, candesartan and EXP 3174 exhibit non-competitive binding to the AT_1 receptor, so the duration of blood pressure-lowering effect is longer than the apparent half-life of the drug.

The angiotensin II antagonists produce similar reductions in blood pressure to other antihypertensive agents, but they seem to be particularly well tolerated with very few side effects, in particular, these drugs are not associated with the dry cough seen with ACE inhibitors. Angiotensin II antagonists may also benefit patients with congestive heart failure and patients with type II diabetes complicated by hypertension and nephropathy.

Other antihypertensive drugs

Drugs with vasodilator properties

Drugs with overt vasodilator activity have been used widely in the past, particularly in combination with beta-blockers and diuretics. This combination is especially effective because the beta-blocker and diuretic attenuate the reflex activation of the sympathetic and renin–angiotensin–aldosterone systems typically provoked with these agents. Direct-acting vasodilators, such as hydralazine and minoxidil, are particularly likely to provoke reflex cardioacceleration and fluid retention and their vasodilator action was also associated with symptomatic adverse effects such as facial flushing and headache.

Hydralazine. In current therapeutic practice hydralazine is reserved for use as a third-line agent in combination with a beta-blocker and a diuretic. An additional complication with hydralazine is that it undergoes hepatic metabolism involving the genetically determined acetylator pathway. Thus, there are 'fast' and 'slow' acetylators with an increased risk of toxicity in slow acetylators, typically a drug-induced lupus syndrome, and a poor anti-hypertensive response in fast acetylators who rapidly metabolize the active drug.

Alpha₁-antagonists. These drugs act via selective blockade of peripheral alpha₁-adrenoceptors to produce their vasodilator effects but they are not widely used first line agents. Instead they tend to be used as third-line agents or where other drugs are poorly tolerated.

Alpha-blockers are associated with a 'first dose' hypotensive effect that constitutes a postural hypotensive response after the initial dosage, accompanied by reflex cardioacceleration and palpitations. In susceptible patients, however, who cannot maintain a rapid heart rate there is the risk of a vago–vagal collapse leading to syncope. This first-dose effect was particularly associated with the short-acting prototype agent prazosin and is less of a problem with longer-acting agents such as doxazosin. However, recent evidence from a controlled trial suggests that the long-term outcome with doxazosin is less good than with a diuretic.

Centrally acting agents

Agents acting on alpha₂-adrenoceptors, or related receptors in the brainstem, are known to reduce sympathetic outflow and lead to a reduction in blood pressure. These agents act upon regulatory and inhibitory neurotransmitter systems but usually are not sufficiently selective or specific to avoid symptomatic adverse CNS effects.

Clonidine is a recognized alpha₂-adrenoceptor agonist that is known to cause sedation and drowsiness, dry mouth, and interference with sexual function in men. In addition, this agent is known to give rise to a rebound hypertensive syndrome on abrupt cessation of treatment, presumably as a consequence of receptor up-regulation.

Alpha-methyldopa, which acts via its active metabolite alpha-methylnoradrenaline, has a profile similar to that of clonidine but in addition is known to give rise to immunological side effects, including pyrexia and hepatitis and, rarely, the precipitation of a haemolytic anaemia.

These centrally acting agents are no longer used widely because of their poor side effect profiles (particularly the CNS depressant effects) and because of the development of newer comparably effective alternative agents. However, alpha-methyldopa is still used to treat hypertension in pregnancy, especially where hypertension precedes pregnancy or is identified in the first or middle trimester. This is justified by the long-term experience of fetal and maternal safety. More recently developed centrally acting agents which preferentially bind to imidazoline binding sites in brain, e.g. moxonidine, are reported to have fewer adverse effects, but this has not yet been confirmed from widespread clinical use. These drugs have not been studied in long-term outcome trials.

Hypertensive emergencies

There are no indications for the rapid (within seconds or minutes) reduction of blood pressure, even where there is severe hypertension and related complications. However, there are some indications for the controlled and progressive reduction of blood pressure (over a period of a few hours) when accelerated or malignant phase hypertension is complicated by hypertensive encephalopathy or acute left ventricular failure, or in other situations such as dissection of the aorta or in eclampsia of pregnancy.

In severe cases, with the above complications, there may be grounds for intravenous treatment that is titrated to produce a gradual and progressive reduction in blood pressure. The preferred agents are glyceryl trinitrate or sodium nitroprusside by infusion where the rate of the infusion can be controlled, minute-by-minute, according to the blood pressure response. The infusion of glyceryl trinitrate is not associated with significant adverse effects beyond those predicted by the blood pressure reduction, but with sodium nitroprusside there is the additional potential complication of thiocyanate accumulation and cyanide poisoning, especially in patients with impaired renal function. For this reason, and especially with sodium nitroprusside, these manoeuvres should only be undertaken in the setting of an intensive care unit with appropriate monitoring facilities.

8.2 Hyperlipidaemia

Aim

The overall aim of lipid-modifying treatment is to reduce the circulating levels of atherogenic lipids in order to slow, or ideally prevent, the development of atherosclerotic vascular lesions and thereby reduce the long-term risk of cardiovascular disease.

Relevant pathophysiology

Cholesterol is a necessary and major component of lipid-containing atherosclerotic plaques. Raised plasma levels of cholesterol—and related lipid disturbances—have been identified as a major risk factor (along with smoking and hypertension) for atherosclerotic cardiovascular disease and its consequences, particularly myocardial infarction. Cholesterol is derived both from the diet and by endogenous synthesis in the liver and it is a necessary component of cell membranes, a precursor of steroid hormones and bile salts, and of glycoproteins and quinones.

The biochemistry and metabolism of cholesterol are complex. Cholesterol, and other lipid fractions, are transported in blood via lipoproteins of different densities. Increased total cholesterol and its major component fraction, low density lipoprotein (LDL) cholesterol, have been linked to accelerated atherosclerosis and increased coronary artery disease. LDL cholesterol is cleared from the circulation by specific receptors on the cell surface and the function of these receptors plays an important role in determining the plasma levels of LDL cholesterol. In contrast, high density lipoprotein (HDL) cholesterol appears to have a protective and antiatherogenic effect because it is involved in the mobilization of cholesterol from tissues and its transportation back to the liver.

Primary and secondary lipid disorders

Disorders of lipid metabolism occur as primary conditions that may be familial, or polygenic in origin, or secondary to an underlying disease state or drug treatment.

Familial hypercholesterolaemia

Very high levels of LDL cholesterol occur in this rare genetic disease which involves the failure to express LDL receptors. It is inherited as an autosomal dominant condition such that homozygotes have no LDL receptors and heterozygotes have only 50% of the normal number of LDL receptors. In this condition LDL cholesterol (and therefore total cholesterol) is very high and in the homozygotes there will be no response to drug treatments which exert their lipid lowering effects via the up-regulation of LDL receptors. In such patients it may be necessary to remove cholesterol by physical techniques such as apheresis using LDL affinity columns.

Polygenic lipid disorders

This is by far the most common type of primary lipid disorder which reflects a variety of factors including a non-specific genetic predisposition, dietary factors such as high calorie and saturated fat intake and lifestyle influences including physical inactivity. In the most common pattern there are moderate increases in LDL and total cholesterol and this is the commonest lipid disorder found in westernized populations. In part, the disturbed lipid profile reflects down-regulation of LDL receptors.

Secondary lipid disorders

These manifest as mixed elevations of cholesterol and triglycerides in response to underlying diseases such as hypothyroidism and diabetes mellitus, or as a manifestation of chronic alcohol abuse, or in response to drug treatments such as thiazide diuretics and beta-blockers.

Risks of hypercholesterolaemia

The central role of cholesterol in the development of atheroma and atherosclerotic cardiovascular disease is well established. The epidemiological evidence from population studies in different countries and from within the same country identify clear associations between LDL and total cholesterol and the development of cardiovascular disease, particularly CHD. There are also weaker associations with elevated triglycerides and an inverse relationship with HDL cholesterol.

Benefits of lipid lowering treatment

A number of large placebo-controlled randomized clinical trials have been performed to examine the effects of cholesterol-lowering therapy in the primary and secondary prevention of cardiovascular disease. Primary prevention refers to patients who might have one or more cardiovascular risk factors, but in whom overt atherosclerotic disease has not presented clinically. Secondary prevention refers to those patients who have, for example, suffered an acute myocardial infarction or who have angina or intermittent claudication. Clinical trials using statins to lower cholesterol have shown 30–40% reductions in coronary heart disease events in both primary and secondary prevention studies. Cholesterol-lowering therapy also reduces the risk of stroke in patients with CHD. The absolute benefits of treatment are proportional to the magnitude of cholesterol reduction and the pretreatment cardiovascular risk in an individual patient. The only statins to be evaluated in mortality studies are simvastatin and pravastatin.

Principles of lipid lowering treatment

1 Detection: hypercholesterolaemia can be detected in patients at risk by the measurement of total cholesterol in a non-fasting blood sample. Thereafter, and to confirm the diagnosis, to give a more accurate assessment of the lipid profile it is then necessary to

obtain a fasting blood sample which can be subfractionated to measure the triglyceride concentration and the HDL and LDL cholesterol fractions.

2 Patients should be counselled about hypercholesterolaemia, and its risk, and the relevance of other concomitant risk factors. The reason for long-term treatment should be carefully explained.

3 As for the treatment of hypertension, hypercholesterolaemia should be treated as part of a management plan for reducing all identifiable cardiovascular risk factors in the 'at risk' patient.

4 Secondary types of lipid disorder: these should be identified in order to undertake the specific treatment and management for the underlying condition. Thus, further investigations should be undertaken to exclude significant renal or hepatic disease, hypothyroidism, diabetes mellitus, or alcohol abuse or relevant drug treatments.

5 Non-pharmacological treatment should be considered initially and this centres around dietary modification.

Lipid lowering treatment

Dietary advice
The principles of dietary advice revolve around the reduced intake of saturated animal fats and, in the obese patient, a reduced total calorie intake. In addition, it is desirable to increase the intake of unsaturated fats and, where possible, increase the level of physical activity. Ideally, dietary modification should be planned in discussion with the spouse, or other members of the family, and it should take account of some of the social, cultural and economic circumstances of each patient. In a compliant and motivated patient total cholesterol may be reduced by about 10% within a few months of adherence to dietary modification but, in the long term, it is unusual for patients to be able to continue dietary restraint in order to maintain this magnitude of change.

Lipid lowering drugs
There are several different drugs available for cholesterol reduction and modification of the plasma lipid profile but currently there are three major classes in widespread use: 3-hydroxy-3-methoxygluteryl coenzyme A (HMG CoA) reductase inhibitors (known as 'statins'); fibrates; and bile acid sequestrant resins (see Table 8.7).

HMG CoA reductase inhibitors
HMG CoA reductase is the rate-limiting enzyme in the hepatic synthesis of cholesterol and inhibition leads to reduced cholesterol production and, as a consequence, an attempt by the liver to compensate by increasing its extraction of LDL cholesterol from plasma by up-regulating its LDL cholesterol receptors. The principal effect, therefore, is a reduction of LDL cholesterol (and, thereby, total cholesterol) by up to 40% and there are only modest

LIPID-LOWERING DRUGS

Drug	LDL	HDL	Triglycerides
HMGCoA reductase inhibitors	↓↓	↑	→
Fibrates	↓	↑	↓
Resins	↓	→	→
Others			
Nicotinic acid	↓	↑	↓
Probucol	↓	↓	→

Table 8.7 Summary of the actions of lipid-lowering drugs.

effects on the other lipid fractions. Some statin drugs (e.g. atorvastatin) also lower triglyceride levels by 15%. Because cholesterol is synthesized mainly during sleep, these drugs are usually administered at night. HMG CoA reductase inhibitors comprise the family of 'statins'—simvastatin, pravastatin, fluvastatin for example—and their principal practical advantage is that they have a relatively low profile of adverse effects. Occasionally there are reports of skin reactions, myalgia, headaches, diarrhoea, nausea, vomiting and non-cardiac chest pain. Myalgia and rhabdomyolisis remain as recognized but very rare serious adverse effects.

Several major clinical trials have been undertaken with different HMG CoA reductase inhibitors. There is evidence from the 4 S study and the CARE study, with simvastatin and pravastatin, respectively, that in secondary prevention the reduction in total and LDL cholesterol leads to reduced cardiovascular morbidity and mortality in high risk patients. A major primary prevention trial with pravastatin in the west of Scotland has also confirmed the benefit of treatment even in patients without overt cardiac disease.

Clinical comment. The impressive clinical evidence from large randomized clinical trials that statin therapy reduces cardiovascular mortality in both primary and secondary prevention has led to a dramatic increase in prescribing. From a public health and cost-effectiveness perspective, the challenge has been to target statin therapy at the highest-risk patients, i.e. those who will benefit most from cholesterol reduction. Current guidelines in the UK advocate statin therapy for patients with total cholesterol levels greater than 4.8 mM following an acute myocardial infarction; and treatment for those patients with angina who have total cholesterol levels above 5.5 mM. For primary prevention the strategy has been to advocate statin therapy for patients who have an absolute risk of a cardiovascular event of more than 3% per year. Various tables have been produced to allow clinicians to quickly risk-stratify an individual patient by entering basic clinical information, e.g. age, smoking status, cholesterol level and blood pressure. Thus, the decision to initiate statin therapy for primary prevention is not based solely on the level of cholesterol, but also on an overall clinical assessment of an individual patients absolute cardiovascular risk.

Fibrates

These drugs lower LDL cholesterol by about 20% and they also cause a significant reduction in total triglycerides and an increase in HDL cholesterol. They have a number of effects on lipid metabolism including the activation of lipoprotein lipase to promote lipolysis of triglyceride-rich particles, which reduces the levels of triglyceride, and they may also inhibit HMG CoA reductase and promote a consequential up-regulation of LDL receptor activity. Bezafibrate and gemfibrozil are examples of fibrates in widespread use and there is evidence (with gemfibrozil) that CHD events can be reduced as part of a primary prevention strategy. As a group, these drugs are absorbed completely from the GI tract and are excreted largely unchanged via the kidney, but they are liable to cause gastrointestinal side effects and they are extensively bound to albumin such that there is potential for drug interactions, most notably with oral anticoagulants.

The side effects most commonly associated with fibrates are gastrointestinal upsets, headaches, fatigue and skin reactions. Less commonly, muscle cramps and loss of libido are reported. The fibrates as a class are thought to increase bile lithogenicity and, although this has not been conclusively demonstrated with the modern agents, these drugs should be regarded as relatively contraindicated in those patients with gall bladder disease or with a strong family history of gallstones.

Bile acid sequestrant resins

These resins such as colestyramine are not absorbed from the GI tract and as a consequence they bind bile salts to prevent their normal enterohepatic recirculation. As a consequence, hepatic cholesterol synthesis increases and the receptor mediated uptake of LDL cholesterol from plasma is also increased. Overall, the resins primarily lower LDL cholesterol and total cholesterol with associated small increases in HDL cholesterol but no effect on triglycerides. Because they are not significantly absorbed the resins are capable of also interfering with the absorption of fat-soluble vitamins (especially vitamin K) and they may also interfere with the absorption of folic acid and with drugs such as digoxin. The adverse gastrointestinal effects of the resins cause major symptomatic problems that few patients are able to tolerate when large doses are administered. For this reason, there is also a significant incidence of poor or non-compliance. Even the taste and texture of the resins are unpleasant and the various devices to conceal these within fruit juices or mixed with sauces and foods have had variable success. Symptomatic adverse effects, although confined to the GI tract with dyspepsia, flatulence and altered bowel habit, may be sufficiently disturbing to cause patient withdrawal from treatment.

Other lipid lowering drugs

There are other agents available for specific indications or where other treatments have proved intolerable or ineffective. Nicotinic acid and its derivatives are potent inhibitors of LDL and VLDL formation; probucol lowers LDL cholesterol but also inhibits the production of HDL cholesterol, although the significance of this latter effect remains to be established; fish oils, high in unsaturated fatty acids, are particularly useful for reducing excessively high triglyceride concentrations.

CHAPTER 9

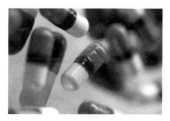

Haemostasis and Thrombosis

9.1 Haemostasis

Vascular injury results firstly in vasoconstriction and formation of a platelet plug at the site of injury (primary haemostasis). The platelet plug is then stabilized by the formation of a fibrin meshwork, resulting from activation of the coagulation cascade. Eventually fibrin is cleared through digestion by fibrinolytic enzymes.

Primary haemostasis

When endothelial integrity is breached, platelets adhere to exposed subendothelial collagen. The adherent platelets become activated resulting in:

1 Exposure of fibrinogen receptors, allowing fibrinogen to bind and cross link adjacent platelets. This process is known as platelet aggregation. The platelet fibrinogen receptor consists of a complex of glycoproteins IIb and IIIa on the platelet membrane.

2 Release of contents of secretory granules including substances such as adenosine diphosphate (ADP) which promote further platelet activation.

3 Synthesis of thromboxane A_2 which also acts to promote further platelet activation and vasoconstriction.

Activation of the coagulation cascade

As shown in Fig. 9.1, the coagulation cascade consists of a series of steps in which precursor proteins in plasma are converted to active enzymes in a sequential series of reactions. For convenience the coagulation cascade can be divided into three parts.

1 The *common* pathway consists of those reactions subsequent to the generation of factor X_a, culminating in the cleavage of fibrinogen by thrombin, with subsequent polymerization of fibrin monomers into fibrin strands. Factor X_a may be generated either by the extrinsic pathway or by the intrinsic pathway.

2 In the *extrinsic* pathway, tissue factor is expressed by cells or released following tissue injury. Binding of tissue factor to factor VII greatly accelerates the activation of factor VII and also the action of factor VII_a in the activation of factor X.

3 The *intrinsic* pathway is initiated by the activation of factor XII by contact of blood with a 'foreign' surface. *In vivo*, this is usually the subendothelial tissues. A sequence of reactions as illustrated in Fig. 9.1 then result in the activation of factor X. Most coagulation factors are synthesized in the liver, and the synthesis of the procoagulant forms of factors II, VII, IX and X is dependent on the availability of vitamin K.

Fibrinolysis

The fibrinolytic system, like the coagulation cascade, also consists of a series of enzymatic steps (see Fig. 9.2), this time resulting in the breakdown of polymerized fibrin by plasmin into small degradation products (FDP).

THE COAGULATION CASCADE

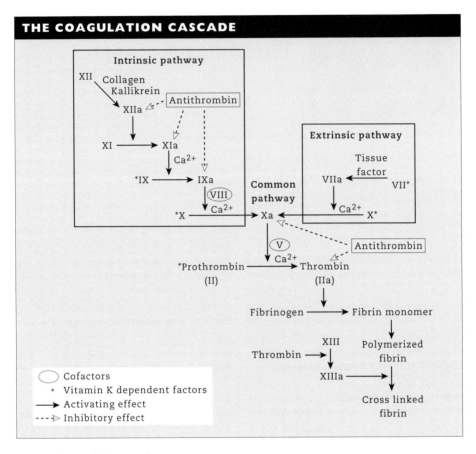

Fig. 9.1 The coagulation cascade.

Plasmin is generated from the plasma protein plasminogen by the action of tissue plasminogen activator (tPA), which is most efficient in activation of plasminogen, when it is bound to fibrin. Furthermore, such localization of fibrinolytic reactions protects plasmin from potent inhibitors present in plasma.

Pathophysiology

Thrombosis is 'haemostasis in the wrong place'. When haemostasis proceeds unchecked within a large vessel, thrombosis occurs and vascular occlusion may result. Thrombi may also break up into small pieces and lodge at distant points within the circulatory system (embolism). The process of thrombosis in a blood vessel is promoted by one or more of three underlying pathological events: (i) abnormalities of the vessel wall; (ii) abnormalities of flow within a vessel; or (iii) abnormalities of blood constituents.

Thrombosis in arteries usually results from rupture of an atheromatous plaque and arterial thrombi consist initially of platelets and subsequently of fibrin. Venous thrombosis often occurs in the context of stasis of blood flow, for example during periods of immobility or during pregnancy when pressure from the gravid uterus may impede venous return, and thrombi in veins are rich in fibrin enmeshing all the cellular constituents of blood.

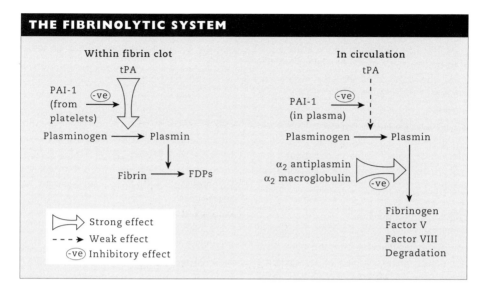

Fig. 9.2 The fibrinolytic system. Exogenous thrombolytic agents act at the same site as tissue plasminogen activator (tPA), but some are not fibrin specific. FDPs, fibrin degradation products.

Approach to the management of thrombosis

Both antiplatelet drugs and anticoagulants are effective in prevention of arterial, cardiac and venous thromboembolism. Antiplatelet drugs are usually preferred, because they are less likely to cause excessive bleeding. However, anticoagulants are more effective in treatment of venous thromboembolism and peripheral arterial embolism. Thrombolytic agents have their main role in the treatment of acute thrombotic arterial occlusion, especially coronary thrombosis. The pharmacology and clinical use of antithrombotic drugs will now be described in detail.

9.2 Antiplatelet agents

There are many potential targets for drug action in the biochemical pathways involved in platelet activation. Aspirin is cheap and effective and hence is usually the drug of choice; clopidogrel and dipyridamole are alternatives.

Aspirin

Pharmacology

All of the pharmacological effects of aspirin (acetylsalicylic acid) are based upon inhibition of prostaglandin synthesis. Aspirin is used as an antiplatelet drug in doses lower than those employed for analgesia. Aspirin acetylates and inactivates cyclo-oxygenase, a key enzyme in the platelet biosynthetic pathway for the pro-aggregatory prostaglandin thromboxane A_2. The interaction of aspirin with cyclo-oxygenase is irreversible. As platelets are anucleate, recovery of thromboxane synthesis is dependent on the appearance of a new platelet population in the circulation. Recovery from the effects of aspirin therefore takes about 10 days. Aspirin also inhibits endothelial cyclo-oxygenase, in this case leading to a reduction in prostacyclin synthesis, an effect which would be theoretically undesirable. A predominant effect on thromboxane synthesis is achieved because the endothelium can regenerate cyclo-oxygenase activity. Differential sensitivity of the platelet and endothelial enzymes, and pre-systemic hydrolysis of aspirin, limiting endothelial exposure to active drug, may also contribute to the achievement of some selectivity of action (see below). The lower the dose of aspirin, the greater the differential effect, but no dose at which useful inhibition of thromboxane synthesis is achieved is absolutely selective. In practice, aspirin doses of 75–300 mg/day appear as effective as higher doses in thrombosis prevention, and have fewer gastrointestinal side effects.

Effects on haemostasis

Administration of aspirin results in prolongation of the skin bleeding time and a characteristic defect on testing platelet aggregation in the laboratory. As would be expected, coagulation tests are unaltered by aspirin. Very large doses of aspirin, e.g. in overdose, can, however, lead to a variable prolongation of the prothrombin time.

Pharmacokinetics

Aspirin, in standard formulation, is rapidly absorbed from the upper gastrointestinal tract including both the stomach and duodenum. Slow-release formulations are available which have delayed and incomplete absorption characteristics. Aspirin undergoes extensive pre-systemic hydrolysis to salicylate. Platelet cyclo-oxygenase may therefore be irreversibly inhibited as platelets pass through the portal circulation, whilst the endothelium on the systemic side of the circulation is exposed to smaller concentrations of active aspirin.

Clinical use of aspirin

Low-dose aspirin has been shown to be clinically beneficial in acute myocardial infarction, unstable angina, and acute ischaemic stroke; in the secondary prevention of arterial thrombosis; and in prevention of arterial, venous and cardiac thrombosis in persons at increased risk (see Table 9.1). There are several general points of importance.

1 'Low-dose' aspirin refers to a range of doses from 75 to 300 mg daily. Doses less than 100 mg require several days to produce their full effects on thromboxane synthesis, hence a loading dose of 150–300 mg/day is given in acute myocardial infarction, unstable angina, and acute ischaemic stroke.

2 Presentation with one form of arterial disease is often associated with risk of another form of vascular disease on which aspirin may have an impact. For example, treatment of a patient with a transient ischaemic attack reduces not only their risk of ischaemic stroke, but also of myocardial infarction and death from other vascular causes.

3 In acute myocardial infarction, it has been shown that administration of aspirin has additive effects with streptokinase in reduction of mortality.

CLINICAL USE OF LOW-DOSE ASPIRIN

Myocardial infarction (acute and chronic)
Unstable angina
Ischaemic stroke (acute and chronic)
Transient cerebral ischaemia
Peripheral vascular arterial disease
Post-coronary artery bypass graft
Post-peripheral arterial surgery
Atrial fibrillation
Prophylaxis of venous thromboembolism
Primary prevention of myocardial infarction in high-risk patients (e.g. risk ≥2% per year)

Table 9.1 Clinical conditions in which low-dose aspirin is of proven benefit.

4 Cerebral haemorrhage should be excluded by brain scanning before administering (or continuing) aspirin to a patient presenting with a stroke.

5 In patients with acute ischaemic stroke who are unable to swallow, aspirin may be given per rectum.

Adverse effects of aspirin

Gastric erosions and gastrointestinal bleeding

1 Gastrointestinal toxicity constitutes the main adverse effect of aspirin. This includes dyspepsia, ulceration and gastrointestinal bleeding (one excess major bleed per 500 patient-years use). It is related to inhibition of prostaglandin synthesis in the gastrointestinal tract as well as to the antiplatelet effects of aspirin. The gastrointestinal effects are dose related, and incidence is reduced but not eliminated by the use of lower doses.

2 Hypersensitivity reactions.

3 Precipitation of asthma.

4 Precipitation of renal failure, especially in patients with renal artery stenosis and in patients taking angiotensin converting enzyme (ACE) inhibitor drugs.

5 Intracranial haemorrhage (one per 2500 patient-years).

Contraindications

1 Peptic ulcer or gastrointestinal haemorrhage.

2 Underlying bleeding disorders, congenital or acquired (including anticoagulant therapy).

3 Severe renal or hepatic impairment.

4 Known hypersensitivity to aspirin.

5 Intracranial haemorrhage or aneurysm.

6 Uncontrolled hypertension (risk of intracranial haemorrhage).

Clopidogrel and ticlopidine

Clopidogrel is a recently introduced antiplatelet drug that has a different mechanism of action on platelets to aspirin. It has an active metabolite that irreversibly modifies the platelet ADP receptor, reducing the aggregability of platelets for the remainder of their lifespan. A dose of 75 mg/day is used clinically, which reduces platelet aggregability and prolongs the skin bleeding time to a similar extent as low-dose aspirin (75–300 mg/day). A recent large study showed that clopidogrel was at least as effective as aspirin in reducing the risk of arterial thrombosis in patients with recent myocardial infarction, recent ischaemic stroke, or chronic peripheral arterial disease. Clopidogrel was also as safe as aspirin, with a lower risk of dyspepsia and gastrointestinal bleeding, but a higher risk of diarrhoea and skin rash. As it is more expensive than aspirin, its main indication is secondary prevention of arterial thrombosis in patients who are intolerant of aspirin or in whom aspirin is contraindicated. The combination of clopidogrel and aspirin appears more effective than aspirin alone (or anticoagulants) in prevention of thrombosis following coronary angioplasty with stenting. Clopidogrel has replaced the related drug, ticlopidine, which has a significant risk of neutropenia requiring monitoring of the white blood cell count.

Dipyridamole

Dipyridamole is a vasodilator drug that provokes myocardial ischaemia and is used in cardiac stress testing: it is therefore contraindicated in patients with angina. It was observed to reduce platelet aggregation in whole blood but not in plasma: it may act by reducing red blood cell uptake of adenosine, a circulating endogenous platelet inhibitor. Dipyridamole (100 mg thrice daily, or 200 mg sustained release twice daily) appears similarly effective to aspirin in secondary prevention of stroke, but has been less extensively evaluated, is more expensive, and has vasodilator side effects including headache. It may be used in secondary prevention of stroke or transient cerebral ischaemia in patients who are intolerant of aspirin or in whom aspirin is contraindicated. Whether or not the combination of dipyridamole and aspirin is more effective than aspirin alone in secondary prevention of cardiovascular events after stroke or transient cerebral ischaemia is controversial.

Glycoprotein IIb/IIIa receptor antagonists

As noted in the introduction to this section, the final common pathway of platelet aggregation is the exposure in activated platelets of membrane glycoprotein IIb/IIIa receptors, which are linked by fibrinogen in platelet aggregation. Several antagonists of this receptor are currently under investigation as antithrombotic agents. Abciximab is a monoclonal antibody that blocks this receptor: it is used as a single intravenous injection in prevention of thrombosis following high-risk coronary angioplasty.

9.3 Anticoagulant drugs

Heparin

Anticoagulation can be achieved rapidly with heparin, and it is therefore the anticoagulant of choice in many acute thrombotic states such as treatment of deep vein thrombosis (DVT) or pulmonary embolism, and in severe unstable angina in which it has an additive effect to aspirin.

Chemistry and pharmacology

Unfractionated heparin is a mixture of naturally occurring glycosaminoglycans with polysaccharide chains of varying length, and molecular weights ranging from 5000 to 30 000. Low molecular weight heparins are manufactured from unfractionated heparin to produce material with an average molecular weight of 4000–6500.

All heparins exert their anticoagulant activity by binding to and greatly accelerating the action of antithrombin as an inhibitor of thrombin (factor II_a), factor X_a, and other serine protease coagulation factors. Binding to antithrombin requires the presence of a specific pentasaccharide sequence on the heparin polysaccharide chain. A further requirement for heparin to enhance the anti-II_a activity of antithrombin is the presence of a minimum chain length of 18 saccharides. As the proportion of chains of this length in low molecular weight heparins is less than in unfractionated heparin, it follows that low molecular weight heparins have a higher ratio of anti-X_a to anti-II_a activity. All heparins must be administered parenterally, either by the intravenous or subcutaneous route. For treatment of thrombosis, unfractionated heparin has traditionally been given by continuous intravenous infusion. The half-life of standard heparin following intravenous administration is 45–60 min, but heparins have complex kinetics, depending on dose, molecular weight and route of administration. Unfractionated heparin can also be given twice daily subcutaneously for treatment of DVT. Low molecular weight heparins demonstrate less binding to cells and to heparin neutralizing proteins than unfractionated heparin. This leads to improved bioavailability and to a longer half-life. These properties allow a more predictable anticoagulant response, once daily subcutaneous administration, and no need to monitor therapeutic doses with coagulation time assays.

Clinical use of unfractionated heparin

Heparin is used in the initial treatment of DVT and pulmonary embolism. In this situation, standard practice has been to administer 5000 IU unfractionated heparin intravenously as a loading dose, followed by a continuous infusion of 30 000–40 000 IU over 24 h, and to monitor the anticoagulant effect. Heparin is also used in unstable angina and in myocardial infarction to prevent coronary reocclusion following thrombolysis, and in the treatment and prevention of mural thrombus. It has a place as an adjunctive treatment to surgery or thrombolysis in the management of acute peripheral arterial occlusion. It is also used to prevent clotting in extracorporeal circulations such as renal dialysis circuits and cardiopulmonary bypass, and at low doses to flush indwelling vascular catheters.

Perioperative subcutaneous administration of low dose heparin (usually 5000 IU bd unfractionated heparin) is effective in reducing the incidence of venous thrombosis and pulmonary embolism following general or orthopaedic surgery, and is also used for this purpose in acutely ill, immobile medical patients.

Clinical use of low molecular weight heparin

Low molecular weight heparins have been evaluated extensively in the prevention of venous thrombosis in patients at risk, including those undergoing general or orthopaedic surgery and high risk medical patients. They have been shown to be of similar efficacy to unfractionated heparin in all of these situations, and the convenience of once daily administration make their use attractive. The increased cost of these agents, however, must be weighed against this. In orthopaedic surgery, particularly hip and knee replacement and hip fractures, there is increasing evidence that use of mechanical methods and aspirin is sufficient prophylaxis and that heparins are not required routinely.

Low molecular weight heparins, administered once or twice daily subcutaneously with dose adjusted for body weight is as effective as unfractionated heparin administered intravenously in the treatment of DVT and pulmonary embolism.

Monitoring of heparin

Administration of therapeutic doses of unfractionated heparin must be monitored in the laboratory. A prolongation of the activated partial thromboplastin time (APTT) and the thrombin time is observed. The APTT, which tests the intrinsic and common pathways of coagulation, is the test usually chosen for therapeutic heparin monitoring. For the treatment of thrombosis, one should aim for an APTT 1.5–2.5 times the mid-point of the normal range, and it is important to achieve this in the first 24 h of treatment. An alternative is to measure plasma heparin levels that are based upon plasma anti-X_a activity. It is not usually necessary to monitor heparin given in low doses for prophylaxis, and such regimens do not lead to prolongation of the APTT.

The APTT is insensitive to the effects of low molecular weight heparin. These may be measured by anti-X_a assays (e.g. in renal failure) but monitoring is usually unneccessary because of the predictability of responses.

Adverse effects

Bleeding

Bleeding is a hazard, especially with full-dose heparin treatment. Bleeding complications are not entirely predictable by the APTT, and patient-related factors are also important. Hopes that low molecular weight heparins would have a substantially better safety profile compared with unfractionated heparin with respect to bleeding have not generally been borne out.

Heparin induced thrombocytopenia

Significant thrombocytopenia occurs in approximately 3% of patients given full-dose unfractionated heparin. Mild early transient thrombocytopenia may be more common and is of no clinical significance. Thrombocytopenia occurring 4–14 days following heparin exposure is of greater significance, as potentially life-threatening thrombosis occurs in a small proportion of such patients. The thrombocytopenia is induced by a heparin-dependent antibody that causes platelet aggregation. Heparin-induced thrombocytopenia can occur with any dose or preparation of heparin, and although it appears to be much less common with low molecular weight heparin, antibody cross-reactivity has been documented. It is mandatory to monitor platelet counts during heparin therapy and prophylaxis from day 5 onwards: a baseline platelet count is useful. If heparin-induced thrombocytopenia is suspected, heparin should be withdrawn immediately and expert haematological advice sought.

Osteoporosis

Reduction in bone density and bone fractures have been described following prolonged administration (usually greater than 20 weeks) and therefore have generally occurred in pregnant women. The mechanism is poorly understood. There appears to be a relationship with dose and duration of treatment, but individual susceptibility is also likely to be important. Monitoring of bone density may be considered in high-risk patients.

Hypersensitivity

Local reactions at injection sites have been reported and, much more rarely, anaphylactic reactions.

Reversal of anticoagulation with heparin

Because of the short half-life of heparin, in the absence of clinical bleeding, it is reasonable simply to withhold therapy temporarily if over-anticoagulation has occurred. In the presence of haemorrhage, protamine should be administered intravenously. Protamine 1 mg neutralizes the effects of 100 IU of unfractionated heparin. Protamine should never be given in doses of greater than 50 mg and should always be administered slowly to avoid hypotension and bradycardia.

Contraindications to heparin

Active bleeding is an obvious contraindication. Others, including relative contraindications, are given below.

Heparinoids and hirudins

These do not cross-react with heparin-dependent antibodies; hence, they can be used in heparin-induced thrombocytopenia. Danaparoid is a heparinoid; desirudin and lepirudin are recombinant hirudins, developed from hirudin, the natural anticoagulant of the medicinal leech.

Warfarin

In practice, warfarin, a derivative of 4-hydroxy-coumarin, is by far the most extensively used oral anticoagulant and is the drug of choice. Acenocoumarol (nicoumalone) and phenindione are also available but are rarely used. All of these drugs act as vitamin K antagonists. The remainder of this section on oral anticoagulants will refer only to warfarin, but similar principles apply to use of the other agents.

Pharmacology

The coagulation factors II, VII, IX and X require gamma carboxylation on glutamic acid residues in order to bind calcium during coagulation reactions. Vitamin K is required for this carboxylation reaction, which is essential for procoagulant activity. Whilst acting as a cofactor, vitamin K is converted to vitamin K epoxide. The epoxide is then recycled via reductase reactions to active forms of vitamin K. Warfarin inhibits the reductase enzymes involved in the recycling of vitamin K, thus leading to a deficiency of procoagulant forms of factors II, VII, IX and X. Because some of these factors have prolonged half-lives, anticoagulation is not achieved for several days

CONTRAINDICATIONS TO HEPARIN

1 Uncorrected major bleeding.
2 Uncorrected major bleeding disorder, e.g. thrombocytopenia, haemophilias.
3 Active peptic ulcer, oesophageal varices, aneurysm, proliferative retinopathy, or organ biopsy.
4 Recent surgery, particularly neurosurgery or ophthalmic surgery.
5 Severe renal or hepatic impairment (not including use for renal dialysis).
6 Recent stroke, intracranial or intraspinal bleed.
7 Severe hypertension.
8 Previous heparin-induced thrombocytopenia or thrombosis.
9 Documented hypersensitivity.

after initiating warfarin therapy, and loading doses are usually given in acute thrombosis. In acute situations, it is necessary to overlap heparin and warfarin therapy.

Warfarin is rapidly absorbed from the gut and is extensively bound to plasma albumin. Elimination of warfarin is by oxidative metabolism in the liver, with a half-life of 15–50 h.

Monitoring of warfarin therapy

Warfarin therapy is monitored by the prothrombin time, which assesses the extrinsic and common pathways of coagulation. In recent years great advances have been made in standardizing the monitoring of warfarin therapy. This has been achieved by calibrating laboratory reagents used for measuring the prothrombin time against an international standard, and assigning an international sensitivity index (ISI) to each reagent. This allows the prothrombin time for the patient on treatment to be converted to an international normalized ratio (INR). The INR is the ratio of the patient's prothrombin time over the mean value in a normal reference population determined using the same batch of reagent and corrected for the ISI of the reagent. The development of the INR system of monitoring oral anticoagulation has allowed comparability of results between laboratories. This is obviously useful if patient care is transferred between centres, but is also very important if results of clinical studies are to be widely applicable.

As a result of the INR system, it has been possible to draw up guidelines for therapeutic ranges for the INR in various clinical situations where warfarin is used. This is discussed in more detail in the following section.

Clinical use of oral anticoagulants

Warfarin is commonly used in the conditions listed at the bottom of the page.

Warfarin is also used long-term in various thrombophilias if there is considered to be a significant risk of thrombosis (e.g. antiphospholipid syndrome, protein C or protein S deficiency). Table 9.2 shows recommended target INR ranges for some common indications for warfarin.

Pregnancy

Warfarin crosses the placenta and is contraindicated in the first trimester of pregnancy because of teratogenicity, and in the last few weeks of pregnancy because of fetal bleeding at delivery. Placental passage of warfarin leads to fetal anticoagulation at any stage in pregnancy, and so warfarin is not generally recommended in the management and prevention of venous thromboembolism during pregnancy. Because of the high risk and potentially catastrophic consequences of embolization from artificial valves warfarin is still the anticoagulant of choice from 12 to 36 weeks of pregnancy in patients with mechanical prosthetic valves.

How to initiate anticoagulation with warfarin

Because of the kinetic considerations described above, anticoagulation with warfarin is not achieved for several days after initiating therapy, and in acute thrombosis loading doses are given at the start of treatment. A baseline coagulation screen should be checked prior to initiating treatment. Common practice for loading would be to administer 5–10 mg warfarin on 2 consecutive days and to check the INR on the third day. Lower doses are used in

CLINICAL USE OF ORAL ANTICOAGULANTS

- Venous thromboembolism—prophylaxis and treatment.
- Atrial fibrillation (high-risk patients).
- Valvular heart disease and prosthetic valve replacements, cardiomyopathy.
- Mural thrombus.

TARGET INR RANGES

INR	Clinical condition
2.0–2.5	Prophylaxis of deep vein thrombosis (DVT) and pulmonary embolism in high-risk patients (e.g. previous DVT, pulmonary embolism or thrombophilias) (for hip surgery 2.0–3.0)
2.0–3.0	Treatment of DVT and pulmonary embolism Prevention of systemic embolism in atrial fibrillation, mitral valve disease, and other cardiac sources of embolism in the presence of previous systemic embolism Bioprosthetic heart valves with embolic risk factors Prevention of cardiac thromboembolism in high-risk patients following myocardial infarction
3.0–4.5	Recurrent venous thromboembolism Mechanical prosthetic cardiac valves Recurrent thrombosis in patients with antiphospholipid syndrome

Table 9.2 Target international normalized ratio (INR) ranges for oral anticoagulation.

congestive cardiac failure, in the presence of abnormalities of liver function or a prolongation of baseline prothrombin time, and in the elderly. It is also necessary to avoid loading doses in patients known to be suffering from familial protein C or protein S deficiency (see below).

Maintenance doses usually lie between 3 and 9 mg warfarin. Daily or alternate day monitoring of the INR should be carried out until stable values are achieved within the target range. In many instances, patients being induced with warfarin will also be receiving heparin for treatment or prevention of thrombosis. It is important to continue heparin until a therapeutic INR is achieved with warfarin.

Once stabilized, all patients, before discharge from hospital, should be enrolled in their local anticoagulant clinic and should receive education (e.g. by a pharmacist), using a national anticoagulant book where warfarin dosage and INR results are documented. The book also contains important information for the patient (or carers) regarding therapy including side effects and information about drug interactions. The following information should always be supplied to the supervising anticoagulant clinic: full personal patient details, indication for anticoagulation, proposed duration of treatment, desired target INR, and full details of all of the patient's medication. The patient should be advised to show the book to all doctors whom they attend, as well as their dentist.

Drug interactions

Drug interactions are the most common reason for loss of anticoagulant control, bleeding and thrombosis in patients previously stabilized on warfarin. Great care should be taken in prescribing any additional medication to patients on oral anticoagulants. Drugs may potentiate the effects of warfarin by inhibiting liver enzymes involved in warfarin metabolism, by competing for protein binding, by reducing vitamin K availability, or by affecting other aspects of haemostasis. Note that alcohol dose-dependently potentiates the effects of warfarin, and patients on oral anticoagulants should keep their alcohol consumption stable and less than 2 units/day. Drugs usually antagonize the effects of warfarin by inducing liver enzymes but in one case (colestyramine) the underlying mechanism is interference with warfarin absorption. Common drug interactions are illustrated in Table 9.3, but this list

WARFARIN DRUG INTERACTIONS

Potentiation	Antagonism
Analgesics	
NSAIDs—azapropazone, phenylbutazone	
Aspirin	
Co-proxamol	
Ketorolac (postoperative)	
Antibiotics	
Co-trimoxazole	Rifampicin
Metronidazole	Griseofulvin
Ampicillin	
Cephalosporins	
Erythromycin	
Aminoglycosides	
Tetracycline	
Miconazole	
Cardiovascular drugs	
Amiodarone	Spironolactone
Fibrates	Colestryramine
	(cholestyramine)
Endocrine agents	
Corticosteroids	
Thyroxine	
Tamoxifen	
Anabolic steroids	
Glucagon	
Gastrointestinal drugs	
Cimetidine	
Omeprazole	
Others	
Allopurinol	Vitamin K
Alcohol	Phenytoin
Chlorpromazine	Carbamazepine
Tricyclic antidepressants	Barbiturates
	Antihistamines

Table 9.3 Important drug interactions with warfarin.

is by no means exhaustive: consult the *British National Formulary* before any change of drugs!

Adverse effects

Bleeding is the most common adverse event encountered in patients on oral anticoagulants. Bleeding is usually related to prolongation of the INR above the therapeutic range, and underlying causes should be sought if bleeding occurs at therapeutic levels (e.g.

endoscopy for gastrointestinal bleeding or haematuria).

Other adverse effects are rare and include alopecia and skin rashes. There was a high incidence of hypersensitivity reactions with phenindione, and so it is now rarely used.

Patients with protein C or protein S deficiency are susceptible to skin necrosis during induction phases of oral anticoagulation. This is a result of the suppression of these vitamin

K dependent coagulation inhibitors by warfarin, which occurs quickly compared with suppression of the procoagulant factors. Adequate heparinization and the avoidance of loading doses of warfarin should help to prevent this complication in patients at risk.

Treatment of haemorrhage and reversal of oral anticoagulation

For elective situations such as surgery including tooth extractions, warfarin should be stopped at least 48 h in advance of the procedure and the INR monitored, with the option of substituting heparin if there is high risk of thrombosis (e.g. mechanical heart valves).

When haemorrhage occurs in patients on oral anticoagulants, there are well-defined guidelines for management. These are shown in Table 9.4. The advice of a haematologist should always be sought. Several general points are important regarding the use of vitamin K. Note that vitamin K takes 6 h to have

any effect, and in an emergency fresh frozen plasma or coagulation factor concentrates must be administered to provide an immediate source of vitamin K dependent factors (these carry small risks of hepatitis and HIV infection). Small doses of vitamin K (0.5–2 mg) are sufficient for reversal of warfarin effects in all but the most extreme cases. Furthermore, caution should be exerted in the administration of vitamin K to patients with prosthetic cardiac valves. The administration of large doses of vitamin K, e.g. 10 mg, makes further use of oral anticoagulants impossible for several weeks.

Contraindications to oral anticoagulants

These are similar to the previously listed contraindications to heparin, except for the following.

1 Lack of patient co-operation for any reason, e.g. mental impairment, alcoholism, or

REVERSAL OF ORAL ANTICOAGULATION	
Condition	Action
Life-threatening bleeding	Give 5 mg vitamin K i.v. slowly, repeated if necessary Give coagulation factor concentrates (factor IX complex and factor VII) or fresh frozen plasma (FFP) according to advice of a haematologist
Less severe bleeding (e.g. epistaxis)	Withold warfarin for 24–48 h Consider vitamin K 0.5–2 mg i.v. slowly or 5–10 mg orally
INR >8.0, no bleeding	Withold warfarin for 24–48 h, consider vitamin K 0.5 mg i.v. slowly or 5 mg orally
INR 4.5–8.0, no bleeding	Withold warfarin for 24–48 h, then repeat INR
Bleeding at therapeutic INR levels	Investigate for underlying cause

Table 9.4 Reversal of oral anticoagulation.

illicit drug use especially injecting, constitutes a contraindication to oral anticoagulants.

2 Oral anticoagulants are teratogenic and are contraindicated in the first trimester of pregnancy except in certain rare circumstances.

3 Heparin induced thrombocytopenia is *not* a contraindication to oral anticoagulants, which may be used as antithrombotic agents when the platelet count increases.

9.4 Thrombolytic agents

Clinical use of thrombolytic agents

Thrombolytic agents have gained an established role in the treatment of acute myocardial infarction. Their early administration leads to angiographically demonstrable coronary artery patency, limitation of infarct size, improved left ventricular function and, most importantly, reduced mortality.

Thrombolysis is also used in selected cases of acute peripheral arterial occlusion (usually by local arterial infusion) and in massive ileofemoral vein thrombosis or massive pulmonary embolism. The role of thrombolysis in venous thromboembolism is more controversial than in coronary thrombosis.

The role of thrombolysis in acute ischaemic stroke has recently been established, under strictly controlled circumstances. In particular, haemorrhage or established infarction must be excluded by brain imaging with computerized tomography (CT) or magnetic resonance (MR), and treatment must be commenced quickly (normally within 3 h of stroke onset); alteplase rather than streptokinase is used.

General aspects of thrombolysis

All thrombolytic agents act by activating plasminogen to plasmin, leading to degradation of fibrin, not only in thrombi but also in haemostatic fibrin plugs, which frequently causes major bleeding (there is a 1% risk of intracranial bleeding which is often fatal or disabling).

Streptokinase

This is a protein produced by group A beta-haemolytic streptococci. Streptokinase requires a complex to be formed with plasminogen before it can cleave other plasminogen molecules to form plasmin. As it is a foreign protein, streptokinase may cause allergic reactions. Many patients already have antibodies to streptokinase because of previous streptococcal infection, but streptokinase administration also frequently leads to antibody formation. Use of an alternative agent such as tPA is recommended if a patient who has previously received streptokinase requires thrombolysis (such patients should carry a card indicating this).

Alteplase (tissue plasminogen activator)

Recombinant tPA (alteplase), is developed from an endogenous fibrinolytic enzyme, release of which initiates physiological fibrinolysis. It lyses thrombi more rapidly, but carries a higher risk of intracranial haemorrhage than streptokinase and is more expensive; hence, its main indication is previous streptokinase therapy. Conversely, after acute ischaemic stroke, streptokinase was associated with excessive intracranial bleeding and increased mortality, whereas alteplase improves outcome in selected patients. Thrombolytic treatment in acute stroke should only be used in specialist centres.

Other thrombolytic agents

Urokinase

Urokinase is another endogenous plasminogen activator originally isolated from human urine, but now made in recombinant form. It is non-antigenic. Although urokinase has been used for thrombolysis, it has been less extensively studied compared with streptokinase and alteplase and its use is limited by its high cost. It is most often used in local peripheral arterial thrombolysis but has also shown benefit after intra-arterial use in acute ischaemic stroke.

Anistreplase (anisoylated plasminogen–streptokinase activator complex)

Anistreplase is a complex of streptokinase with plasminogen that has been rendered inactive by reversible chemical protection of its active site. Streptokinase antibodies cross react with antistreplase and clinical superiority to streptokinase has not been demonstrated by clinical trials.

9.5 Reference

Scottish Intercollegiate Guidelines Network (SIGN) (1999) *Antithrombotic Therapy. A National Clinical Guideline.* SIGN, Edinburgh.

CHAPTER 10

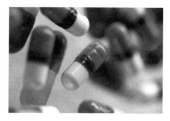

Antimicrobial Therapy

Aim
The aim is to control infection without damage to the patient.

10.1 Principles of drug treatment

One of the greatest of all therapeutic advances was the introduction of drugs to treat bacterial infections in man. The introduction of sulphonamides in 1936 and penicillin in 1941 dramatically reduced mortality from infections. During the decades since then there has been a vast increase in the number of antimicrobial agents available for clinical use. This ready availability of drugs has enhanced the likelihood that a suitable agent can be found for a particular infection, but it has also resulted in a confusing range of choice and a readiness to prescribe antimicrobial agents even when the presence of bacterial infection is poorly documented. The newer antibiotics are expensive and not necessarily better than established agents: they should be prescribed only after careful consideration of the issuses identified in Table 10.1.

The patient

Documentation of infection
Whenever possible the clinical suspicion of infection should be supported by laboratory diagnosis. Appropriate specimens, e.g. sputum, urine, pus, blood, etc., should be obtained before treatment is commenced.

ANTIMICROBIAL THERAPY

Patient	Organism	Drug
Document infection	Culture	Absorption
Factors altering kinetics: age; renal/hepatic function	Identification Typing Antimicrobial susceptibility	Tissue distribution Route of elimination Adverse reactions
Previous drug sensitivity	Drug interactions	
General health (resistance to infection)		
Pregnancy		

Table 10.1 General principles of antimicrobial therapy.

Age

Drug kinetics are influenced by age dependent changes in pathways of elimination (Chapter 4). Clinically important examples involving antimicrobial agents include:

1 Relative deficiency of hepatic glucuronyl transferase in neonates, leading to an accumulation of chloramphenicol with a likelihood of cardiovascular collapse if serum concentration exceeds 25 mg/l.

2 Physiological decrease in renal function with age, leading to an accumulation of aminoglycosides in the elderly with a likelihood of toxicity: dose modification is necessary. Other antimicrobials contraindicated in specific age groups are:

3 Sulphonamides in the neonate (displacement of bilirubin, leading to kernicterus).

4 Tetracyclines in growing children (tooth discoloration).

Renal and hepatic function

(Chapter 3, Section 3.2)

Many commonly used antimicrobials are eliminated by the kidney while a few undergo hepatic metabolism. Dose modification is likely to be necessary if renal function is moderately or severely impaired (Table 10.2). Drug level monitoring is mandatory for antimicrobials with concentration-related toxicity.

Drug sensitivity

Always ask about previous exposure to drugs. Penicillins and cephalosporins are the antimicrobials most frequently associated with sensitivity reactions and there is a 5–10% cross-sensitivity between these two drug groups because they both contain the beta-lactam ring. Sulphonamides also frequently cause allergic reactions.

Diminished resistance to infection

Patients with malignant disease or who are receiving cytotoxic or immunosuppressant drugs are susceptible to infections with commensal bacteria as well as less common organisms, e.g. some viruses, yeasts, fungi and protozoa. In particular, granulocytopaenia (less than 500×10^6/l) is accompanied by a high risk of septicaemia. Fever in such patients must be assumed to have an infective aetiology and should be treated aggressively before a definitive bacteriological diagnosis is available.

Pregnancy (Chapter 5, Section 5.1)

Penicillins and cephalosporins are not harmful to the fetus. Fetal damage has been associated

RENAL FAILURE AND LIVER DISEASE

Renal failure			
Mild	Moderate	Severe	Liver disease
Aminoglycosides	Metronidazole	Co-trimoxazole	Clindamycin
Amphotericin B	Ticarcillin	Penicillins	Isoniazid, cephalosporins, rifampicin, ethambutol
	Acyclovir		Avoid: Erythromycin estolate, pyrazinamide, talampicillin
Flucytosine			
Vancomycin			
Avoid: Cephalothin, cephaloridine, nalidixic acid, nitrofurantoin, talampicillin, tetracyclines			

Table 10.2 Antimicrobials for which dose modification is required in mild, moderate or severe renal failure and in liver disease.

definitely with streptomycin and the tetracyclines. Possible adverse fetal effects have been ascribed to gentamicin, kanamycin and cotrimoxazole.

Comment. The patient's age, sex and general state of health must be considered when choosing both the drug and its dose.

The organism

Bacteria

Sensitivity
Bactericidal drugs kill the organisms against which they are effective. Bacteriostatic drugs do not kill the organism but inhibit its ability to replicate. Use of a bacteriostatic drug assumes that body defences can destroy the organisms whose replication has been prevented. Testing *in vitro* is available for most antibacterial drugs. Application of *in vitro* findings to the patient assumes that adequate drug concentrations are achieved at the site of infection.

Resistance
Some bacteria have always been resistant to the effects of certain drugs, while others have developed resistance in the course of repeated exposure to antimicrobials. The two major mechanisms by which resistance is produced are gene mutation and DNA exchange between bacteria. Resistance may take three main forms:
1 An alteration in the bacterial component on which the drug acts, e.g. changes in the 30S ribosomal subunit in organisms developing resistance to aminoglycosides.
2 The drug might be destroyed by the organisms, as in the case of penicillins which are inactivated by beta-lactamases produced by resistant bacteria.
3 Cell membrane permeability to drugs is reduced, as in resistance to tetracyclines.
 The development of resistance can be reduced if antimicrobials are not given indiscriminately. Additionally, the use of drug combinations should limit the appearance of resistant organisms in conditions such as tuberculosis (TB) where prolonged treatment is necessary.

Viruses and fungi
The range of effective drugs is more limited and in many cases treatment is still experimental. Consequently, information about sensitivity or resistance to treatment is far less complete than for bacteria.

Comment. Antimicrobial treatment must take appropriate account of the organism's susceptibility to drugs and the patient's intrinsic ability to combat infection.

The drug

Absorption
Certain antimicrobials, e.g. the aminoglycosides, can only be given parenterally because absorption from the gastrointestinal tract is negligible. Where a choice exists between oral and parenteral drug formulations, the decision must rest on the severity of the illness and the need to achieve high tissue concentration.

Tissue distribution
The principles determining drug distribution are described in Chapter 1, Section 1.2. In addition to these general considerations of blood concentration, protein binding, lipid solubility, etc., a further factor influencing antimicrobial distribution is the presence of inflammation, which tends to improve tissue penetration. However, it must not be assumed that the presence of inflammation greatly transforms the penetration of drugs. For example, gentamicin and cephalosporins cross poorly into the cerebrospinal fluid (CSF) even in the presence of meningitis. Table 10.3 indicates those agents with high penetration to CSF, bile and urine.

Route of elimination
This is usually renal or hepatic metabolism (or rarely biliary excretion); see Chapter 3 and the section above on renal and hepatic function.

CSF, BILE AND URINARY CONCENTRATIONS

CSF	Bile	Urine
Chloramphenicol	Penicillins	Penicillins
Erythromycin	Cephalosporins	Cephalosporins
Isoniazid	Erythromycin	Aminoglycosides
Pyrazinamide		Sulphonamides
Rifampicin		Nitrofurantoin
Flucytosine		Nalidixic acid
		Ethambutol
		Flucytosine

Table 10.3 Antimicrobials for which high concentrations are achieved.

Adverse effects

These are of two general types:

1 Hypersensitivity reactions that are either immediate or delayed. The former produce anaphylaxis while the latter manifest themselves in various ways, the most common being rashes. Hypersensitivity reactions usually occur with no prior warning and are most commonly seen with penicillins, cephalosporins and sulphonamides.

2 The other type of adverse reaction is usually predictable in being concentration related; aminoglycoside ototoxicity is an example. Fortunately, the toxic concentrations of most antimicrobials in common use greatly exceed the required therapeutic concentrations. Where this is not the case, e.g. gentamicin, drug level monitoring is mandatory. Adverse reactions to antimicrobials are summarized in Table 10.4 and discussed in more detail under specific agents.

Drug interactions

These can be either kinetic, e.g. enzyme induction or inhibition, or dynamic, e.g. two drugs adversely affecting the same organ. Examples include:

1 Aminoglycosides and furosemide have an additive nephrotoxic effect.

2 Rifampicin induces the same enzymes that metabolize the contraceptive pill and can cause failure of contraception.

3 Sulphonamides inhibit the enzymes that metabolize phenytoin and can cause phenytoin toxicity.

4 Tetracyclines form insoluble complexes in the gut lumen with both antacids and iron, leading to treatment failure.

5 Quinolones may trigger side effects of theophylline as a result of its decreased elimination.

6 Amphotericin B and aminoglycosides or vancomycin display increased nephrotoxicity and ototoxicity.

Antimicrobial prophylaxis

Antimicrobial agents are sometimes given to people who do not have an infection but who are considered to be at risk from a specific organism. Examples include the use of minocycline or rifampicin in close contacts of patients with meningococcal meningitis, the administration of penicillin before and following dental procedures in people at risk of endocarditis and the long-term use of cotrimoxazole in children with repeated urinary tract infections and evidence of vesicoureteric reflux. Perioperative prophylaxis in certain types of surgery where the risk of infection is high (e.g. colorectal) or the consequences of infection are life-threatening (e.g. open heart) is now standard practice, e.g. cefotaxime and metronidazole or ciprofloxacin and metronidazole.

ADVERSE REACTIONS OF ANTIMICROBIAL DRUGS

Organ system	Drug	Comment
Kidney	Aminoglycosides	Concentration related
	Cephalosporins	Mainly earlier drugs of this group
	Sulphonamides	
	Methicillin	Other penicillins rarely
	Amphotericin B	
	Polymyxins	Limits use
Bone marrow	Antiviral agents	
suppression	Amphotericin B	
	Flucytosine	
	Chloramphenicol	
	Sulphonamides	Rare
Haemolytic anaemia	Sulphonamides	Two distinct mechanisms: immune and glucose-6-phosphate deficiency
	Nitrofurantoin	
	4-Fluoroquinolones	
	Penicillins	Rare
	Cephalosporins	Rare
Thrombocytopenia	Sulphonamides	Rare
	Cephalosporins	Rare
	Latamoxef	Dose dependent
	Rifampicin	Intermittent therapy
Neutropenia	Penicillins	Rare: mainly ampicillin, carbenicillin
	Cephalosporins	Rare
	Sulphonamides	Rare
	Chloramphenicol	
Neurological eighth nerve	Aminoglycosides	Concentration related
	Vancomycin	
Optic nerve	Ethambutol	
Peripheral neuropathy	Isoniazid	Prevented by pyridoxine
	Metronidazole	Prolonged treatment
	Nitrofurantoin	
Convulsions	Penicillins	Large intrathecal or massive intravenous doses
	Cephalosporins	Large intrathecal doses
	4-Fluoroquinolones	Large doses
Benign intracranial hypertension	Tetracyclines	
	Penicillins	
	Nalidixic acid	
Neuromuscular blockade	Aminoglycosides	
Gastrointestinal system		
Liver	Isoniazid	More often rapid acetylators
	Rifampicin	Usually mild—worse in alcoholics/ preceding damage
	Tetracyclines	Massive doses
	Erythromycin estolate	
	Nitrofurantoin	

continued on p.108

ADVERSE REACTIONS OF ANTIMICROBIAL DRUGS

Organ system	Drug	Comment
Transient rise in transaminases	Penicillins Cephalosporins	
Diarrhoea	Penicillins Tetracyclines	Specially ampicillin
	Clindamycin	Pseudomembranous colitis (*Clostridium difficile*)
Other adverse reactions		
Hypersensitivity	Penicillins Sulphonamides	10% cross-sensitivity
Stevens–Johnson syndrome	Sulphonamides Penicillins	
Bone development/tooth staining	Tetracyclines	Contraindicated in childhood and pregnancy
Pulmonary fibrosis	Nitrofurantoin	
Rashes	Commonly penicillins and sulphonamides but virtually any drug can cause rashes	

Table 10.4 Major adverse reactions of antimicrobial drugs.

Comment. An antimicrobial agent might be quite ineffective, or even dangerous, unless its clinical pharmacology is viewed in relation to the whole clinical situation. The drug chosen must reach the site of infection, in an effective concentration, without producing toxicity or adversely influencing any concurrent therapy.

10.2 Antibacterial drugs

Penicillins

Mechanism
Penicillins have a bactericidal action. They inhibit cell wall synthesis by preventing the formation of peptidoglycan cross-bridges in actively multiplying bacteria.

Pharmacokinetics

Oral absorption
Not absorbed: carbenicillin, ticarcillin, mecillinam.

Moderately absorbed: benzylpenicillin (penicillin G), ampicillin, cloxacillin.
Well absorbed: phenoxypenicillin, amoxicillin, bacampicillin, pivampicillin, talampicillin, ciclacillin, flucloxicillin, pivmecillinam.

Even relatively well-absorbed penicillins are destroyed to some extent by gastric acid and should therefore be given at least 30 min before meals.

Distribution
The penicillins have good penetration to most tissues but poor entry to CSF. Giving large doses intravenously when treating meningitis compensates for this effect.

Elimination
Penicillins undergo enterohepatic circulation: drug is excreted via bile and reabsorbed. The major route of elimination after reabsorption is active secretion in the renal tubules. This tubular secretion can be blocked by probenecid with doubling of penicillin blood levels. Dose modification is necessary in severe renal failure.

Adverse effects

Immediate hypersensitivity
This occurs in 0.05% of patients with manifestations ranging from urticaria or wheezing to a life-threatening anaphylactic response.

Delayed hypersensitivity
This occurs in <5% of patients, mainly as rashes. Rare manifestations are haemolytic anaemia, leukopenia, interstitial nephritis (mainly reported with methicillin). Cross-sensitivity with cephalosporins occurs in around 10% of patients.

Toxicity
Convulsions follow large (>15 mg) intrathecal or very high intravenous doses of penicillin. Patients with renal insufficiency can develop cation overload following large doses of potassium penicillin or sodium carbenicillin. Diarrhoea is commonly reported, particularly with ampicillin (20%). Ampicillin has a unique adverse effect comprising a rash in up to 90% of patients with infectious mononucleosis or chronic lymphocytic leukaemia.

Drug interactions
Ampicillin can lead to oral contraceptive failure. This is probably because of diminished enterohepatic circulation. The anticoagulant effect of warfarin is potentiated.

Antibacterial spectrum
The major factor limiting efficacy is the production by certain organisms of enzymes (beta-lactamases or penicillinases) that destroy the beta-lactam ring of the penicillin molecule. This structure is essential to the antibacterial action of penicillins. Several synthetic penicillins incorporate side chains that protect the beta-lactam ring against these enzymes. These types of beta-lactamase resistant drugs therefore are generally less effective than their beta-lactamase sensitive counterparts and are indicated only for the treatment of infection caused by beta-lactamase-producing staphylococci. An alternative approach has been to combine amoxicillin with clavulanic acid, which itself has very little antibacterial activity but inhibits beta-lactamase activity.

Penicillinase-sensitive penicillins
Benzylpenicillin and phenoxypenicillins are active against streptococci, pneumococci, gonococci and meningococci, *Treponenma pallidum*, *Actinomyces israelii* and many anaerobic organisms, but not *Bacteroides fragilis*.

Ampicillin has a broader spectrum and is effective against some strains of *Escherichia coli*, *Proteus mirabilis*, *Shigella*, *Salmonella*, *Haemophilus influenzae* and various enterococci. Several derivatives of ampicillin are better absorbed but have the same antibacterial spectrum: amoxicillin, bacampicillin, pivampicillin and talampicillin. The main indications are acute exacerbations of chronic bronchitis, urinary tract infection, cholecystitis and, parenterally (ampicillin), *Haemophilus influenzae* meningitis (depending on the sensitivity of the organism).

Carbenicillin and ticarcillin are active against *Pseudomonas aeruginosa* and *Proteus* species. At least *in vitro*, ticarcillin is more effective than carbenicillin and azlocillin is more effective than ticarcillin against *Ps. aeruginosa*. All three drugs must be given parenterally. The phenyl ester of carbenicillin (carfecillin) achieves antibacterial concentrations in the urine when given orally. Drug resistance is encountered in some strains. Mecillinam and its orally active ester pivmecillinam are effective against *Salmonella* species.

Penicillinase-resistant penicillins
Cloxacillin, flucloxacillin and methicillin are indicated only in the treatment of infections caused by penicillinase-producing staphylococci. Flucloxacillin is better absorbed from the gut than cloxacillin. More cases of interstitial nephritis have been reported following methicillin therapy than with any other penicillin.

Co-amoxiclav

The amoxicillin/clavulanic acid combination is mainly used in treating urinary tract infections caused by beta-lactamase-producing coliforms.

Tazocin

This combination of piperacillin with tazobactam is used mainly in the treatment of patients with impaired host defences (e.g. following bone marrow transplantation) where infection with beta-lactamase producing coliforms is suspected.

Cephalosporins

Mechanism

Cephalosporins are bactericidal. They contain a beta-lactam ring and their mechanism of action is similar to penicillins.

Pharmacokinetics

Six cephalosporins are effective orally: cefalexin, cefradine (cephradine), cefaclor, cefixime, cefadroxil and cefuroxime. They distribute widely. Cefuroxime and cefotaxime are used in meningitis. Cephaloridine does not cross the blood–brain barrier. The drugs are eliminated renally, partly by glomerular filtration and partly by tubular secretion, with the contribution of each route varying with individual cephalosporins.

Adverse effects

Hypersensitivity is the main adverse effect, with around a 10% cross-reactivity with penicillin-sensitive patients. Cephaloridine can cause renal tubular necrosis, particularly in doses above 6 g/day. A positive Coombs' test occurs in about 5% of patients receiving cephalothin but haemolytic anaemia is rare. Cephalosporins, particularly latamoxef, can reduce prothrombin concentration and bleeding has been described. Several cephalosporins, including those commonly used orally, cause false positive urinalysis tests for glucose, as measured by reducing substances.

Drug interactions

The nephrotoxicity of cephaloridine is potentiated by loop diuretics and aminoglycoside antibiotics.

Antibacterial spectrum

The early cephalosporins were broad spectrum but with limited activity against Gram-negative organisms. Cephamandole and cefuroxime are more resistant to beta-lactamases and are effective against a number of Gram-

DOSES OF PENICILLINS

1 Benzylpenicillin: intramuscular 300–600 mg 2–4 times daily (children 10–20 mg/kg daily); intravenous up to 14.4 g daily; intrathecal 6–12 mg daily.
2 Phenoxymethylpenicillin: oral dose 250–500 mg 6-hourly (children, 125–250 mg 6-hourly).
3 Ampicillin: oral dose 250–1000 mg 6-hourly; intravenous or intramuscular 500–1000 mg 6-hourly (children, half doses).
4 Amoxicillin: oral 250–500 mg 8-hourly (children, half dose).
5 Bacampicillin: 400 mg 8- to 12-hourly.
6 Ciclacillin: 250–500 mg 6-hourly.
7 Pivampicillin: 500 mg 12-hourly.
8 Talampicillin: oral 250–500 mg 8-hourly.
9 Carbenicillin: intravenous (rapid infusion) 5 g 4- to 6-hourly (children, 250–400 mg/kg daily

divided doses); intramuscular 2 g 6-hourly (children, 50–100 mg/kg divided doses).
10 Ticarcillin: intravenous infusion (rapid) or intramuscular 15–20 g daily divided doses.
11 Azlocillin: 2 g 8-hourly by intravenous injection; up to 5 g 8-hourly by infusion.
12 Carfecillin: 0.5–1 g 8-hourly.
13 Mecillinam: slow intravenous injection or intramuscular 5–15 mg/kg 6-hourly.
14 Pivmecillinam: oral 1.2–2.4 g daily in salmonellosis.
15 Cloxacillin: intramuscular 500 mg 6-hourly; intravenous 500–1000 mg 6-hourly (children, quarter to half dose).
16 Flucloxacillin: oral 250 mg 6-hourly.
17 Co-amoxiclav: oral 1–2 tablets (of 250 mg amoxicillin, 125 mg clavulanic acid) 8-hourly.

DOSES OF CEPHALOSPORINS

Oral
Cefalexin and cefradine: 250–500 mg 6-hourly
  (children, 25–50 mg/kg daily in divided doses).

Cefaclor: 250 mg 8-hourly (children, 20–40 mg/kg
  daily in divided doses).
Cefadroxil: 0.5–1 g 12-hourly.

Intravenous
Cefradine: 500–1000 mg 6-hourly (children,
  50–100 mg/kg daily in 6-hourly doses).
Ceftazidime: 1–2 g 8- to 12-hourly.
Cefazolin (cephazolin): 500–1000 mg 6-hourly
  (children, 125–250 mg 8-hourly).

Cefuroxime: 1.5 g 6-hourly (children, 30–100
  mg/kg daily in divided doses).
Cephamandole: 500–2000 mg 6-hourly
  (children, 50–100 mg/kg daily in divided doses).
Cefsulodin: 1–4 g daily in divided doses
  (children, 20–50 mg/kg daily).
Cefotaxime: 1 g 12-hourly to 3 g 6-hourly,
  depending on severity (children, 100–200
  mg/kg daily in divided doses).
Cefoxitin: 1–2 g 8-hourly (children, 80–160
  mg/kg daily in divided doses).
Ceftriaxone: 1–1.2 g daily (children 20–50 mg/kg
  daily as a single dose).

negative bacilli. Cefotaxime is more effective than cephamandole or cefuroxime against Gram-negative bacilli but less effective against Gram-positive organisms. Cefsulodin and ceftazidime are active against *Ps. aeruginosa*. Cefoxitin is closely related to the basic cephalosporin structure and is active against Gram-negative and anaerobic bacteria. Ceftriaxone has modest antistaphylococcal activity with variable resistance shown by Gram-negative bacilli.

Comment. The cephalosporins are used extensively but, in most infections for which a cephalosporin might be considered, another antibiotic is usually at least as effective, at least as safe and almost certainly much less expensive.

Aminoglycosides

Mechanism
Aminoglycosides are bactericidal. They bind to the 30S subunit of bacterial ribosomes, leading to misreading of m-RNA codons.

Pharmacokinetics
Oral absorption is negligible. They have poor penetration into CSF and only moderate penetration to bile. Otherwise, there is good entry to inflamed tissue. Elimination is mainly by glomerular filtration.

Adverse effects
There are two major adverse reactions, both concentration related: nephrotoxicity and ototoxicity. The renal lesion consists of tubular destruction. Eighth nerve damage can be mainly vestibular (streptomycin, gentamicin) or mainly auditory (kanamycin).

The severity of these reactions is related to aminoglycoside serum concentration, which in turn is related to dose and rate of elimination. Accumulation of drug occurs when glomerular filtration is decreased by renal disease or at the extremes of age. Doses must be modified in these situations and drug concentration monitoring is mandatory. Aminoglycosides cross the placenta and can cause eighth nerve

DOSES OF AMINOGLYCOSIDES

Gentamicin: if renal function is normal, the intramuscular dose is 2–5 mg/kg daily given at 8-hourly intervals. Various nomograms and formulae are widely available for calculating dose modifications in renal impairment. A rough guide, based on creatinine clearance, is: >70 ml/min 8-hourly; 30–70 ml/min 12-hourly; 10–30 ml/min 24-hourly; 5–10 ml/min 48-hourly.

It must be emphasized that rules of thumb are not a substitute for drug level monitoring.
Tobramycin: 3–5 mg/kg daily given in divided doses 8-hourly. Modify dose in renal failure.
Amikacin: 15 mg/kg daily in 12-hourly doses. Modify dose in renal failure.
Netilmicin: 4–6 mg/kg daily in divided doses.

damage in the fetus. An uncommon effect of aminoglycosides is neuromuscular blockade occurring after rapid intravenous injection; this is marked in patients with myasthenia gravis.

Drug interactions

Nephrotoxicity is enhanced by co-administration with cephaloridine or polymyxin. Similarly, ototoxicity is enhanced by loop diuretics. The neuromuscular blockade of curare-like drugs can be prolonged by aminoglycosides.

Antibacterial spectrum

Gentamicin is the most widely used aminoglycoside and is active against all aerobic Gram-negative rods, including pseudomonas and proteus, and also against staphylococci. Most streptococci are resistant because gentamicin cannot penetrate the cell. However, penicillin and aminoglycosides have synergistic effect against some streptococci. All anaerobic organisms are resistant. Tobramycin is 2–4 times more active against pseudomonas but is otherwise very similar to gentamicin. Amikacin is resistant to most of the bacterial enzymes that inactivate gentamicin, and is only indicated for infections caused by aerobic Gram-negative rods against which gentamicin is no longer effective. Netilmicin has a similar antibacterial spectrum to gentamicin, but is claimed to be less ototoxic: confirmatory evidence is limited. Neomycin is given orally to decrease the bacterial content of the colon in liver failure or before bowel surgery. If there is severe liver or renal failure or inflammatory bowel disease, sufficient neomycin can be absorbed to cause ototoxicity. Streptomycin is effective against tubercle bacilli and is discussed later.

Comment. The major role of aminoglycosides is the parenteral treatment of serious infection caused by sensitive organisms. These drugs are popular for the initial management of life-threatening septicaemia of uncertain aetiology. In this situation an aminoglycoside is usually combined with metronidazole and/or an extended spectrum penicillin.

Sulphonamide–trimethoprim combinations

Mechanism

These drugs are bactericidal. Co-trimoxazole contains a sulphonamide, sulfamethoxazole (sulphamethoxazole), and trimethoprim in the ratio 5 : 1. The basis of the action of sulphonamides is that bacterial cells are impermeable to folic acid so must synthesize their own from p-aminobenzoic acid, with which sulphonamides have a strong similarity. Thus, competitive inhibition of folic acid synthesis occurs. Trimethoprim blocks the next synthetic step, from folic acid to tetrahydrofolate, by inhibiting the enzyme dihydrofolate reductase.

Pharmacokinetics

Co-trimoxazole is well absorbed following oral administration and is also available for intravenous use. There is wide tissue distribution and elimination is by renal excretion.

Adverse effects

The sulphonamide component can cause rashes and, much less commonly, Stevens–Johnson syndrome, renal failure and blood dyscrasias. Trimethoprim can also cause rashes and impaired haemopoiesis and can produce gastrointestinal symptoms. The trimethoprim component has been implicated in teratogenesis. In the newborn, sulphonamides can displace bilirubin from protein binding sites and cause kernicterus.

Drug interactions

The sulphonamide component competes for hepatic enzyme binding sites and can decrease the clearance of phenytoin, tolbutamide and warfarin sufficiently to produce phenytoin toxicity, hypoglycaemia and enhanced anticoagulation, respectively. Displacement of methotrexate from protein binding sites can also lead to toxicity.

Antibacterial spectrum

These drugs have a broad spectrum, including Gram-positive cocci, Neisseria gonorrhoeae,

Haemophilus influenzae, *Escherichia coli*, *Proteus mirabilis*, *Shigella* species, *Salmonella* species, *Pneumocystis carinii* and *Brucella* species.

Dose
Co-trimoxazole: 960 mg (two tablets of 400 mg sulfamethoxazole, 80 mg trimethoprim) 12-hourly for oral or intravenous administration (children, 120–480 mg 12-hourly depending on age).

Comment. The combination of sulphonamide and trimethoprim is the treatment of first choice in urinary tract infections but is also a good alternative regimen in several other conditions, including typhoid fever, exacerbation of chronic bronchitis and gonorrhoea in penicillin-sensitive patients.

Trimethoprim alone is also used in treating urinary tract and respiratory tract infections. Dose: 300 mg daily or 100 mg daily for prophylaxis.

Tetracyclines

Mechanism
Tetracyclines are bacteriostatic, binding to the 30S ribosomal subunit with consequent misreading of information needed for protein synthesis.

Pharmacokinetics
Tetracyclines are adequately absorbed following oral administration. Tissue distribution is good and the drugs are eliminated mainly unmetabolized by biliary excretion.

Adverse effects
Tetracyclines bind to calcium in bones and teeth, leading to impaired bone growth and discoloration of teeth during active mineralization (up to 7 years). Tetracyclines cross the placenta and are contraindicated in pregnancy. Following large doses, both hepatic necrosis and renal failure have been reported. Except for doxycycline and minocycline, these drugs are contraindicated in renal failure because they impair protein synthesis and so

enhance the effects of catabolism. Many patients develop diarrhoea on tetracycline therapy.

Drug interactions
Milk, antacids, calcium, magnesium and iron from insoluble complexes with tetracyclines in the gut lumen, leading to treatment failure, the exception being minocycline.

Antibacterial spectrum
The tetracyclines are effective against a wide range of bacteria but resistance is increasing, and they should no longer be considered useful broad-spectrum antibiotics. The importance of tetracyclines is based on their efficacy against chlamydia (e.g. non-specific urethritis, psittacosis), rickettsia (e.g. Q fever, typhus, Rocky Mountain spotted fever), mycoplasma, brucella and cholera. In these infections, tetracyclines are the drugs of first choice. Tetracyclines are also useful adjuncts to the treatment of acne by preventing the growth of *Propionibacterium acnes* in the blocked sebaceous ducts. The other specific indication for a tetracycline is the use of minocycline in meningococcal prophylaxis.

Dose
Tetracycline and oxytetracycline: 250–500 mg 6-hourly. Minocycline: 200 mg then 100 mg 12-hourly.

Other antibacterial drugs

Metronidazole
Metronidazole was initially used in protozoal infections, but was later found to be very effective against anaerobic bacteria, including *Bacteroides fragilis*. It is currently popular in treating serious anaerobic infections. In addition, metronidazole is often combined with gentamicin in treating serious mixed infections or septicaemia of uncertain aetiology. The other major uses are in treating trichomonal vaginitis, amoebiasis and giardiasis. Metronidazole is often combined with gentamicin or ciprofloxacin as prophylaxis in abdominal

surgery. The only major adverse effects are peripheral neuropathy following prolonged therapy and seizures following high doses.

Dose

For severe infections, intravenous infusion of metronidazole is given at the rate of 500 mg every 8 h in adults and 7.5 mg/kg 12-hourly in children for 7 days.

Oral: 200 mg 8-hourly for 7 days for trichomoniasis and 2 g daily for 3 days in amoebiasis and giardiasis. If appropriate, suppositories can be used in circumstances where intravenous infusion might be considered: similar blood levels but much cheaper. Dose: 1 g 8-hourly.

Erythromycin

Erythromycin has an antibacterial spectrum similar to penicillin and is a suitable second-line drug for patients allergic to penicillin. It is currently the drug of choice for *Legionella pneumophilia*, it is of some value in whooping cough prophylaxis and is effective against mycoplasma. It is also used in chlamydial non-specific urethritis and campylobacter enteritis. The only major adverse effect is cholestatic jaundice associated primarily with the estolate formulation. This formulation is therefore contraindicated in liver disease.

Dose

Oral: 250–500 mg 6-hourly for adults, 125–250 mg 6-hourly for children. Intravenous: 300 mg by infusion 6-hourly, children, 30–50 mg/kg daily in divided doses 6-hourly.

Clarithromycin

Clarithromycin has similar antibacterial spectrum but causes less nausea, vomiting and abdominal cramps than erythromycin. It has been shown to be effective in eliminating gastric *Helicobacter pylori* usually in combination with amoxicillin and omeprazole (a proton pump inhibitor).

Dose

Oral: 500 mg 12-hourly for adults.

Chloramphenicol

Chloramphenicol is a very effective broad-spectrum bacteriostatic antibiotic but use is restricted because of bone marrow suppression, which occurs as a rare complication of treatment. Chloramphenicol is indicated in life-threatening infections for which other agents are unsuitable because of bacterial resistance or patient allergy. The drug is particularly useful in *H. influenzae* meningitis and typhoid fever. Chloramphenicol is contraindicated in neonates because of cardiovascular collapse (Chapter 4).

Dose

Intravenous: 1 g 6-hourly in adults. Children require 50–100 mg/kg daily, divided into 6-hourly doses.

Fusidic acid

This drug has a narrow spectrum and is indicated in combination with another antistaphylococcal drug only in serious penicillin-resistant staphylococcal infections, e.g. those of bone.

Dose

Fusidic acid is given at a dose of 500 mg 8-hourly by intravenous infusion or orally.

Clindamycin

Clindamycin is effective against penicillin-resistant staphylococci and many anaerobic organisms. It is indicated only in serious conditions where other agents are contraindicated, or ineffective, notably staphylococcal bone and joint infections. However, an adverse effect is pseudomembranous colitis caused by toxinogenic strains of *Clostridium difficile*.

Dose

0.6–2.7 g clindamycin daily are given in divided doses by slow intravenous infusion; children, 15–40 mg/kg daily in divided doses.

Nitrofurantoin

Nitrofurantoin, an orally administered drug that achieves antibacterial concentrations only in urine, is effective against many organisms infecting the urinary tract. However, it is a second-line drug for this indication because of frequent adverse effects, including gastrointestinal symptoms and rashes. It precipitates haemolytic anaemia in glucose-6-phosphate deficiency and can cause peripheral neuropathy and pulmonary fibrosis.

Vancomycin

Vancomycin is effective against *Clostridium difficile* and can be used to treat pseudomembranous colitis. It is also used intravenously in the prophylaxis and treatment of endocarditis caused by Gram-positive cocci. Increasingly vancomycin treatment is necessary in the treatment of catheter-associated infections resulting from coagulase-negative staphylococci. Because of possible nephrotoxicity, serum levels need to be monitored.

Dose
Intravenous: 1 g 12-hourly.

Teicoplanin

Teicoplanin is an alternative to vancomycin. Serum levels need not be monitored.

Quinolones

Nalidixic acid, the first quinolone, has been available for 30 years. Administered orally, it achieves low tissue concentrations and its use is restricted to the treatment of uncomplicated urinary tract infections. Chemical modifications have produced a series of improved drugs and the most recent are the 4-fluoroquinolones; ciprofloxacin is the first agent in this group available in the UK.

Ciprofloxacin

Mechanism
Bactericidal in action, ciprofloxacin inhibits DNA-gyrase activity by binding to chromosomal DNA strands. This interferes with DNA replication and prevents supercoiling within the chromosome.

Pharmacokinetics
It is well absorbed after oral administration and is distributed rapidly into body tissues. Most of the drug is eliminated unaltered by the kidneys; the remainder is excreted by hepatic metabolism or unchanged in the faeces.

Adverse effects
The most frequently reported side effects are minor gastrointestinal upsets, and severe systemic adverse reactions are rare. However, central nervous system disturbances such as insomnia, confusion and convulsions have been reported. Because it can cause damage to cartilage in young animals, ciprofloxacin is contraindicated in children and growing adolescents.

Drug interactions
Its absorption is reduced significantly by the coadministration of aluminium and magnesium antacids. It interferes with the metabolism of theophylline, caffeine and warfarin so that the toxic effects of these drugs may be encountered if they are given along with ciprofloxacin.

Antibacterial spectrum
It is active against aerobic Gram-negative bacteria, including *Pseudomonas aeruginosa*, and less active against Gram-positive bacteria: staphylococci are more sensitive than streptococci. Anaerobes, in general, are resistant. Ciprofloxacin is particularly useful for pseudomonas infections where oral therapy is preferred, such as respiratory tract infection in patients with cystic fibrosis. It is very effective in gastrointestinal infections ranging from traveller's diarrhoea to typhoid fever.

Dose
Oral: 250–750 mg 12-hourly; intravenous: 100–200 mg 12-hourly.

Comments. Ciprofloxacin has been available for 10 years but there is no reason why it should replace established, effective and much less expensive antibiotics for many urinary and respiratory tract infections.

Ofloxacin

Similar spectrum to ciprofloxacin but with less resistance developing among staphylococci and *Pseudomonas* sp.

Several new 4-fluoroquinolones are being developed.

Dose

Oral: 200–400 mg 12-hourly; intravenous 200–400 mg 12-hourly.

10.3 Antituberculous drugs

Isoniazid

Mechanism

The precise mechanism is unknown, but it is bactericidal.

Pharmacokinetics

Isoniazid is well absorbed following oral administration and is widely distributed through the body, including the CSF where concentrations equal those in blood. Isoniazid is inactivated in the liver by pathways including genetically dependent acetylation. The same metabolic pathway is involved in the acetylation of hydralazine, procainamide and dapsone (Chapter 1, Section 1.3). About 50% of Caucasians are slow acetylators but the proportion varies widely in other populations, and slow acetylation is very common in people of Asian ethnic origin.

Adverse effects

Peripheral neuropathy occurs mainly in slow acetylators and can be prevented by coadministration of pyridoxine (20 mg/day). Hepatotoxicity occasionally occurs and is more frequent in the elderly and those with a large alcohol intake. Very high doses of isoniazid can lead to psychosis, convulsions or coma.

Drug interactions

Isoniazid inhibits enzymes that metabolize phenytoin and warfarin; thus phenytoin con-

centrations and anticoagulation level should be carefully monitored.

Dose

Oral: 3 mg/kg adults or 6 mg/kg daily in children, i.e. children require more on a weight basis; for tuberculous meningitis, 10 mg/kg daily. Also available for parenteral use.

Rifampicin

Mechanism

It is bactericidal, and inhibits the DNA-dependent RNA polymerase of *Mycobacterium* sp.

Pharmacokinetics

Rifampicin is well absorbed following oral administration and widely distributed, including the CSF. It is deacetylated in the liver and eliminated by biliary excretion.

Adverse effects

There is often a transient elevation of liver enzymes but serious hepatotoxicity is uncommon. The risk of liver damage is increased by alcoholism and pre-existing liver disease. Intermittent treatment is associated with more frequent and serious adverse effects, including renal failure and thrombocytopaenia. Rifampicin causes red urine, tears and sputum.

Drug interactions

Rifampicin induces hepatic enzymes and, because of increased clearance, can cause treatment failure with oral contraceptives, sulphonylureas, warfarin, steroids and barbiturates.

Dose

Rifampicin is given at a dose of 10 mg/kg daily before breakfast.

Ethambutol

Mechanism

The mechanism is uncertain but bacteriostatic.

Pharmacokinetics

Ethambutol is well absorbed following oral administration. It has poor penetration of CSF but otherwise is adequately distributed. Excretion of unchanged drug is mainly renal.

Adverse effects

The most important reaction is retrobulbar neuritis with loss of visual acuity and colour vision. This is largely preventable by using doses below 25 mg/kg daily. The visual defect usually reverses over several months after stopping the drug.

Drug interactions

Aluminium hydroxide can decrease absorption.

Dose

A daily dose of 15–25 mg/kg is given.

Pyrazinamide

Mechanism

Pyrazinamide is bactericidal.

Pharmacokinetics

It is well absorbed following oral administration and has good penetration to CSF. It is eliminated by renal excretion.

Adverse effects

Pyrazinamide causes hepatotoxicity and arthralgia. Dose modification is required in patients with renal impairment.

Dose

A daily dose of 20–30 mg/kg is given up to a maximum of 3 g.

Second-line drugs

Streptomycin is now infrequently used. It is an aminoglycoside that is eliminated by the kidneys. Ototoxicity is the main adverse reaction. Streptomycin could particularly be considered for use in patients with liver disease. Several other agents are available for use in situations of bacterial resistance or adverse reactions to first-line drugs, e.g. capreomycin, cycloserine, ethionamide and p-aminosalicylic acid.

Comment. Mycobacterium tuberculosis multiplies slowly and the long periods of treatment required encourage the emergence of resistant strains. Combination chemotherapy is thus the basis of treatment. Initially, isoniazid, rifampicin and either ethambutol or pyrazinamide are administered for 8 weeks. Subsequently, isoniazid and rifampicin are given. Six months of treatment with this regimen is adequate for pulmonary TB. If other drugs are used, 9 months of therapy is necessary. If TB occurs elsewhere, or if intermittent therapy is used, 12–18 months is required.

10.4 Antifungal drugs

Amphotericin B

Mechanism

Amphotericin B combines with sterols in the plasma membrane, with a resulting increase in permeability and cell death.

Pharmacokinetics

Absorption is negligible following oral administration. In practice it is usually given intravenously. It is highly protein bound with apparently poor penetration to tissues and body fluids. It is not removed by haemodialysis. The mode of elimination is unknown but it is not influenced by renal function.

Adverse effects

These are very common. Most patients develop fever, chills and nausea. Nephrotoxicity (distal tubular destruction and calcification) usually occurs during prolonged treatment at or above 1 mg/kg daily and manifests as hypokalaemia, loss of concentrating ability and renal tubular acidosis; nephrotoxicity reverses if detected early.

Drug interaction
It is additive with other nephrotoxic drugs. Concurrent digoxin therapy can become toxic if hypokalaemia develops.

Antifungal spectrum
It is currently the drug of choice for most systemic mycoses: active against *Cryptococcus*, *Candida* and other yeasts, *Aspergillus*, *Coccidioides* and other fungi. Resistance has not been reported.

Dose
A 1-mg test dose is given, then 250 μg/kg daily, increasing to 1–1.5 mg daily depending on disease severity and appearance of nephrotoxicity. Hydrocortisone can reduce febrile reactions and chlorpromazine can reduce nausea.

A liposomal preparation is also available that shows better bioavailability and better efficacy.

Comment. Amphotericin B is an example of the need to carefully weigh the risks and benefits of treatment. It is highly toxic but untreated systemic mycoses are invariably fatal.

Flucytosine

Mechanism
It is deaminated inside the fungal cell to 5-fluorouracil, which inhibits nucleic acid synthesis with cell death.

Pharmacokinetics
It is well absorbed following oral administration and is widely distributed, including the CSF. Elimination is mainly renal. Clearance is decreased in patients with renal impairment.

Adverse effects
Concentration related bone marrow suppression is the only major problem. This can usually be avoided by drug level monitoring.

Antifungal spectrum
It is only active against yeasts; efficacy is limited by rapid emergence of resistance.

Dose
150–200 mg flucytosine are given daily in divided doses.

Comment. Although much less toxic than amphotericin, flucytosine is of limited value because of its narrow spectrum and the existence of resistant organisms. It is usually administered together with amphotericin B.

Imidazoles and related compounds

Mechanism
Imidazoles increase permeability by preventing ergosterol formation in cell membranes. They also produce cell necrosis by inhibiting peroxidative enzymes.

Miconazole, clotrimazole, econazole

Pharmacokinetics
These drugs are poorly absorbed following oral administration and are usually restricted for topical use.

Antifungal spectrum
They are active against a wide range of yeasts and fungi. Their main use is topical, e.g. athlete's foot or vaginal candidiasis.

Fluconazole, itraconazole, ketoconazole

Pharmacokinetics
Following oral administration these drugs are widely distributed; adequate CSF levels are obtained with the exception of ketoconazole. Fluconazole is eliminated by the kidneys; itraconazole and ketoconazole are metabolized by the liver.

Antifungal spectrum
They are active against a wide range of yeasts and fungi; fluconazole is particularly effective against yeasts and itraconazole against filamentous fungi, e.g. *Aspergillus*.

Adverse effects

Hepatotoxicity is associated particularly with ketoconazole, which requires monitoring of liver function.

Doses

Fluconazole: 100–400 mg orally or by i.v. infusion, daily single dose.
Itraconazole: 100–200 mg orally, daily single dose.
Ketoconazole: 200–400 mg orally, daily single dose.

Nystatin

Nystatin is used topically in the treatment of yeast infections of the skin and mucous membranes. It is not used parenterally because of high toxicity.

Griseofulvin

Griseofulvin is active only against dermatophytes and is given orally in the treatment of skin or nail infections. It is fungistatic so must be given for weeks or months. It diminishes the anticoagulant effect by enzyme induction. Barbiturates lead to griseofulvin treatment failure by enzyme induction. Griseofulvin can precipitate porphyria.

10.5 Antiviral drugs

These are the least developed as a group of antimicrobial agents: viruses use the biochemical system of their host cells, and it is therefore difficult to prevent viral multiplication without seriously damaging the patient. However, effective therapy is now available for a number of virus infections of clinical importance.

Acyclovir

Mechanism

The pharmacological effect of acyclovir depends on its conversion to an active metabolite by a herpes simplex coded enzyme, thymidine kinase. It is phosphorylated only in herpes infected cells and normal cellular processes are unaffected. The resulting acyclovir triphosphate inhibits herpes-specified DNA polymerase, preventing further viral DNA synthesis. The herpes genome in latently (non-replicating) infected cells is not altered during antiviral therapy. Varicella zoster virus is also susceptible to acyclovir but its action is not thymidine kinase dependent.

Pharmacokinetics

Acyclovir is adequately absorbed orally in patients with normal gut function. It is eliminated by renal clearance involving glomerular filtration and tubular secretion. Acyclovir penetrates the blood–brain barrier passively to enter CSF.

Adverse effects

Renal impairment occasionally follows intravenous administration.

Drug interactions

No clinically important interactions have been observed yet.

Clinical use

Acyclovir is indicated for herpes simplex and varicella zoster infections of the skin and mucous membranes, the brain and in lung disease and in prophylaxis against herpes infections in immunocompromised hosts. An intravenous route is required for serious disease manifestations and in immunocompromised patients.

Dose

For herpes simplex: oral, 200 mg five times per day for 5 days; intravenous, 5 mg/kg over 1 h, repeated every 8 h (10 mg/kg in herpes encephalitis). A dose modification is necessary in renal failure. For varicella zoster: oral, 800 mg five times per day for 7 days; intravenous, 10 mg/kg 8-hourly.

Idoxuridine

Idoxuridine is a thymidine analogue that inhibits DNA synthesis. It is highly toxic when given systemically and is therefore only used topically in the treatment of herpes simplex infections of the eye, as an aqueous solution, and in dimethyl sulfoxide (dimethyl sulphoxide) for skin eruptions. Shingles can be treated similarly.

Vidarabine

Vidarabine inhibits DNA but does not target a specific virus. It has been used systemically in the treatment of chicken pox or herpes zoster infections in immunocompromised hosts but has been largely superseded by acyclovir owing to the low toxicity of acyclovir. It has been shown to decrease the early mortality in herpes simplex encephalitis. The major adverse reactions are suppression of bone marrow and a wide range of neurological effects.

Amantadine

Amantadine (including its analogue, rimantadine) prevents entry of influenza A to host cells and is used predominantly in prophylaxis but also in the treatment of infections caused by this virus. Influenza B virus is not susceptible. Amantadine can produce neurological side effects but usually only if high concentrations are achieved, e.g. in renal failure.

Ribavirin

Ribavirin inhibits a number of DNA and RNA viruses. Its antiviral action has been demonstrated *in vitro* and *in vivo* against a number of important viruses, including respiratory syncytial virus (RSV), influenza A and B viruses, parainfluenza 1 and 3 and Lassa fever virus. The mechanism of action is not completely understood but involves the action of ribavirin triphosphate interfering with the binding of viral messenger RNA to ribosomes. It is predominantly used in the form of a nebulized aerosol in the treatment of bronchitis in infancy as a consequence of RSV infection.

Zidovudine (azidothymidine, AZT)

Mechanism

AZT is phosphorylated in both infected and uninfected cells by thymidine kinase and subsequently by other kinases to triphosphate, which is a chain terminator in DNA synthesis. Human immunodeficiency virus (HIV) is not eradicated during or following treatment.

Pharmacokinetics

It is well absorbed from the gut; CSF levels are 50% of plasma levels. It is eliminated by glucuronidation.

Adverse effects

There is serious haematological toxicity: anaemia and neutropenia are seen in up to one-third of patients treated with AZT.

Clinical use

AZT is indicated in:
1 Serious manifestations of HIV infections in patients with acquired immunodeficiency syndrome (AIDS) or AIDS-related complex. It has been shown to prolong life in this group of patients.
2 Early symptomatic or asymptomatic HIV infection, with markers indicating risk of disease progression.

Dose

200 mg AZT 4-hourly for symptomatic disease.
500 mg AZT daily for asymptomatic patients.
Dose modification is required in anaemia, myelosuppression, renal and hepatic impairment, pregnancy and the elderly.

Ganciclovir

Mechanism

Ganciclovir is an acyclic analogue structurally related to acyclovir. It acts as a substrate for viral DNA polymerase and as a chain terminator aborting virus replication.

Pharmacokinetics

It is excreted primarily unchanged in the kidneys and is largely unbound in plasma. Renal impairment leads to altered kinetics.

Adverse effects

Neutropenia occurs in 40% of patients but is usually reversible. It occurs after 1 week of induction therapy. There is occasional rash, nausea and vomiting.

Drug interactions

No drug interactions have been observed as yet.

Clinical use

Ganciclovir is indicated for life-threatening cytomegalovirus (CMV) infections in immuno-compromised individuals, particularly with AIDS or transplanted organs, and in the treatment and prevention of CMV retinitis in these patients.

Dose

Intravenous: 5 mg/kg over 1 h every 12 h for 14 days.

Dose reduction is required in patients with impaired renal function.

CHAPTER 11

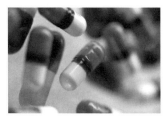

Drugs and Respiratory Disease

11.1 Drugs and airflow obstruction

Aims

The aim of treatment in airflow obstruction is to ease ventilation by reducing bronchial smooth muscle tone and by reducing the underlying inflammatory and allergic response.

Relevant pathophysiology

Bronchial smooth muscle tone depends on a complex balance between different bronchoconstrictor and bronchodilator influences; the autonomic nervous system is an important regulator of smooth muscle tone in the airways.

Bronchoconstrictor influences

1 Cholinergic efferent vagal nerves release acetylcholine which acts on muscarinic receptors on airway smooth muscle. This is the main motor nerve supply to the airways.
2 Non-cholinergic excitatory nerves are thought to release tachykinins such as substance P. The importance of these nerves in man is unknown.
3 Humoral factors such as histamine and leukotrienes are released in the inflammatory/allergic response seen in asthma.

Bronchodilator influences

1 Circulating catecholamines which stimulate beta$_2$-adrenoceptors on airway smooth muscle and mast cells.

2 Sympathetic nerve supply to the airway smooth muscle is sparse, but these nerves may reduce airway tone via an inhibitory effect on presynaptic cholinergic efferent vagal nerves.
3 Non-adrenergic non-cholinergic (NANC) inhibitory nerves; the neurotransmitter is unknown but may be nitric oxide.

In normal individuals there is a degree of resting airway tone as a result of cholinergic vagal nerve input. Abnormalities in neural control of the airways may contribute to the increase in airflow resistance in airway diseases, though there is no direct evidence so far.

Asthma

Asthma is characterized by airflow obstruction that is reversible either spontaneously or as a result of treatment. The increase in airflow resistance is a consequence of contraction of airway smooth muscle, mucosal oedema and increased airway secretions. In some asthmatic patients attacks can be provoked by specific triggers, such as allergens, some occupational agents or drugs, e.g. non-steroidal anti-inflammatory drugs (NSAIDs). Non-specific triggers, such as exercise, irritants or cold air, will produce asthma in most, if not all, asthmatic patients.

Asthma developing in childhood is usually associated with increased levels of allergen-specific IgE antibodies and there is often a family or personal history of hayfever or eczema. This type of asthma is often termed extrinsic or early-onset asthma. Late-onset asthma characteristically develops in adults, usually in middle age, and symptoms tend to be persistent. Serum eosinophil levels may be raised, whilst allergen-specific IgE levels may be normal. This type of asthma is sometimes termed intrinsic asthma.

Chronic airflow obstruction

Chronic obstructive airways disease is usually associated with cigarette smoking and is characterized by a progressive decline in airways calibre over many years. The airways obstruction is predominantly irreversible. The separation between asthma and chronic airflow obstruction is not always easy and some patients have features of both. Of more practical importance is the functional response to bronchodilator and steroid drugs, which can be determined by measuring their effect on peak flow rate or spirometric measurements. In difficult cases a trial of steroids (prednisolone 30 – 40 mg/day for 10 – 14 days) may be necessary fully to assess the reversibility of their airflow obstruction.

Drugs used in the treatment of airways obstruction

Beta₂-adrenoceptor agonists

Short-acting (e.g. salbutamol, terbutaline) and long-acting (e.g. salmeterol, formoterol (eformoterol))

Mechanism. These selective beta₂-adrenoceptor stimulants act on airway smooth muscle and mast cells. Relaxation of bronchial smooth muscle is mediated by increased intracellular cyclic adenosine monophosphate (cAMP). Beta₂-stimulants are best given by inhalation as this delivers the drug directly to the airways thus increasing their selective bronchodilator effect and minimizing generalized systemic effects. The dose required by aerosol is very much lower than that required by mouth or intravenously, further limiting dose-related adverse effects. Duration of action is: short-acting beta₂-agonists (salbutamol, terbutaline) 4–6 h; long-acting beta₂-agonists (salmeterol, formoterol) 8–12 h.

Adverse effects. Hypokalaemia caused by beta₂-mediated stimulation of the Na^+/K^+ pump. This may be serious and can be potentiated by concurrent use of theophylline, steroids, diuretics or by hypoxia. Other dose-dependent adverse effects include tremor (beta₂) and tachycardia (beta₁). These effects are relatively rare with the aerosol route of administration but may be seen with higher doses. Paradoxical bronchospasm may occur with the longer acting drugs.

Clinical use and dose. Short-acting beta₂-agonists (salbutamol, terbutaline) are used in asthma and chronic airflow obstruction for relief of symptoms (pressurized or dry powder aerosol ideally; tablets cause increased side effects) or in acute attacks when they may be given by nebulizer. (Typical recommended dosage is: by aerosol inhalation,

---

MAIN GROUPS OF DRUGS USED TO TREAT AIRFLOW OBSTRUCTION

1 Beta-adrenoceptor agonists, which increase cAMP in airway smooth muscle cells and mast cells.
2 Theophylline and related methylxanthines, which also increase intracellular cAMP by inhibiting phosphodiesterase, the enzyme that breaks down cAMP (whether this is their main mode of action is less certain).
3 Antimuscarinic drugs, which inhibit cholinergic (vagal) bronchoconstriction.

4 'Anti-allergy' drugs, which inhibit the production, release or effects of bronchoconstrictor or inflammatory mediators.
5 Corticosteroids, which reduce the inflammatory response in asthma in particular; the precise mechanisms(s) underlying their action are unknown but reducing the release of inflammatory cytokines is probably important.

salbutamol 0.1–0.2 mg, terbutaline 0.25–0.5 mg as needed up to 4- to 6-hourly; by nebulizer, 2.5–10 mg four times daily.) There is some evidence that asthma may be less well controlled if patients take beta$_2$-agonists regularly rather than as required so patients should be encouraged to take them only 'as necessary'.

Salmeterol or formoterol, the long-acting beta$_2$-agonists, are used in patients with asthma who continue to have symptoms despite moderate or high doses of inhaled corticosteroids. They are normally given by pressurized aerosol or dry powder inhaler and have a slower onset of action than salbutamol so should not be given more than twice daily and should not be given to acutely ill patients.

Other selective beta$_2$-stimulants
A number of other beta$_2$-agonists are available, including isoetharine, rimiterol, reproterol and pirbuterol. These agents are either less selective or shorter acting and have no clear advantages.

Comment. Beta$_2$-adrenoceptor agonists given by aerosol inhalation relieve bronchospasm with minimal adverse cardiac effects in patients with reversible airways obstruction. Response depends on the patient using the pressurized aerosol correctly. Even when used correctly, only about 10% of the metered dose reaches the airways, and 10–20% from a dry powder inhaler, although this amount is usually sufficient to produce near maximum bronchodilatation for that patient. Some patients have difficulty in using a pressurized aerosol inhaler correctly, despite instruction; a variety of other devices are available including dry powder inhalers, spacing devices attached to a metered dose inhaler and nebulizers.

Theophylline

Mechanism
Theophylline is 1,3-dimethyl xanthine. The alkyl group at the 3-position is responsible for its bronchodilator effect; that at the 1-position (which it shares with caffeine and theobromine) produces central nervous system (CNS) stimulation and a weak diuretic effect. It is a non-selective inhibitor of phosphodiesterase isoenzymes and hence increases intracellular cAMP concentrations.

Pharmacokinetics
Theophylline is ineffective when given by inhalation and has to be given orally or intravenously. It is absorbed nearly totally from the gut, but is then metabolized extensively by the liver. Differences in hepatic metabolism are the principal reason for the wide variability in pharmacokinetics between individuals and within the same individual during the course of an illness (Chapters 1 and 2). There is a well-defined relationship between serum theophylline concentration and effect, but response varies from individual to individual. Theophylline has a small therapeutic window and in some patients adverse effects, particularly nausea, occur at plasma concentrations in the therapeutic range and before near maximum bronchodilatation has been achieved. Theophylline should be given as slow-release preparations to minimize the differences between peak and trough concentrations; the average elimination half-life in adults is about 8–12 h, so they are usually given two or three times daily by mouth. The exact dosage schedule depends on the assessment of clearance in individual patients (see Chapter 2). Theophylline clearance is relatively high in children and young adults, who therefore need higher daily doses than elderly patients, particularly those with congestive cardiac failure where theophylline clearance may be significantly reduced (Chapters 2 and 3).

Drug interactions are very important with theophylline because it is metabolized by the liver and because of its small therapeutic window. Drugs that increase its half-life include erythromycin, fluvoxamine and ciprofloxacin; drugs that reduce its half-life include rifampicin and phenytoin.

Adverse effects

Tachycardia, palpitations, nausea, vomiting, arrhythmias and convulsions are associated with increased plasma levels, particularly above 25–30 mg/l. Nausea may occur at therapeutic plasma levels.

Clinical use and dose

Oral theophylline is used to treat some patients with asthma and chronic airflow obstruction long-term. Several slow-release tablet formulations are available. The dose should be adjusted according to therapeutic response, adverse effects and, if available, pharmacokinetic information based on plasma theophylline concentrations.

Aminophylline contains theophylline and ethylenediamine to increase its solubility (2 : 1); only the theophylline has a therapeutic effect. Aminophylline can be given orally or intravenously for severe acute asthma (status asthmaticus) not responding to nebulized beta$_2$-agonists. It should be considered only in patients not previously taking an oral xanthine preparation to avoid problems with toxicity. It is advisable to monitor serum theophylline concentrations.

Comment. Oral theophylline preparations can be useful as second-line bronchodilators in the treatment of asthma and chronic airflow obstruction. Their small therapeutic window, large variation in metabolism and vulnerability to drug interactions limit their value. Adverse effects can be minimized by measuring plasma theophylline concentrations.

Anti-allergy drugs

Sodium cromoglicate (sodium cromoglycate), nedocromil sodium

Mechanism. These drugs are not bronchodilators. Their mechanism of action in the treatment of asthma is unclear. They stabilize sensitized mast cells and inhibit the release of bronchoconstrictor mediators such as histamine and prostaglandins; in addition, they inhibit neural reflexes in the lung.

Clinical use and dose. These drugs are used to prevent exercise-induced asthma and for the prophylaxis of asthma where benefit is only seen after repeated, regular administration. They are of no value in acute asthma or in patients with chronic airflow obstruction. Both drugs are more useful in extrinsic asthma, particularly in children and young adults, and in preventing exercise-induced asthma. Response in late-onset asthma is usually disappointing.

Sodium cromoglicate can be administered by inhalation as a dry powder from a spinhaler (20 mg four times daily), from a metered dose pressurized inhaler as an aerosol (10 mg/2 puffs) four times daily or as a nebulizer solution (10 mg/ml); the latter is useful for young children unable to use an inhaler.

Nedocromil sodium appears to have similar indications to sodium cromoglicate. It is administered from a metered dose inhaler (4 mg/2 puffs) two to four times daily. Both drugs are less effective than inhaled corticosteroids.

Corticosteroids (Chapter 14)

The actions of corticosteroids on the bronchi are not fully understood, but they have anti-inflammatory activity and probably reduce mucosal oedema. It is likely that several mechanisms contribute to this effect including a reduction in the production of proinflammatory cytokines. Most of the effects of corticosteroids are the result of an intracellular effect that involves transcription of messenger RNA, which is one reason for their slow onset of action.

Corticosteroids are given by the following routes to patients with airways obstruction:

1 By inhalation.
2 Orally.
3 Intravenously.

Inhalation. Topical steroid aerosols represent a significant advance in the management of asthma because the generalized adverse effects associated with systemic routes of administration are reduced. This is in part a result of the mode of administration but also because the drugs administered by inhalation have a high first-pass hepatic metabolism (around 90% compared to 20% for prednisolone); thus the proportion of drug from an inhaler that is swallowed (80–90% from a metered dose inhaler) is largely metabolized before entering the systemic circulation. Beclometasone (beclomethasone), budesonide and fluticasone are administered by regular aerosol inhalation, the dose depending on the particular drug. They do not act acutely. All are available as a metered dose and dry powder inhaler. Patients using a metered dose inhaler should inhale the steroid through a large spacing device; this reduces impaction on the back of the throat and markedly reduces the incidence of candidiasis (it also reduces particle size so that more is inhaled and much less is swallowed).

Adverse effects of inhaled steroids can be divided into local and systemic effects. Local effects include candidiasis of the pharynx and larynx and laxity of the vocal cords causing hoarseness. High doses of inhaled steroids (beclometasone dipropionate or budesonide >1 mg/day, fluticasone >500 μg/day) have some systemic activity, as shown by measures of adrenal suppression and bone metabolism. The effect seen is small but the long-term effect in patients who take the drugs for several decades is not certain. The inhaled drugs clearly have a much better safety profile than oral steroids.

Intravenous corticosteroids. Patients with acute severe asthma should be given a high dose of oral prednisolone or a single intravenous dose of hydrocortisone (200 mg) followed usually by regular oral prednisolone. The dose can be repeated every 6 h though 40 mg prednisolone daily is usually adequate; it is important to note that steroids take several hours to work and other measures should be pursued aggressively at the same time, i.e. nebulized bronchodilators and supplementary oxygen.

Oral corticosteroids. Patients with a severe exacerbation of asthma require high doses of prednisolone, e.g. 40 mg/day by mouth after intravenous hydrocortisone. Prednisolone should be continued at this dose until asthma symptoms are controlled; this may take 5–7 days and sometimes longer. Thereafter, the steroid dose can be discontinued or tailed down until the minimal dose required to control symptoms has been reached. Other anti-asthma treatment must be reviewed to assess whether such attacks can be prevented, e.g. by increasing the dose of inhaled steroid therapy. A written asthma management plan for the patient is helpful to ensure that they know what to do as and when their asthma deteriorates.

Comment. Inhaled corticosteroids should replace long-term oral corticosteroid therapy whenever possible, as the benefits of drug treatment can be obtained with far fewer long-term adverse consequences than systemic steroid treatment.

Antimuscarinic drugs

Ipratropium bromide, oxitropium bromide
Mechanism. Parasympathetic cholinergic bronchoconstrictor tone can be blocked by atropine-like drugs. The effect of antimuscarinic drugs on airway resistance is usually less than that of the beta$_2$-agonists, being restricted to abolishing the bronchoconstrictor effect of vagal tone. Ipratropium bromide, a synthetic derivative of atropine, is very poorly absorbed and, hence, has fewer adverse effects than atropine when administered by inhalation. When given by nebulizer it can cause glaucoma, probably as a consequence of the drug escaping from round the sides of the face mask. Oxitropium bromide, a quaternary ammonium compound derived from scopolamine, has similar activity to ipratropium.

Clinical use and dose. Ipratropium is given as 40–80 μg three or four times daily by pressurized aerosol or from a nebulizer (500 μg four times daily). Oxitropium is given in a dose of 200 μg (2 puffs) two to three times daily by pressurized aerosol.

Leukotriene receptor antagonists

Montelukast, zafirlukast
Mechanism of action. Leukotriene D_4 (LTD$_4$) is a potent bronchoconstrictor in human airways. Montelukast and zafirlukast are antagonists at the LTD$_4$ receptor and produce improvements in lung function.

Clinical use and dose. Montelukast (10 mg daily) and zafirlukast (20 mg twice daily) are given orally. Their role in national guidelines remains to be defined. At present they are used as additional treatment for patients uncontrolled on inhaled steroids. Because they are orally active they may be helpful in people unable to use inhalers and may be particularly useful in asthmatics sensitive to NSAIDs.

The management of airways obstruction

Asthma

1 Patients with asthma should avoid known allergens when possible, e.g. animals. This is usually difficult and often proves to be of little therapeutic value.
2 Remember occupational causes of asthma, e.g. isocyanates and flour. These are an important and underdiagnosed cause of asthma.
3 All asthmatic patients should avoid beta$_2$-adrenoceptor antagonists (e.g. propranolol) including beta-blocking eye drops (timolol—given for glaucoma). Even selective beta$_1$-adrenoceptor antagonists such as atenolol can be dangerous. Aspirin-sensitive asthmatics (approximately 5% of all cases of asthma) should avoid all NSAIDs.

4 Drug treatment is considered in a stepwise approach (see p. 128). Patients should be on the lowest step that provides adequate asthma control, including asthma-free nights.
5 Patients are encouraged to alter their treatment themselves within limits. Serial peak expiratory flow rate measurements help patients and doctors to assess the adequacy of asthma control.
6 Short courses of oral prednisolone (see section on oral corticosteroids) should be given for exacerbations of asthma which are not severe enough to require emergency hospital admission.
7 Remember to check inhaler technique; 20–40% of patients cannot use a metered dose inhaler correctly. If there is a problem, another inhaler device should be used.
8 Patient education about asthma is essential, and this should include written instructions for most patients on what the patient should do if their asthma control deteriorates.

Comment. Asthma is a common condition affecting 10% of children and 5% of the adult-population. Recent surveys indicate that it is frequently underdiagnosed and undertreated.

Acute severe asthma (status asthmaticus)

1 Clinical assessment may be misleading. Repeated blood gas measurements and peak expiratory flow rate should be used to assess the severity of the attack and the response to treatment.
2 Initial treatment normally has three components—oxygen, beta$_2$-agonist and corticosteroids.
  (a) High concentration oxygen therapy is indicated because hypoxia is acute.
  (b) A beta$_2$-agonist is best administered from a nebulizer given with oxygen. This route is usually more effective than the intravenous route.
  (c) Intravenous hydrocortisone (200 mg) or prednisolone (40 mg) should be given to all

DRUG TREATMENT OF ASTHMA

Step 1. This is the use of an inhaled $beta_2$-receptor agonist (1 or 2 puffs a day) for patients with very mild or occasional asthma.

Step 2. For patients needing more than one or two doses of an inhaled $beta_2$-agonist per day, is the addition of inhaled prophylactic therapy, i.e. low dose of an inhaled steroid, sodium cromoglicate or nedocromil sodium. Inhaled steroids are the most effective of these prophylactic agents.

Step 3. If symptoms persist a higher dose of an inhaled steroid or a long-acting $beta_2$-agonist is given.

Step 4. If symptoms still persist, a long-acting $beta_2$-agonist, inhaled ipratropium or oral theophylline should be tried.

Step 5. Despite the use of the above drugs, a small percentage of patients with severe chronic asthma will require in addition a daily maintenance dose of oral prednisolone.

patients; followed by regular oral prednisolone.

3 If patients do not respond to this regimen consider

(a) adding intravenous aminophylline (as a loading dose, followed by an intravenous infusion) if they are not taking oral theophylline; or

(b) combine nebulized ipratropium bromide with the nebulized $beta_2$-receptor agonist.

4 Exacerbations are rarely due to bacterial infections so antibiotics should not be routinely given.

5 Serum potassium should be checked as steroids, beta-agonists and theophylline all lower serum potassium levels.

6 Sedatives, anxiolytics, opiate analgesics and hypnotics should never be given, as central depression of ventilation may worsen respiratory failure.

7 Intermittent positive pressure ventilation should be considered if the Pco_2 starts to rise, or if exhaustion or circulatory collapse occurs.

Comment. Severe asthma is a serious condition and may be life-threatening. Severity is difficult to assess clinically. Failure to respond to the patient's usual treatment is an indication for aggressive intervention with careful monitoring of ventilatory function.

Chronic airflow obstruction

1 Patients should stop smoking.

2 Patients with predominantly irreversible airflow obstruction usually obtain some symptomatic benefit from an inhaled bronchodilator ($beta_2$-receptor agonist or anticholinergic drug).

3 Oral slow-release theophylline with monitoring of plasma concentrations can be given to patients shown to respond to it. But remember drug interactions.

4 Exacerbations resulting from intercurrent chest infections should be treated with a broad spectrum antibiotic, e.g. amoxicillin.

5 If fluid retention (cor pulmonale) develops diuretic therapy is indicated. Venesection may be indicated for secondary polycythemia if the haemoglobin level is above 18 g/dl.

6 Acute ventilatory failure (high $Paco_2$ with a low pH) is a medical emergency. Patients may be drowsy and confused and should be treated as given at top of p. 129.

7 Patients with chronic ventilatory failure due to severe chronic airflow obstruction (oxygen and carbon dioxide tensions <7.5 kPa and >6 kPa; FEV_1 <1.5 l) should be considered for long-term oxygen therapy. When given as recommended in low concentration (24%) continuously for at least 15 h each day it is most conveniently administered by an oxygen concentrator.

TREATMENT OF ACUTE VENTILATORY FAILURE

- Vigorous physiotherapy.
- Antibiotics.
- Bronchodilators.
- Controlled 24% oxygen (see below).
- Doxapram, a respiratory stimulant, can be helpful though its beneficial effects are limited and it has non-specific stimulant effects producing agitation in particular.

- IPPV—patients may be helped by nasal intermittent positive pressure ventilation (IPPV) on the ward or may need to be intubated for IPPV in the Intensive Care Unit, if appropriate.

FACTORS AFFECTING CARBON DIOXIDE OXYGEN EXCHANGE

1 Alveolar ventilation.
2 Pulmonary blood flow.
3 The matching of ventilation and perfusion.

4 The quantity of haemoglobin in the blood and its affinity for oxygen.

INDICATIONS FOR HIGH OXYGEN CONCENTRATIONS

1 Pneumonia.
2 Acute pulmonary oedema.
3 Pulmonary thromboembolism.
4 Fibrosing alveolitis.
5 Acute severe asthma.

6 Acute circulatory failure.
7 Severe anaemia.
8 Cyanide and carbon monoxide poisoning.
9 Adult respiratory distress syndrome.

11.2 Oxygen

The efficiency of carbon dioxide and oxygen exchange in the alveoli of the lungs depends on many factors (see above).

Alveolar ventilation is regulated centrally by a complex mechanism that responds to arterial hypercapnia and hypoxaemia. When oxygen is given to supplement that present in inspired air it should be regarded as a drug. Oxygen is given either in high concentrations (usually around 60%) or in low (24–28%) controlled concentrations.

High oxygen concentrations

High oxygen concentrations should be given to patients with acute hypoxaemia apart from those with hypercapnia (type 2 respiratory failure). An oxygen flow rate of 4 l/min or more with an appropriate mask will supply a high concentration of oxygen in the inspired

gas. Masks with a dead space volume under 100 ml do not cause appreciable carbon dioxide rebreathing; nasal cannulae cause none at all.

Low (controlled) oxygen concentrations

Low concentration oxygen therapy is reserved for patients with an exacerbation of chronic airflow obstruction who have type 2 respiratory failure (ventilatory failure). These patients have become insensitive to CO_2 and depend on their hypoxic drive to maintain ventilation. High concentrations of oxygen remove the hypoxic drive suppressing ventilation further; further carbon dioxide accumulation can then produce narcosis and death. Low concentrations are most accurately administered by masks using the Venturi entrainment principle; these supply a calibrated inspired oxygen concentration of 24 or 28% irrespective of oxygen flow rate between 2 and 6 l/min. Nasal cannulae with an oxygen flow rate of 2 l/min will usually give around 24% oxygen, but this is slightly more dependent on the patient's ventilation.

Comment. Oxygen therapy should be individually selected on the basis of clinical features and arterial gas measurements. Subsequent clinical progress should be closely monitored. Most patients will require high oxygen concentrations. Low concentration oxygen should be used only in patients with type 2 respiratory failure and CO_2 retention.

CHAPTER 12

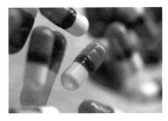

Drugs and Inflammatory Joint Disease

Aims

In inflammatory joint disease, the aims are as follows.
1 To reduce pain.
2 To reduce stiffness and improve mobility.
3 To prevent chronic deformity by minimizing the inflammation that results in synovial membrane proliferation and bone erosions.

Relevant pathophysiology

Anti-inflammatory analgesic drugs are used to relieve the painful symptoms of joint diseases, including those listed below.

The aetiology of these diseases is varied and in most cases not entirely clear, but with the exception of gout and possibly osteoarthritis there seems to be a disturbance in immune responses. In rheumatoid arthritis, for example, activated T cells and cytokine release from macrophage result in a cascade of events which result in lysosomal enzyme release which damage cartilage while prostaglandins promote synovial vasodilatation and exacerbate pain. Thus there are a number of areas where an anti-inflammatory drug might be effective:

1 Immunosuppression.
2 Inhibition of cell migration.
3 Inhibition of enzyme release.
4 Inhibition of prostaglandin synthesis.
5 Inhibition of proinflammatory cytokines.

12.1 Principles of drug treatment

The chronicity of inflammatory joint disease such as rheumatoid arthritis necessitates long-term follow-up and management within a multidimensional framework aimed at preserving the patient's quality of life. This is achieved by attempting to improve functional ability, mental and social health and vocational status and reduce disease activity. While drugs are an important part of the treatment of patients with inflammatory joint disease, other non-pharmacological aspects demand careful consideration. These include rest, exercise and psychological management.

Rest

Inflammatory arthritis is typically a disease of exacerbation and remission. During an acute

JOINT DISEASES

Rheumatoid arthritis.	Gout.
Osteoarthritis.	Reactive arthritis (including Reiter's syndrome).
Psoriatic arthritis.	Arthritis associated with systemic lupus
Ankylosing spondylitis.	erythematosus.

attack it may be necessary to recommend bedrest, with local support and splinting of the affected joints.

Exercise

After an acute attack, carefully graded exercises in the form of physiotherapy and hydrotherapy are required to ensure an early return to normal activities. Exercise also has psychological goals. It can enhance a feeling of well-being and provide active recreation. Excessive exercise, however, can be harmful.

Psychological management

Psychological factors are implicated in pain perception. The intensity of pain is in part related to patients' beliefs in their ability to cope with or control the effect of their disease. Counselling about employment is also important as the patient's self-esteem often depends on useful and purposeful work. The development of support groups for various inflammatory arthritides has an important role in improving patients' education and these 'group therapies' encourage self management behaviour and better adaptation to a chronic incurable disease, often leading to psychological, social and perhaps financial well-being.

Various physical aids are available to allow those with disabilities to maintain independence while protecting the affected joints.

The traditional treatment of inflammatory arthritis is represented by a pyramid starting with non-steroidal anti-inflammatory drugs (NSAIDs) and progressing to disease controlling antirheumatic therapies (DCARTs) such as antimalarials, sulfasalazine (sulphasalazine), gold, D-penicillamine, methotrexate, azathioprine and other immunosuppressive agents; oral corticosteroids are usually used as a 'bridge treatment' between the NSAIDs and DCARTs. Over the past decade, there has been increasing use of DCARTs, especially early in the course of the disease, together with an NSAID because the majority of patients who develop joint damage do so in the first 2 years.

12.2 Symptom modifying antirheumatic therapies (SMARTs)

Simple analgesics

Simple analgesics such as paracetamol may be used to supplement other therapy, but they are relatively ineffective when used alone in rheumatoid arthritis. They do not retard the progress of the disease and cannot provide adequate pain relief. They may be adequate in the management of some patients with osteoarthritis.

NSAIDs

NSAIDs act in a variety of ways but their prime mode of action is via the inhibition of cyclooxygenase (Cox), which exists in two isoforms—Cox-1 and Cox-2. It is now known that Cox-1 is the constitutive form and that Cox-2 is the inducible form of the enzyme. Most currently available NSAIDs primarily inhibit Cox-1 but there are now several highly selective Cox-2 inhibitors available. Although lysosome stabilizing effects and inhibition of cellular migration have also been demonstrated, the clinical significance of this observation is unclear. The available NSAIDs come in a variety of chemical classes (Table 12.1). Differences in physicochemical characteristics may influence their pharmacokinetics and give rise to differences in their efficacy and adverse effects.

Aspirin and related salicylates

Aspirin is the longest established and most traditional of the anti-inflammatory drugs and is relatively cheap. However, in the UK its role has been supplanted by other NSAIDs. Benorilate (benorylate) is a compound in which aspirin is linked with paracetamol, and diflunisal is a difluorophenyl salicylic acid derivative.

Pharmacokinetics

The pharmacokinetics of aspirin are complex and when used in relatively high doses for long periods of time plasma levels should be monitored. Aspirin is readily absorbed from the

NON-STEROIDAL ANTI-INFLAMMATORY DRUGS		
Drug	Dose* (mg)	Dosage interval (h)
Salicylates		
Aspirin	900	4†
Diflunisal	500	12
Benorilate (benorylate)	4000	12
Pyrazolones		
Phenylbutazone	100	8
Azapropazone	300	8
Indoles		
Indometacin (indomethacin)	50	8
Sulindac	200	12
Etodolac	400	8
Fenamates		
Mefenamic acid	500	8
Flufenamic acid	200	8
Propionates		
Ibuprofen	400	8
Naproxen	250	8
Ketoprofen	50	6
Phenylacetates		
Diclofenac	50	8
Oxicams		
Piroxicam	20	Daily
Tenoxicam	20	Daily
Other		
Nabumetone	1000	Daily
Cox-2 inhibitors		
Rofecoxib	25	Daily
Celecoxib	200	Daily

Table 12.1 Examples of the principal groups of non-steroidal anti-inflammatory drugs.

* These doses are near the upper limit and therapy should be commenced with approximately half doses.
† Adjust according to serum concentration.

gastrointestinal tract and is given orally. Elimination normally follows first-order kinetics, but after very large doses the enzymes that metabolize aspirin become saturated.

Adverse effects

1 Gastrointestinal effects. Nausea and vomiting follow high doses of aspirin. Dyspepsia, gastric irritation and occult or frank blood loss are common adverse effects, particularly when aspirin is associated with alcohol ingestion. Blood loss results from superficial gastric erosions or peptic ulceration. Inhibition of prostaglandin synthesis is probably responsible because some prostaglandins increase gastric mucosal blood flow and have other protective

effects. Gastrointestinal blood loss occurs even with parenteral aspirin or aspirin by suppository. However, fewer erosions and ulcers are found with these and more recent enteric coated formulations. Newer NSAIDs have been claimed to cause less gastric irritation. These comparisons have not usually been made with enteric coated aspirin. At present there appears to be a dose-dependent relationship between anti-inflammatory analgesic effect, prostaglandin synthetase inhibition and the frequency of gastric irritation. Less active analgesics cause less gastric irritation.

2 Prolonged bleeding time may result from the inhibition of thromboxane synthesis and impaired platelet aggregation (Chapter 9) or reduced hepatic clotting factor synthesis.

3 Bronchospasm, urticaria or hayfever may rarely occur in sensitive individuals and appear to result from release of immune mediators secondary to prostaglandin synthesis inhibition.

4 Tinnitus, dizziness and deafness are dose and plasma level related adverse effects. Vomiting and tachypnoea may also occur.

5 In overdose, confusion, convulsions and hyperpyrexia are seen. Forced diuresis may speed elimination of aspirin in cases of poisoning (Chapter 23).

Dose
Aspirin tablets of 300–900 mg are given 4- to 6-hourly. In rheumatoid arthritis, up to 4.5 g/day may be required in divided doses.

Phenylbutazone
This belongs to the pyrazolone class and has analgesic, antipyretic and potent anti-inflammatory actions. However, unfortunately, it can cause serious and sometimes fatal marrow depression. Its use is now limited to ankylosing spondylitis and is available on hospital prescription only.

Azapropazone
Azapropazone is chemically related to phenylbutazone but it does not apparently give rise to the marrow depression that led to the severe restrictions on the use of phenylbuta-

zone. As well as acting as a non-steroidal anti-inflammatory agent, it also has a uricosuric effect and is used in the treatment of gout. In the treatment of osteoarthritis, rheumatoid arthritis and ankylosing spondylitis, dosage in elderly patients with a creatinine clearance of less than 60 ml/min should not exceed 300 mg twice daily. If creatinine clearance in these patients is greater than 60 ml/min, dosage may be increased to 900 mg daily. In younger patients who have normal renal function, the standard dose is 1200 mg daily.

Drug interactions
Azapropazone increases plasma concentrations of phenytoin and combined use should be avoided. It also potentiates the action of warfarin and should not be used with this anticoagulant. It should be used with great caution, if at all, with any other oral anticoagulants. Combination with oral hypoglycaemics may result in excessively low blood sugars and, again, concurrent use should be avoided if possible.

Adverse effects
Skin rashes, fluid retention, angioneurotic oedema, dyspepsia and gastrointestinal bleeding have been reported.

Indometacin and related drugs
Indometacin has been used widely in inflammatory and non-inflammatory joint diseases for years. It is given by mouth or by suppository and is generally very effective. Gastric adverse effects are a predictable problem, but headache, mental confusion and dizziness may also present problems. Salt and water retention with oedema may aggravate cardiac failure or hypertension and reduce the efficacy of antihypertensive drugs. Rectal administration may be associated with pruritus, discomfort and bleeding. Sulindac is chemically related to indometacin and is a pro-drug, reversibly metabolized by the liver into its active metabolite. This might explain its relatively lower incidence of gastric side effects. Etodolac, another member of this group, is

extensively metabolized and excreted in both urine and bile. The kinetics of etodolac are unchanged in the elderly and in renal impairment.

Dose

Indometacin

Oral: 25–50 mg two to three times daily. The 75-mg sustained release capsule is designed to deliver 25 mg of the drug immediately and the remaining 50 mg over the next 8–12 h. Rectal suppository: 100 mg at night; this may be repeated in the morning.

The recommended dose for sulindac is 200 mg twice daily and that of etodolac, 200–400 mg every 6–8 h.

Propionic acid derivatives

A large number of agents from this group of drugs have been marketed. They are well absorbed orally and have fewer gastric adverse effects than plain aspirin. This has led some rheumatologists to favour them as first-line therapy. This group consists of the drugs listed below.

Note that fenbufen is a pro-drug with no direct effect on the stomach. None of these propionic acid derivatives has been shown to interact significantly with oral anticoagulants, and if a patient must also receive warfarin this group of drugs is preferable.

Phenylacetic acid derivatives

Diclofenac is very similar to the propionic acid derivatives. It may sometimes cause hepatitis.

Fenamates

The long-established mefenamic acid and flufenamic acid are effective in inflammatory joint disease, but they share the problems of salicylates to which they are chemically related. Thus, they share the gastric adverse effects but, in addition, they cause diarrhoea, a dose related phenomenon for which the basis is not clear.

Piroxicam and related oxicams

Piroxicam is an anti-inflammatory agent that is chemically unrelated to other drugs. It does, however, share their propensity to cause gastrointestinal adverse effects, and potentiates the effect of oral anticoagulants. It is contraindicated in asthmatic patients who cannot tolerate aspirin. It may cause fluid retention, a particular hazard in the elderly. Tenoxicam is reported to have less gastric toxicity.

Nabumetone

This is a non-acidic compound and a poor inhibitor of prostaglandin synthesis. After absorption, it is metabolized rapidly by the liver into an acidic metabolite that has effective anti-inflammatory actions. In comparison to other NSAIDs, nabumetone is less gastrotoxic. The recommended dose is 1000 mg daily.

Comment. This group of drugs forms the first-line and mainstay of treatment aimed at symptom modification in inflammatory joint disease. There is now a bewildering array of strongly promoted agents. Despite this, no drug has been shown to be clearly superior to the remainder in terms of symptomatic relief, disease suppression or toxic effects. It is important that a constant vigilance is maintained for side effects and drug interactions, particularly in elderly patients. It is advisable to become familiar with a few drugs and restrict use to them. Unfortunately, individual

PROPIONIC ACID DERIVATIVES	
Ibuprofen	Flurbiprofen
Fenoprofen	Fenbufen
Ketoprofen	Tiaprofenic acid
Naproxen	

response to a particular drug is unpredictable and the choice of drug is inescapably empirical.

Cox-2 inhibitors. Two inhibitors of Cox-2 celecoxib and rofecoxib have recently been released for the treatment of rheumatoid (RA) and osteo-(OA) arthritis. Rofecoxib is currently available in the UK for the treatment of OA only. These drugs are claimed to reduce gastrotoxicity because of their Cox-2 selectivity but the results of long-term trials to establish whether there is a decreased frequency of perforations, ulcers and bleeds are still awaited.

12.3 Disease controlling antirheumatic therapies (DCARTs)

DCARTs are used in the management of inflammatory arthritis to achieve disease remission and slow down the progression of joint erosions. These antirheumatic agents comprise a group of widely different chemical entities, including hydroxychloroquine, sulfasalazine, gold, D-penicillamine, immunosuppressant drugs (methotrexate, azathioprine, cyclophosphamide, chlorambucil and ciclosporin), and corticosteroids. Mechanisms of action of these drugs are not clear. There is a lag between starting therapy and observing an effect. They are indicated in the earlier years of the disease and it is conventional to begin with drugs with the least toxicity, for example, hydroxychloroquine. It is usual to continue with conventional anti-inflammatory drugs. Unlike NSAIDs, DCARTs may influence the underlying disease process. For example, in RA, decreasing erythrocyte sedimentation rate (ESR) and rheumatoid factor titre will be associated with an increase in haemoglobin in patients who respond.

Chloroquine and hydroxychloroquine

These drugs, originally developed as antimalarials, have been used to treat RA and systemic lupus erythematosus (SLE) since the 1950s and responses in RA are similar but somewhat less than those observed with other DCARTs except for auronofin (oral gold). However, they have a major advantage in their lack of life-threatening toxicity compared to other DCARTs and are increasingly being used early in the course of disease and in combination regimens with other DCARTs. The mechanisms of action of these preparations may be by lysosome stabilization and inhibition of phagocytic functions.

They are well absorbed orally, taken up by many tissues and then very slowly excreted in the urine. The most disturbing toxic effect is a retinopathy as a result of gradual accumulation of the drug in the retina and is dose dependent. Irreversible retinal damage with permanent blindness has been reported in patients taking high doses of chloroquine. Rashes and marrow toxicity are rarely seen. Neuropathies and myopathies have been reported.

Clinical use

Hydroxychloroquine in the usual doses employed is less likely to be associated with adverse effects and has largely superseded chloroquine in clinical practice. Initially 400 mg daily is given and this dose can be reduced after 6–12 months depending on response. Careful ophthalmological screening at baseline and 6 monthly is mandatory to identify retinal damage, which is reversible if diagnosed early, although this complication is rare provided dosage is kept below 6.5 mg/kg.

Sulfasalazine

Sulfasalazine is an effective and relatively safe antirheumatic drug in RA and also in ankylosing spondylitis and HLA-B27 related arthropathies such as reactive arthritis and psoriatic arthritis. It consists of 5-aminosalicylic acid joined to sulfapyridine (sulphapyridine) by an azo bond. In the gut, these two moieties are liberated following bacterial reduction of the azo bond. Sulfapyridine is thought to be the principal antirheumatic agent while 5-aminosalicylic acid is the active anti-inflammatory moiety when sulfasalazine is used in the treatment of inflammatory bowel disease.

Adverse effects

These include skin rashes, nausea, headache and occasional leucopenia, neutropenia and thrombocytopenia. The blood abnormalities usually occur early on in the course of treatment (within 6 months) and reverse if the drug is stopped. Other side effects are mentioned in Chapter 16.

Clinical use and dose

Sulfasalazine ranks with antimalarials and auronofin as the best tolerated of the DCARTs. The oral dose is initially 500 mg daily, usually increased by 500 mg at 1-week intervals to a maximum of 2–3 g daily. Blood counts are performed fortnightly in the first 12 weeks, 3-monthly thereafter.

Gold salts

These have been used for over 40 years in the management of RA. Previously, gold salts were thought to act by reducing macrophage activity. A potentially important new finding is that gold salts affect the immune system by regulating gene expression and consequent protein synthesis. One-third of patients derive considerable benefit, one-third have only a modest response and one-third have adverse effects which require interruption of treatment.

Adverse effects

1 Pruritic rashes are common and present in many forms, including mouth ulcers.
2 Proteinuria secondary to a membranous glomerulonephritis occurs in 10% of patients but it resolves on stopping gold treatment.
3 Vasodilatation with orthostatic hypotension may acutely follow drug dosing.
4 Neutropenia and thrombocytopenia may occur suddenly or develop slowly.

Recovery is usually assured provided no more gold is given. Aplastic anaemia is extremely rare now gold treatment is closely supervised with haematological checks before each dose. If it occurs, it has a high fatality rate.

Clinical use and dose

An intramuscular injection of sodium aurothiomalate is given initially as a 10-mg test dose followed by 50 mg weekly for up to 6 months or until a response or toxic effects are observed. Dose frequency may be reduced to monthly and continued for years. An oral preparation (auronofin) is also available. It is safer and less toxic than injectable gold, but is commonly associated with diarrhoea and lower abdominal discomfort. It is also much less effective than other DCARTs. Gold is indicated commonly in rheumatoid arthritis and occasionally in psoriatic arthritis.

D-penicillamine

First introduced as a copper chelating agent in Wilson's disease, D-penicillamine modifies the formation of immunoglobulin. It has a similar action to gold salts but relapse may occur with continuing therapy.

Adverse effects

These are similar to those with gold. Cross-toxicity with gold has been reported but is disputed.
1 Skin rashes are common.
2 Taste disturbance is usually transient.
3 Proteinuria, as with gold.
4 Marrow toxicity is similar to gold, consisting of thrombocytopenia and neutropenia. As these changes develop gradually, routine fortnightly haematological monitoring is essential during the initial stages of therapy.
5 Immunological effects. Up to 50% of patients develop positive antinuclear antibodies. Rarely, systemic lupus erythematosus or myasthenia gravis may be precipitated.

Clinical use and dose

D-Penicillamine is given as a 125 mg dose initially followed by monthly increments of 125 mg until response is satisfactory or a dose of 1000 mg is achieved.

Cytotoxic drugs

Methotrexate, azathioprine, cyclophosphamide and chlorambucil are increasingly widely used in inflammatory arthritis. Their use as immunosuppressants is discussed in Chapter 13. In rheumatic diseases, these drugs are indicated in resistant inflammatory joint disease, and commonly used together with corticosteroids in the presence of potentially serious extra-articular disease involvement, systemic vasculitis and connective tissue diseases such as systemic lupus erythematosus and dermatomyositis.

Methotrexate

Methotrexate is currently considered by many as the DCART of choice after NSAIDs, especially in early aggressive inflammatory joint disease. It works quickly and significant improvement in the disease is observed within the first 4–6 weeks. It shares similar side effects with other cytotoxic agents. In addition, hypersensitivity pneumonitis is seen in 2–6% of patients. This can be serious but if detected early, is reversible on stopping the drug. Liver toxicity leading to raised transaminase levels is common and reversible on reducing the dose or stopping the drug, although progressive hepatic fibrosis can occur rarely.

Clinical use and dose

Methotrexate is given by a weekly oral pulse regimen, starting at 7.5 mg, increasing by 2.5 mg every 6 weeks to 15–25 mg weekly depending on disease response. Lower doses should be used in the frail elderly or if there is significant renal impairment. Folic acid 5 mg given 3 days after each dose may reduce the incidence of toxicity, in particular oral ulceration. Cotrimoxazole should be avoided in patients taking methotrexate.

Azathioprine, cyclophosphamide and chlorambucil

A number of controlled trials have shown these drugs to be effective in inflammatory arthritis. Azathioprine is a pro-drug that is metabolized to its active form, 6-mercaptopurine. The starting dose is usually 100 mg/day orally, with increments of 25 mg every 3 months depending on disease response, or

until a maximum recommended dose of 2.5 mg/kg per day (about 175 mg) has been reached. Cyclophosphamide is usually reserved for more life-threatening conditions such as systemic vasculitis and SLE because of its toxicity. It can be given orally or intravenously, and either as regular daily doses or as weekly/monthly pulses. One of the most serious complications of cyclophosphamide therapy is haemorrhagic cystitis related to its metabolite, acrolein. The coadministration of mesna (mercaptoethane sulphonate) reduces acrolein urotoxicity (Chapter 13, Section 13.1).

Chlorambucil has been used as an alternative to cyclophosphamide, but most clinicians regard it as an inferior drug for the majority of rheumatic conditions. In addition, chlorambucil appears to be associated with a higher incidence of leukaemia and other malignancies. These drugs are discussed in greater depth in Chapter 13.

Combination therapy

Rheumatologists are now using selected DCARTs in combination with clinical evidence of a synergistic effect. Two combinations have been shown to be efficacious: (i) ciclosporin with methotrexate, and (ii) methotrexate with sulfasalazine and hydroxychloroquine. The incidence of side effects is not increased when these drugs are used in combination.

Immunotherapy

Ciclosporin

Ciclosporin is effective in improving inflammatory joint disease but is limited by its potential nephrotoxicity. New onset hypertension is a common side effect seen in about a third of rheumatoid and psoriatic patients, possibly requiring antihypertensive therapy.

Further details are given in Chapter 13.

Corticosteroids

Corticosteroids have potent immunosuppressant activity (Chapter 13) and a range of other effects (Chapter 14). They are the most powerful anti-inflammatory drugs available.

In rheumatoid arthritis there is little evidence that high doses are more effective than low doses. For chronic use, not more than 7.5 mg prednisolone per day (or on alternate days) or the equivalent can be given without the development of serious adverse effects (Chapter 14, Section 14.1). Steroids are particularly useful in SLE and are essential in polymyalgia rheumatica and giant cell arteritis.

Where one or two joints are particularly troublesome in an otherwise reasonably controlled patient, an intra-articular injection of corticosteroid is widely used.

Leflunomide
Leflunomide is a pyrimidine synthesis inhibitor with a plasma half-life of 2 weeks and has recently been released for the treatment of RA. It has a rapid onset of action within 4–6 weeks and is given as a loading dose of 100 mg for 3 days followed by 20 mg daily. Trials published to date show that it is equipotent with methotrexate and is superior to sulfasalazine. Important side effects are hepatotoxicity and immunosuppression.

Anti-cytokine therapy
Two monoclonal antibodies Etanercept and Infliximab are now available for the treatment of RA and juvenile idiopathic arthritis (JIA). They both block the actions of the pro-inflammatory cytokine tumour necrosis factor alpha (TNFα) and have been shown to be of clinical benefit and to delay joint damage as measured by X-ray. Etanercept is given by twice weekly subcutaneous injections and Infliximab by one or two monthly intravenous infusions. They should be avoided in patients with a past history of serious infections.

Comment. Inflammatory joint disease remains an important and difficult therapeutic challenge. The chronicity of the disease, its variable expression, with remissions and exacerbations, and its implications for the patient's life must all be considered. Therapeutic decisions must be tailored to individual patients at any particular time. The most log-ical approach to choosing a DCART is to work through the drugs available, continuously weighing the risk of serious toxicity against their benefits in terms of pain relief and minimization of joint destruction and deformity, moving from one to the next only when there is convincing evidence of therapeutic failure.

12.4 Drugs used in gout

It is important to distinguish the following.
1 Management of the acute attack.
2 Long-term management.

Management of the acute attack
An acute attack of gout is extremely painful and effective anti-inflammatory drugs should be given at once. The drugs used are:
1 NSAIDs such as indometacin, naproxen, diclofenac, piroxicam in large doses for 24–48 h.
2 Colchicine: this drug can still be used in acute gout (orally or intravenously) or in the early months of treatment with allopurinol. Adverse effects—nausea, vomiting, abdominal pain and diarrhoea—can be less common with low-dose regimens.

Long-term management
As the underlying mechanism in gout involves excess production of uric acid and/or reduced renal excretion of urate, long-term management aims at reducing uric acid in the body in two ways:
1 Inhibition of uric acid formation from purines by xanthine oxidase inhibition.
2 Promotion of urate excretion in the urine.

Xanthine oxidase inhibition

Allopurinol

Pharmacokinetics
Allopurinol is well absorbed from the gastrointestinal tract and is rapidly cleared from the plasma with a half-life of 2–3 h. It is converted to alloxanthine and this metabolite in turn

inhibits the metabolism of the parent drug. Alloxanthine is also a xanthine oxidase inhibitor.

Adverse effects
These are not common. Hypersensitivity reactions, which subside on withdrawing the drug, consist of a skin rash accompanied by fever, malaise and muscle pain. Rarely, leukopenia or leukocytosis with eosinophilia occur.

Drug interactions
Drugs depending on xanthine oxidase for their metabolic conversion should be given with caution in association with allopurinol. This applies to 6-mercaptopurine and azathioprine. Inhibition of warfarin metabolism may also occur; anticoagulant control should be monitored closely in circumstances such as these.

Clinical use and dose
Allopurinol must not be used in an acute attack of gout because this will be prolonged. Initially, 100 mg allopurinol is given daily as a single dose increasing to about 300 mg daily depending on serum uric acid levels. The aim is to keep serum uric acid levels in the bottom half of the normal range. Colchicine or indometacin may be given concurrently over the first 2 months to prevent acute gout.

Allopurinol should be considered in:
1 Urate overproduction, primary or secondary.
2 Acute uric acid nephropathy (tumour lysis syndrome).
3 Nephrolithiasis of any type.
4 Renal impairment (dose 100 mg/day per 30 ml/min glomerular filtration rate).
5 24 h urinary uric acid >0.42 g.
6 Intolerance or allergy to uricosuric agents.
7 Chronic tophaceous gout.

Uricosuric drugs

Probenecid
Probenecid inhibits the transport of organic acids across lipid membranes including the renal tubule. Whereas this leads to an increase in the plasma concentration of a number of acidic drugs, the uric acid concentration falls because its reabsorption from tubular fluid is inhibited.

Pharmacokinetics. Probenecid is well absorbed from the gastrointestinal tract and peak concentrations are achieved in 2–4 h. Metabolism and renal excretion result in a half-life of about 9 h; a large proportion of the parent drug is actively secreted by the proximal tubules.

Adverse effects. About 25% of patients experience dyspepsia and this limits its use in peptic ulceration. Hypersensitivity reactions occur occasionally as skin rashes. Drug-induced nephrotic syndrome has been reported.

Drug interactions. The uricosuric effect of probenecid may be inhibited by large doses of salicylates. Aspirin should therefore be avoided in patients receiving probenecid.

Dose. A 250-mg dose of probenecid is given twice daily initially, increasing to a maximum of 2 g daily over 2–3 weeks, depending on serum uric acid concentrations.

Sulfinpyrazone (Sulphinpyrazone)
Sulfinpyrazone inhibits the tubular reabsorption of uric acid when given in sufficient dose. Like probenecid, it reduces the renal tubular secretion of many other organic acids.

Pharmacokinetics. Sulfinpyrazone is well absorbed from the gastrointestinal tract. It is strongly bound (98–99%) to plasma albumin; 90% is excreted unchanged in the urine; 10% is metabolized to the N-p-hydroxyphenyl metabolite, itself a potent uricosuric.

Adverse effects. Ten to fifteen percent of patients receiving sulfinpyrazone develop gastrointestinal symptoms; as a rule it should be avoided in patients with a history of peptic ulceration. Rarely, it causes skin rashes and fever.

Drug interactions. As with probenecid, salicylates inhibit the uricosuric effect of sulfinpyrazone and more than occasional doses of aspirin should be avoided. Decreased excretion of oral hypoglycaemic agents may lead to hypoglycaemia and sulfinpyrazone may enhance the effect of warfarin.

Dose. A 100–200 mg dose of sulfinpyrazone is given daily, increasing over 2–3 weeks to about 600–800 mg daily, depending on serum uric acid concentrations.

Azapropazone

Azapropazone has a uricosuric effect and is used in acute attacks of gout and in long-term prophylaxis.

Dose. During the first 24 h of an acute attack, 2400 mg azapropazone is given in divided doses, then 1300 mg daily until acute symptoms subside followed by 1200 mg daily until symptoms have disappeared. In chronic gout, 600 mg twice daily are given unless the patient is elderly (over 65 years of age; see above).

Comment. The management of gout aims to reduce uric acid formation prophylactically by xanthine oxidase inhibition with allopurinol and thus prevent arthritis and renal damage. If acute arthritis occurs it should be managed symptomatically with high doses of NSAIDs and allopurinol therapy begun after symptoms subside. The uricosuric drugs are now used less commonly and indicated mainly in patients who are intolerant to allopurinol. They are ineffective in patients with poor renal function and contraindicated in renal failure and in patients with uric acid stones or a history of uric acid stones.

CHAPTER 13

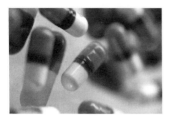

Cytotoxic Drugs and Immunopharmacology

Drugs that modify the growth of cells are used in the treatment of cancer, in the control of immune responses after organ transplantation and in the management of autoimmune diseases.

13.1 Cytotoxic drugs and cancer chemotherapy

Aims
Drug therapy is used in patients with cancer to:
1 Eradicate the disease.
2 Induce a remission.
3 Control symptoms.

In most situations the drugs used to treat cancer are cytotoxic agents. However, some cancers (breast and prostate cancer) can be treated with hormonal agents.

Relevant pathophysiology
Chemotherapy, or the use of drugs in the management of cancer, was introduced in the 1890s with non-specific cell poisons. More specific agents became available with the discovery in the 1940s of nitrogen mustard, an alkylating agent, and methotrexate, an antimetabolite. There are now 30–40 drugs used in the management of a variety of different forms of cancer.

Treatment was initially restricted to patients with leukaemia and lymphomas, but drugs are now used in patients with solid tumours, in

adults and in children. Considerable progress has been made towards curative treatment of some of the childhood cancers and rarer solid tumours. Nevertheless, there are still many forms of cancer that are difficult to treat with chemotherapy. In order to obtain maximum therapeutic benefit it is important to clearly define the aims of therapy at the outset. This often dictates the choice and duration of therapy and potential adverse effects that may be acceptable to patients.

Chemotherapy represents only one component of cancer management. Surgery and radiotherapy are of considerable value, especially in treating localized tumours. Chemotherapy has the potential to treat more widespread disease. Increasing use is made of 'combined modality therapy', or the integration of several different approaches to cancer treatment.

Cytotoxic drugs are used:
1 As potentially curative therapy either before (neoadjuvant) or after (adjuvant) surgery or radiotherapy for the primary tumour. The aim is to eradicate micrometastatic disease. Such treatment significantly prolongs survival for certain groups of women with early breast cancer (Table 13.1).
2 In the treatment of metastatic disease. In rare cases this may be curative; in others, life may be significantly prolonged. Commonly, disease control rather than cure is the aim, and symptomatic benefit and achievement of

CHEMOTHERAPY—PRIMARY TUMOURS

Breast	Colon	Osteogenic and Ewing's sarcoma	Bladder, cervix, head and neck
Premenopausal axillary nodes positive for cancer	Stage Duke's C	Preoperative	Locally advanced disease (trial only)

Table 13.1 Chemotherapy as part of combined modality treatment of primary tumours.

CHEMOTHERAPY—METASTASES

Curative	Prolongs survival	Useful palliation	Benefit unlikely
Testis	Ovary	Breast	Pancreas
Lymphoma	Small cell lung	Bladder, cervix	Renal
Acute leukaemia	Chronic leukaemia	Head and neck	Brain
Certain childhood cancers	Myeloma	(Colon, gastric)* (Non-small cell lung)	
Choriocarcinoma			

* Lower overall prospect of response.

Table 13.2 Chemotherapy for the management of metastatic cancer.

improved quality of life become important considerations (Table 13.2).

Principles of drug treatment

Although cytotoxics can be given as single agents it is more common to use a combination of two to six drugs (see below). With a few important exceptions, combinations of drugs are more effective than single agents.

Most drug combinations have been developed empirically. As the number of drugs used increases, so does the potential for toxicity.

Myelosuppression is the commonest dose limiting toxicity of most cytotoxic agents. When chemotherapy is given at standard doses, treatment is usually given intermittently as pulses administered at 3- to 4-weekly intervals, allowing time for marrow recovery. The coadministration of haemapoietic growth factors (granulocyte colony-stimulating factor (G-CSF) and granulocyte–macrophage colony-stimulating factor (GM-CSF)) allows drugs to be given at significantly higher doses, or more frequently, by reducing the risk of significant neutropenia. However, other toxicities become dose limiting and the place of growth factors in routine treatment has not yet been defined.

Much higher doses of drugs such as cyclophosphamide, melphalan, etoposide and

DRUG COMBINATIONS

This is achieved by combining drugs:
1 That are active when used alone.
2 With different mechanisms of action.
3 That have different toxicities.
4 At doses close to their maximum tolerated levels.

carboplatin have been used with the aim of eliminating the tumour completely. These high-dose chemotherapy regimens are used in association with bone marrow transplantation or peripheral blood stem cell transfusion. Such treatment is used in the management of leukaemias and lymphomas and experimentally in some other solid tumours. When giving high-dose chemotherapy it is essential that supportive measures, such as platelet transfusions, are available to deal with marrow failure, infection and bleeding.

Measurement of plasma concentrations (therapeutic drug monitoring) allows administration of agents with minimal toxicity of doses that would otherwise be lethal, e.g. methotrexate. Methotrexate is a potent but reversible inhibitor of the enzyme dihydrofolate reductase, a key enzyme for DNA synthesis. Enzyme inhibition and the toxic effects of methotrexate can be reversed by the subsequent administration of folinic acid. It is possible to give methotrexate at doses of 100–1000 times those used previously, measure plasma methotrexate levels and calculate the amount of folinic acid required for 'rescue'. This method of treatment may be of considerable therapeutic value in some situations.

In addition to oral or intravenous dosing, cytotoxics are occasionally given:

1 Intrathecally, to achieve effective concentration in the cerebrospinal fluid (CSF), particularly for drugs that do not readily cross the blood–brain barrier.

2 Intra-arterially into a limb, the head and neck or the liver.

3 Intraperitoneally or intrapleurally to increase the local concentration of drug, particularly where rapidly accumulating ascites or pleural effusions present clinical problems.

4 Topically onto lesions of the skin, vagina or buccal mucosa.

If a drug requires metabolic activation by the liver, e.g. cyclophosphamide or azathioprine, it is of little value to administer it locally, intraperitoneally or intrathecally.

Drugs used in cancer chemotherapy

Most cytotoxic drugs have a narrow therapeutic index; they are active only at doses close to those causing significant toxicity. A common attempt to tailor treatment to the individual patient adjusts doses for surface area (mg/m^2).

Cytotoxic drugs

The majority of cytotoxic drugs act by interfering with the synthesis and replication of DNA. The molecular basis of action of some widely used agents is shown in Fig. 13.1. Currently, much research is directed at identifying novel targets for cancer treatment such as intracellular signalling pathways.

Mechanisms

Cytotoxic drugs can be classified as follows.

1 Alkylating agents, including drugs such as nitrogen mustard, cyclophosphamide, chlorambucil and melphalan. These are highly reactive molecules when activated and bind irreversibly to macromolecules in the cell, notably DNA, RNA and proteins.

2 Antimetabolites, which are closely related analogues of the normal components of intermediary metabolism or DNA synthesis. Methotrexate inhibits folic acid metabolism and the nucleotides (5-fluorouracil, cytosine arabinoside, 6-mercaptopurine) inhibit DNA synthesis.

3 Natural products. A wide range of drugs has been developed from plants, bacteria, yeasts and fungi. Some act to inhibit cell division, by preventing spindle formation. Others inhibit DNA synthesis through intercalation into the helix or binding to nuclear topoisomerase I or II, enzymes that control conformational changes in DNA. They include:

(a) Mitosis inhibitors: the vinca alkaloids (vincristine, vinblastine and vindesine) disrupt the mitotic spindle. The taxanes (taxol and taxotere) inhibit mitosis by stabilizing the spindle.

(b) Anthracyclines, such as doxorubicin, epirubicin and daunorubicin intercalate into DNA and also form highly reactive

CYTOTOXIC DRUG MECHANISM

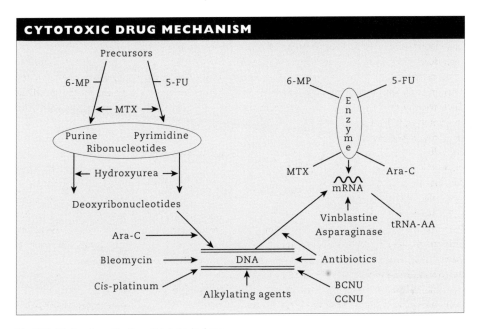

Fig. 13.1 Mechanism of action of cytotoxic drugs.

free radicals. However, their principal action appears to be as inhibitors of the enzyme topoisomerase II.

(c) Podophyllotoxins: etoposide and teniposide bind to tubulin but their major action is to inhibit topoisomerase II.

(d) Bleomycin: binds to DNA and may also form free radicals.

(e) Actinomycin D: binds to DNA to inhibit RNA transcription.

4 Others: several drugs have been identified, often by random synthesis and screening, whose mechanism of action is not fully established but are thought to interact with DNA synthesis or replication. They include the nitrosoureas, hydroxycarbamide (hydroxyurea), dacarbazine, procarbazine, cisplatin and its analogue carboplatin. Inhibitors of the enzyme topoisomerase I, such as topotecan, are a promising new group of drugs that are under development.

5 Steroid hormones: these are widely used in cancer management. They are particularly cytotoxic against lymphoid tumours but are

also used in the treatment of symptoms such as anorexia and vomiting. The drug most commonly used is prednisolone.

For clinical purposes, cytotoxic drugs are generally grouped according to their mechanism of action as above, but they may also be classified according to their effect on the cell cycle, as demonstrated in tissue culture. Actively dividing cells pass through several phases. Mitosis is followed by a gap or delay (G1), then a synthetic phase (S), a second gap (G2) and mitosis again. Cells may cycle continuously or enter a quiescent phase. Some drugs act at all phases of the cell cycle, others exert effects specifically at certain of these phases.

Class I drugs are non-specific and act on cells whether or not they are actively dividing, e.g. nitrogen mustard. Class II drugs act only at specific phases of the cell cycle, e.g. vincristine, methotrexate, cystosine arabinoside. Class III drugs act on cells in division and at all phases of the cycle, e.g. cyclophosphamide, actinomycin D and the nitrosoureas.

Pharmacokinetics

Pharmacokinetic aspects of cytotoxic drugs may present drug-specific or general problems. Some cytotoxic drugs are excreted unchanged by the kidney (cisplatin, carboplatin and methotrexate). When using these drugs in patients with renal impairment, dose modification is important. With carboplatin, dose-limiting thrombocytopenia is more common in patients with renal impairment and related to an increase in the area under the concentration-time curve (AUC). As total body clearance of carboplatin is directly correlated with glomerular filtration rate (GFR), it is possible to relate drug exposure (AUC) to dose and GFR using the equation:

$$AUC = dose/GFR \qquad \text{(Eqn. 13.1)}$$

This equation, rearranged as:

$$dose = \text{'target' } AUC \times GFR \qquad \text{(Eqn. 13.2)}$$

is widely used to calculate carboplatin dose.

Other drugs such as doxorubicin and vincristine are predominantly excreted via the biliary tract. In the presence of hepatic impairment, dose reduction of these drugs is recommended. By contrast, some drugs are metabolized to their active forms. Cyclophosphamide is converted to an active metabolite in the liver. Similarly, inactive azathioprine is converted to the antimetabolite 6-mercaptopurine in the liver. There is a theoretical risk that efficacy of these drugs may be impaired in patients with impaired liver function.

There are other clinical pharmacokinetic problems with cytotoxic drugs:

1 The problem of the 'third space'. Many patients with cancer have pleural effusions or ascites. Administration of a cytotoxic drug to such a patient may result in the sequestration of the drug into this compartment with slow release back into the circulation. This may aggravate toxicity.

2 Sanctuary sites. For many purposes, cancer can be considered to be a systemic disease. It is essential therefore that the administered drug reaches all parts of the body. Some drugs do not cross the blood–brain barrier and may not therefore act on tumour cells in the brain. Another important sanctuary site appears to be the testes: lymphomas in particular may relapse there. Clinically, perhaps the most important sanctuary site is the large tumour with a poor blood supply into which the drug cannot adequately penetrate.

Adverse effects

Reactions to chemotherapy are secondary to cell death both in the tumour and in other rapidly dividing cells of bone marrow, gastrointestinal tract, germinal epithelium, etc. These can be divided into:

1 General adverse reactions to chemotherapy.

2 Specific adverse reactions to individual agents.

General adverse reactions

1 Nausea and vomiting may be severe with many drugs, especially cisplatin, and is related to the direct actions of cytotoxic drugs on the chemoreceptor trigger zone (Chapter 16, Section 16.4). Anticipatory vomiting can be a major problem in patients after repeated treatments. The selective $5HT_3$ receptor antagonists are highly effective in preventing acute emesis. They have largely replaced high dose metoclopramide, which was reasonably effective but associated with dystonic reactions, as a result of unwanted dopamine antagonism, particularly in young patients.

2 Alopecia is a common adverse effect of some, but not all, cytotoxic drugs. Hair regrows after the course of chemotherapy has been completed.

3 Hyperuricaemia, with precipitation of clinical gout or renal failure may complicate treatment of highly chemosensitive tumours when there is rapid tumour lysis, e.g. leukaemias and lymphomas. Allopurinol, the xanthine oxidase inhibitor, may be used to prevent gout (Chapter 12) but care should be taken when azathioprine or mercaptopurine are given at the same time (see drug interactions below).

4 Mucositis can occur with some drugs, causing ulceration in the mouth. When there is coexistent neutropenia there is increased risk of opportunistic infections.

5 Bone marrow depression. The bone marrow is particularly sensitive to many cytotoxic drugs (Chapter 17, Section 17.2). Neutropenia is common and opportunistic infections occur as a result of impaired humoral and cell-mediated responses. Unusual infection with fungi and protozoa, in addition to more common pathogenic bacteria and viruses, may occur. Thrombocytopenia may result in an increased risk of haemorrhage.

Specific adverse reactions

Specific effects of some of the more widely used cytotoxic drugs are shown in Table 13.3. Some have a specific pharmacological basis. Haemorrhagic cystitis with cyclophosphamide is a consequence of urinary excretion of the irritant metabolites, e.g. acrolein. This can be prevented by maintaining a high fluid output or giving the drug mesna (mercaptoethone sulphonate) that conjugates these metabolites, to promote safe excretion.

Drug interactions

Drug interactions may occur between cytotoxics but more important are interactions with non-cytotoxic agents.

Methotrexate and salicylates

As methotrexate is highly protein bound it is readily displaced from the binding site by aspirin and other salicylates. This may increase the risk of adverse effects of methotrexate. Other acidic drugs which are highly protein bound may show similar effects.

6-Mercaptopurine and allopurinol

These two drugs are frequently used together. Allopurinol is a competitive inhibitor of xanthine oxidase (Chapter 12, Section 12.4) and also inhibits the breakdown of 6-mercaptopurine. The dose of 6-mercaptopurine must be halved at least or toxicity ensues. Azathioprine, which is metabolized to 6-mercaptopurine, should also be given in lower doses if used with allopurinol.

Procarbazine and alcohol

Hot flushing may occur and patients should be warned of this before treatment. Procarbazine

EFFECTS OF CYTOTOXIC DRUGS

Drug	Mechanism	Specific adverse effects	Indications
Cyclophosphamide	Alkylating agent	Haematuria, cystitis	Haematological malignancy, solid tumour
Doxorobicin	Antibiotic	Alopecia, cardiac failure, local tissue necrosis	Wide range of haematological and solid tumours
Cisplatin	Interacts with DNA	Neurotoxicity Nephrotoxicity Vomiting	Wide range of solid tumours, including lung, ovarian and testicular carcinoma
Bleomycin	Topoisomerase II inhibition	Pulmonary fibrosis, skin rashes	Lymphomas, testicular teratoma, squamous cell carcinoma
Methotrexate	Antimetabolite	Mucositis	Leukaemia

Table 13.3 Effects of cytotoxic drugs.

is a monoamine oxidase inhibitor and tyramine-containing foods should be avoided (Chapter 19, Section 19.3).

Comment. Cytotoxic drugs should be given by physicians who have experience and facilities for managing malignant disease and the problems associated with chemotherapy. Haemorrhage and opportunistic infections secondary to marrow and immune suppression may shorten life rather than prolong it if they are not aggressively managed.

Hormones and antihormones

Oestrogens and progestogens

Surgical removal of endocrine organs, such as the ovaries, testes, adrenals and pituitary gland, has been used for many years in the treatment of breast and prostatic cancer. Treatment with hormones and antihormones aims to achieve the same effect of changing the hormonal environment. Hormonal effects are mediated by receptors on the cell surface or within the cell. These receptors, notably oestrogen receptors, can be identified within tumours and allow a prediction of the response to endocrine manipulation in breast cancer. Patients whose breast cancer contains oestrogen receptors are more likely to respond to anti-oestrogen therapy than those without oestrogen receptors. The synthetic anti-oestrogen, tamoxifen, is now widely used both as adjuvant treatment and in advanced breast cancer and has very few adverse effects. Second-line therapy includes aminoglutethimide, a non-specific inhibitor of adrenal steroid synthesis. More specific inhibitors of the aromatase enzyme, that are better tolerated than aminoglutethimide, are entering clinical use. Progestogens, such as medroxyprogesterone acetate, are also active in breast cancer.

In cancer of the prostate, treatment aimed at reducing testosterone levels may be very effective. This includes orchidectomy and the use of diethylstilbestrol (stilboestrol), but oestrogens may have cardiovascular side effects. An alternative is the use of synthetic luteinizing hormone releasing hormone (LHRH) analogues that inhibit testosterone release and have an effect equivalent to that of orchidectomy.

Glucocorticoids

The corticosteroids cortisol, hydrocortisone and prednisolone are used in drug combinations in the management of leukaemia and lymphomas. Dexamethasone is used in the management of raised intracranial pressure associated with intracerebral primary or secondary tumours, and is also a useful antiemetic agent, often in combination with other agents.

Steroids can also be useful to stimulate appetite in patients with advanced cancer. Progestogens can also be used in this way and to improve the quality of life.

13.2 Immunopharmacology

Relevant pathophysiology

The immune system is a host defence network of different cell types and molecules that protect against invasion by pathogens. Immune responses occur at different levels of specificity.

Innate or natural immunity

Innate immunity is mediated by phagocytic cells (neutrophils, macrophages), eosinophils and natural killer cells together with complement proteins. It is a rapid response system. It does not rely on specific recognition of organisms and has no 'memory' of previous infecting agents. Micro-organisms are recognized through the 'toll-like' receptor system. Production of cytokines, such as interleukin (IL)-12 and IL-18, during innate responses is critical to efficient generation of subsequent acquired immunity.

Acquired or adaptive immunity

Acquired immunity is mediated by lymphocytes and their secreted products, notably cytokines and antibodies. Acquired immunity is highly specific and re-exposure to a previously encountered antigen produces a greatly augmented and more efficient immune response. T lymphocytes are of primary importance in regulating acquired immune responses. CD4$^+$ T-helper (Th) cells initiate and define the nature of the subsequent response and as such represent important therapeutic targets. T cells possess highly specific cell-surface receptors that recognize foreign proteins only after they have been broken into peptide antigens and attached to major histocompatibility complex (MHC) molecules expressed on the surface of specialized antigen-presenting cells, e.g. dendritic cells. Th cells may be functionally subdivided into two distinct populations—Th1 cells produce interferon-γ and thereby promote a *cell-mediated immune response*. Th2 cells produce IL-4 and IL-5 and promote B cell maturation into plasma cells, leading to antibody formation and thus *humoral responses*. CD8$^+$ T cells function predominantly as cytotoxic effector cells able, for example, to kill virus-infected cells or tumours. A critical role of the immune system is to distinguish self proteins from those belonging to invading micro-organisms—this process is called *tolerance*. There are a variety of immunological diseases in which the immune system inflicts damage on normal cells and body tissues, representing a 'breach' of tolerance.

Immune responses have historically been classified according to the principal effector mechanism responsible.

Type I: Immediate hypersensitivity
Antigen binds to antibody (IgE) attached to mast cells or basophils and provokes release of inflammatory mediators such as vasoactive amines, proteases and prostaglandins. This results in increased vascular permeability, smooth muscle contraction and local inflammation. The clinical manifestations, especially in atopic individuals are:
1 Allergic asthma.
2 Hayfever.
3 Eczema.
   In extreme cases anaphylactic shock may result.

Type II: Antibody-mediated hypersensitivity
Autoreactive or crossreactive antibodies (IgG and IgM) bind to antigens found on cells or tissues and cause damage by activating complement or recruiting inflammatory cells. This may result in tissue or organ specific autoimmune diseases (e.g. pernicious anaemia, autoimmune haemolytic anaemia or thrombocytopenic purpura and glomerulonephritis). Alternatively, antibodies directed against cell-surface receptors may either stimulate or block target cell function (e.g. anti-TSH receptor antibodies in Graves disease and anti-acetylcholine receptor antibodies in myasthenia gravis). Antibody-mediated cytotoxicity is also responsible for hyper-acute (immediate) organ allograft rejection in sensitized renal transplant recipients who have preformed antidonor antibodies.

Type III: Immune complex-mediated hypersensitivity
Circulating antibody–antigen complexes are deposited in tissues where they produce local activation of complement and leucocytes. Immune complex deposition occurs mainly in the glomeruli resulting in nephritis but other tissues may also be affected. Administration of large amounts of protein antigen intravenously may result in serum sickness.

Type IV: Cell-mediated hypersensitivity
CD4$^+$ effector T cells release proinflammatory cytokines (particularly interferon-γ, i.e. Th1 type) and recruit activated macrophages to produce a delayed-type hypersensitivity (DTH) reaction. DTH is responsible for contact sensitivity after topical exposure to chemicals. T-effector cells are suspected of causing several autoimmune diseases (e.g. insulin-dependent diabetes mellitus, multiple sclerosis and rheumatoid arthritis). This form of hypersensitivity is responsible for causing acute rejection of organ allografts and is also likely to be important in organ specific autoimmunity.

Drugs that suppress immune responses

Excess immune activity has clinical importance in several areas, particularly transplantation and autoimmune disease (Table 13.4). Most immunosuppressive drugs currently in use are relatively non-specific and therefore increase the risk of both opportunistic and conventional infections. They may also increase the risk of lymphoproliferative disorders and of solid tumours. In addition to the problem of non-specific immunosuppression, individual agents have drug-specific side effects.

It is common practice after organ transplantation to use combinations of agents to maintain adequate overall immunosuppression and minimize drug-specific complications. Regimens employed differ in the UK and in the USA. In UK, a triple approach consisting of ciclosporin, azathioprine and prednisolone is preferred, whereas in the USA, inductive antibody administration may be added to ciclosporin, azathioprine and prednisolone to achieve T-cell depletion. Mycophenolate and tacrolimus may be used to substitute azathioprine or ciclosporin respectively. Tacrolimus may also be preferred after liver transplant.

Recently, combination drug approaches have been developed to treat autoimmune diseases, particularly rheumatoid arthritis. In the latter a combination of sulfasalazine, methotrexate and hydroxychloroquine, with or without low-dose prednisolone, has been shown to be beneficial in resistant disease.

Antimetabolites

Antimetabolites and alkylating agents are used as immunosuppressives but given at lower doses than when used in cancer chemotherapy. They inhibit actively dividing cells and at low doses are relatively selective for activated lymphocytes.

Azathioprine

This prodrug is metabolized in the liver to 6-mercaptopurine, a purine nucleotide analogue, which inhibits DNA and RNA synthesis. It is widely used in organ transplantation and in several autoimmune diseases. Side effects include leucopenia and thrombocytopenia.

Mycophenolate mofetil

This new drug appears more selective than azathioprine and may find a use in organ transplantation. It inhibits inosine monophosphate dehydrogenase, the rate-limiting enzyme for the *de novo* pathway of purine synthesis. Because lymphocytes have no salvage pathway for purine synthesis they are selectively inhibited.

IMMUNOSUPPRESSIVE DRUGS	
Induction/maintenance of immunosuppression	Treatment of rejection
Ciclosporin (cyclosporin) monotherapy *or*	High-dose prednisolone *or*
Ciclosporin + prednisolone *or*	Polyclonal/monoclonal antibody
Ciclosporin + prednisolone + azathioprine (triple therapy) *or*	
Polyclonal/monoclonal antibody + ciclosporin + prednisolone + azathioprine (quadruple therapy)	

Table 13.4 Immunosuppressive drugs used to prevent graft rejection.

Methotrexate

Methotrexate is used as prophylaxis for graft vs. host disease following bone marrow transplantation and increasingly, as a disease modifying antirheumatic drug for rheumatoid arthritis, psoriasis and psoriatic arthritis. It is not used directly in organ transplantation.

Mizoribine and brequinar sodium

These two new antimetabolites may prove useful in preventing transplant rejection, but are not currently widely used.

Alkylating agents

Cyclophosphamide and chlorambucil

These drugs are used to treat some types of glomerulonephritis, e.g. complicating systemic lupus erythematosis or systemic vasculitis, and occasionally other types of autoimmune disease but are not used in organ transplantation.

T-cell targeting agents

Ciclosporin

Mechanism. Ciclosporin acts predominantly on T-helper cells. It selectively impairs production of cytokines, particularly IL-2 and inhibits IL-2 receptor expression, thereby blocking T-cell growth. This prevents T-cell activation and stops the generation of the cell-mediated immune responses responsible for allograft rejection, or tissue damage in autoimmune diseases.

Pharmacokinetics. Ciclosporin is poorly absorbed following oral administration but this problem has been reduced by a new microemulsion formulation. It is a highly lipophilic compound and is distributed widely in body tissues. It is metabolized in the liver and small bowel by the cytochrome P-450 system and then excreted in the bile. Because of variation between individuals in ciclosporin pharmacokinetics, measurement of whole blood ciclosporin levels is used as a guide to dose requirements.

Side effects. Nephrotoxicity is the major drug specific side effect of ciclosporin. Other side effects include hypertension, convulsions, mild elevation of hepatic transaminases, anorexia, nausea, vomiting, hypertrichosis, gingival hyperplasia, tremor and paraesthesia. Toxicity is usually managed by lowering the dose.

Drug interactions. A large number of drug interactions with ciclosporin have been reported. There are two major types:
1 Drugs which are nephrotoxic themselves. Examples are the aminoglycosides and amphotericin, which may enhance the nephrotoxicity of ciclosporin.
2 Drugs which alter the pharmacokinetics of ciclosporin.

Cytochrome P-450 inhibitors such as erythromycin and ketoconazole lead to increased ciclosporin blood levels. Conversely, drugs which induce cytochrome P-450 such as carbamazepine, phenytoin and rifampicin reduce ciclosporin blood levels

Clinical use and dose. The introduction of ciclosporin revolutionized organ transplantation allowing greater than 80% 1-year graft survival for kidney, heart and liver transplantation. Nearly all immunosuppressive protocols for organ transplantation include ciclosporin although treatment regimens vary widely between centres (Table 13.4).

The daily oral dose in the immediate post-transplant period is usually 10–15 mg/kg and this is gradually reduced to a maintenance dose of 3–5 mg/kg, guided by ciclosporin blood levels and clinical assessment. Ciclosporin is used in the prophylaxis and treatment of graft vs. host disease after bone marrow transplantation and increasingly in some types of autoimmune disease. It has been used either alone, or in combination with methotrexate to treat severe rheumatoid arthritis.

Tacrolimus

This fungal macrolide acts in a very similar way to ciclosporin, although it has a different structure. Its clinical role is not yet clear but it is sometimes used in organ transplantation as an alternative to ciclosporin. Drug specific side effects are broadly similar to those of ciclosporin. Gingival hypertrophy and hypertrichosis are not seen but neurological side effects may occur.

Sirolimus

This new drug is similar in structure to tacrolimus but acts at a different site within the lymphocyte. It may synergize with ciclosporin and has the potential advantage of reduced nephrotoxicity.

Leflunomide

Leflunomide inhibits the mitochondrial enzyme, dihydroorotate dehydrogenase (DHODH), involved in synthesis of pyrimidines. It thereby inhibits lymphocyte activation and growth. This drug has recently been shown to exhibit efficacy and disease-modifying activity in rheumatoid arthritis.

Glucocorticoids

Prednisolone and other glucocorticoids have both anti-inflammatory and immunosuppressive properties (Chapter 14, Section 14.1). They have many different effects on the immune system and interfere with the following:

1 Lymphocyte recirculation.
2 T-cell activation.
3 Generation of cytotoxic lymphocytes.
4 Cytokine release.
5 Macrophage and monocyte function.

Steroids are widely used as immunosuppressives but long-term use in high dose is associated with an unacceptable incidence of adverse effects, and it is therefore preferable to use low dose steroids combined with other immunosuppressive agents.

Biological therapies

Biological therapies consist usually of antibodies or receptors that can specifically bind soluble or cell bound molecules of demonstrable importance in pathological immune responses. They are usually developed following elucidation of pathophysiologic-

ally important pathways that appear amenable to immunomodulation. Broadly they can target cells mediating immune responses, or their soluble products, usually cytokines.

13.3 Targeting cells

Polyclonal anti-T-cell antibodies are raised by injecting animals (e.g. goats or rabbits) with human lymphocyte or thymocyte preparations. OKT3 is a mouse monoclonal antibody to the CD3 complex on T lymphocytes. These antibody preparations are given intravenously and cause profound immunosuppression by depleting T cells from the circulation. They are used in transplantation either as prophylaxis or to treat steroid-resistant acute graft rejection. Polyclonal antibody preparations often cause fever and thrombocytopenia and rarely serum sickness or anaphylaxis. OKT3 may result in the cytokine release syndrome (pyrexia, rigors, nausea, wheeze, diarrhoea and rash).

Several other monoclonal antibodies are currently being assessed for treatment of graft rejection and autoimmune disease. Monoclonal antibodies directed against CD4 and the IL-2 receptor are being tried in organ transplantation. Genetic engineering technology is being used to 'humanize' relevant mouse monoclonal antibodies to render them less immunogenic and therefore more effective.

Targeting cytokines

A chimeric antibody (part mouse/part human immunoglobulin) against tumour necrosis factor (TNF) (infliximab) has been successfully used to treat rheumatoid arthritis and Crohn's disease. Similarly, a soluble TNF receptor fused to the Fc portion of human immunoglobulin (etanercept) has similar efficacy in rheumatoid arthritis. These agents induce significant clinical responses in up to 70% of patients. The risk of potential side effects, which theoretically will include infection and development of lymphoproliferative diseases or solid tumours, is as yet poorly defined although early clinical studies appear promising. Soluble decoy receptors to IL-1 (IL-1 receptor antagonist) are also being tested in patients with rheumatoid arthritis. Numerous other biological agents (monoclonal antibodies and soluble receptors) targeting cytokines, chemokines and pro-angiogenic factors implicated in autoimmune responses are in development.

Antihistamines

These block classical histamine (H_1) receptors and interfere with the actions of histamine released in type I immune reactions.

They are used in hayfever, allergic rhinitis, urticaria and other acute allergic reactions. The vascular effects of histamine including flare, wheal and itch are prevented. They are of no use in asthma.

Older antihistamines like promethazine and diphenhydramine have sedative and anticholinergic side effects. These are less prominent with cyclizine and chlorphenamine (chlorpheniramine). New agents like terfenadine cause little or no sedation, have non-reversible antagonist properties and can be given once daily.

Antihistamines are also used to treat motion sickness and vestibular disease (Chapter 16).

Drugs that block mediator release

Drugs that increase intracellular cyclic adenosine monophosphate (cAMP) stabilize the mast cell and prevent degranulation and mediator release. This reduces or attenuates the symptoms of IgE-mediated hypersensitivity reactions.

Beta$_2$-adrenoceptor agonists

Drugs like adrenaline, terbutaline or salbutamol (Chapter 11, Section 11.1) increase intracellular cAMP, reduce mediator release and improve symptoms.

Theophylline derivatives

These block phosphodiesterase, prevent cAMP breakdown, increase local levels and thus reduce mediator release.

Disodium cromoglicate and ketotifen

These agents stabilize the mast cell membrane and reduce mediator release. The precise mechanism is unknown but it may be related to inhibition of phosphodiesterase.

Non-steroidal anti-inflammatory drugs (NSAIDs)/Cox-2 selective inhibitors

Indometacin and related agents block synthesis of eicosanoids including prostaglandins and also leukotrienes. NSAIDs are useful in the management of some autoimmune diseases, particularly rheumatoid arthritis, but the interference with prostaglandin synthesis may interrupt normal homeostatic prostaglandin-dependent functions, in the lung, kidney and gut. NSAIDs may provoke acute asthma in some sensitive individuals, promote nephrotoxicity or lead to gastrointestinal perforation.

Cyclo-oxygenase (Cox) exists in two isoforms—Cox-1 is primarily involved in normal homeostatic function, whereas Cox-2 is upregulated during inflammatory responses. Agents that specifically inhibit Cox-2 have recently been developed that show promising efficacy in treating arthritis (e.g. rofecoxib, celecoxib), with improved gastrointestinal toxicity profiles. Effects on renal function may persist.

Immunostimulatory and immunomodulatory agents

Effective strategies for stimulation of the immune system have proved elusive although there has been some recent progress.

Cytokines

Cytokines are soluble proteins produced by a wide variety of cells and act primarily in an autocrine or paracrine manner. They have many important and complex actions and play a particularly important role in the regulation of immune and inflammatory responses. Recombinant DNA technology has allowed the large-scale production of many cytokines and these are being used increasingly to modify the biological response to malignancy and infection. Interferon alpha is an effective therapy for hairy cell leukaemia (a rare form of chronic leukaemia) and is useful for Kaposi's sarcoma in patients with acquired immunodeficiency syndrome (AIDS). Selected patients with chronic hepatitis B or C infection may also respond to interferon alpha therapy. Interferon alpha and IL-2 have been used in the treatment of metastatic renal carcinoma and malignant melanoma but response rates are disappointing and, in view of the cost of therapy and side effects, this is a controversial area. Interferon beta has been employed successfully in multiple sclerosis and is being developed in rheumatoid arthritis. G-CSF and GM-CSF are being used to shorten the duration of neutropenia after cytotoxic therapy for non-myeloid malignancies, and also in bone marrow transplantation (Chapter 17, Section 17.2). The use of cytokines as biological response modifiers is at an early stage of development and holds much promise for the future. This may be of particular relevance in immune stimulation in patients with human immunodeficiency virus (HIV)/AIDS.

Other immunostimulatory agents

Bacille Calmette–Guérin (BCG) and other agents, e.g. levamisole and *Corynebacterium parvum*, have been tried as immunostimulants in a wide variety of malignancies because of their potential ability to enhance cell-mediated immunity. Results have been disappointing and they are not in widespread use. Recently adaptive transfer of live dendritic cells to recipients has been used to stimulate immune responses against tumours. These exciting studies remain at an early stage.

CHAPTER 14

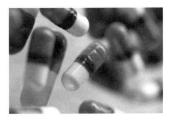

Corticosteroids

Corticosteroids are usually given for one of three reasons:
1 Suppression of inflammation.
2 Suppression of immune responses.
3 Replacement therapy.

They are hormones normally synthesized from cholesterol by the adrenal cortex and have a wide range of physiological functions. Pharmacologically, they are divided according to the relative potencies of their physiological effects into:
1 Glucocorticoids that principally affect carbohydrate and protein metabolism (type II receptor).
2 Mineralocorticoids that principally affect sodium balance (type I receptor). Production of the naturally occurring glucocorticoid, cortisol (hydrocortisone) is stimulated by the release of adrenocorticotropic hormone (ACTH) from the anterior pituitary. Production of the major naturally occurring mineralocorticoid, aldosterone, is controlled by other factors in addition to ACTH, including the activity of the renin–angiotensin system and plasma potassium. Synthetic steroids have largely replaced the natural compounds in therapeutic use as they are usually more potent, may be more specific with regard to mineralocorticoid and glucocorticoid activity and can be given orally. Prednisolone, betamethasone and dexamethasone are widely used as anti-inflammatory and immunosuppressant drugs.

14.1 Glucocorticoids

Cortisol and its derivatives

Pharmacological effects

1 Inflammatory responses. Irrespective of the injury or the insult, corticosteroids interfere non-specifically with all components of the inflammatory responses. This includes reduced capillary dilatation and exudation, inhibition of leucocyte migration and phagocytic activity and reduced fibrin deposition with diminution of subsequent scar formation (Chapter 12, Section 12.3). It has been suggested that glucocorticoids induce the production of lipocortins in cells taking part in the inflammatory response. These proteins inhibit phospholipase A2 and, hence, the production of arachidonic acid and both cyclo-oxygenase and lipo-oxygenase products.

2 Immunological response. In high doses lymphocyte mass and immunoglobulin production are reduced as are monocyte and macrophage function. This results in impaired immunological competence (Chapter 13, Section 13.2).

3 Carbohydrate and protein metabolism. Steroids promote glycogen deposition in the liver and gluconeogenesis, an increase in glucose output by the liver and a decrease in glucose utilization by peripheral tissues. There is a concomitant increase in protein catabolism with mobilization of amino acids from peripheral tissues.

4 Fluid and electrolyte balance. Even glucocorticoids have some mineralocorticoid activity and can act on type I receptors. The principal effect is of enhanced sodium reabsorption from the distal tubule of the kidney, with an associated increase in the urinary excretion of potassium and hydrogen ions. Oedema is rare but moderate hypertension is not uncommon.

5 Lipid metabolism. Corticosteroids facilitate fat mobilization by adrenaline and redistribution of body fat to 'centripetal' areas: face, neck, shoulders.

6 Mood and behaviour changes. Mild euphoria is quite common with higher doses.

7 Increase in the number of red cells, platelets and polymorphs but a decrease in the number of eosinophils and lymphocytes.

8 Increased production of gastric acid and pepsin.

9 Reduction in bone formation, a decrease in calcium absorption from the intestine and an increase in calcium loss from the kidney. There is also reduced secretion of growth hormone and antagonism of its peripheral effects, so that in children there may be growth retardation.

Adverse effects

The adverse effects of corticosteroids are largely predictable from the wide range of known physiological and pharmacological effects.

Toxicity

1 Metabolic effects. Patients on high-dose steroid therapy quickly develop a characteristic appearance: a rounded, plethoric face (moon face), deposits of fat over the supraclavicular and cervical areas (buffalo hump), obesity of the trunk with relatively thin limbs, purple striae typically on the thighs and lower abdomen, and a tendency to bruising. Disturbed carbohydrate metabolism leads to hyperglycaemia and glycosuria and rarely proceeds to overt diabetes mellitus.

In addition to the loss of protein from skeletal muscle, patients also develop muscular weakness, which particularly affects the thighs and upper arms (proximal myopathy).

2 Fluid retention may be associated with hypokalaemic alkalosis and hypertension.

3 Increased susceptibility to infection.

4 Osteoporosis, which may cause compression fractures of the vertebral bodies and avascular necrosis of the head of the femur.

5 Psychosis. A sense of euphoria frequently accompanies high dosage steroid therapy and this may rarely proceed to overt manic psychosis. The increased sense of well-being leads to an improved appetite and contributes to weight gain.

Steroids may precipitate a depressive illness.

6 Cataract. This is a rare complication, usually in children, reflecting prolonged high dosage therapy.

7 Gastrointestinal symptoms. Dyspepsia frequently accompanies high-dose oral steroid therapy. Signs of peritonitis, which would complicate a perforated peptic ulcer, may be masked by the anti-inflammatory effect of steroids.

These predictable and serious adverse effects should lead to particular caution in the use of steroid therapy in patients who have pre-existing peptic ulceration, severe hypertension, congestive cardiac failure and osteoporosis.

Adrenal suppression

The administration of exogenous corticosteroids results in negative feedback to the anterior pituitary, with inhibition of ACTH release and the consequent withdrawal of trophic stimulation to the adrenal cortex. In time, the adrenal cortex atrophies and when long-term steroid therapy is finally stopped it may be 6–12 months before normal pituitary–adrenal function recovers. An alternate day steroid regimen may cause less adrenal suppression than daily treatment. Adrenal suppression has two consequences:

1 Impairment of patient's response to 'stress' (illness, injury, surgery) and susceptibility to infection. Chicken pox may be particularly severe: passive immunization with varicella zoster immunoglobin should be given to non-immune patients.

2 The withdrawal of corticosteroid therapy must be slow and supervised.

Short-term therapy (4–6 weeks) can be reduced quickly and stopped abruptly without difficulty. Long-term therapy, particularly with more than 7.5 mg prednisolone daily, or equivalent, carries the risk of adrenal and hypothalamic–pituitary suppression. Withdrawal must be undertaken cautiously and gradually. Assuming that there is no flare-up of the systemic disease for which the steroid therapy was originally prescribed, the daily dose should be reduced by 5 mg of prednisolone, or equivalent every 1–2 weeks until the total daily dose is at the physiological replacement level of 5 mg daily. This dosage should be converted to a single morning administration, and at intervals of 2 weeks decrements of 1 mg should be made. The safety of this gradual withdrawal can be monitored by the endogenous plasma cortisol level; full recovery can be verified by a Synacthen (ACTH) test. All these patients require supervision and advice for 6 months after steroid withdrawal.

Patients on long-term steroid therapy, and particularly those undergoing steroid withdrawal, require a temporary increase in dose of steroid during periods of stress because of the inability of the hypothalamic–pituitary–adrenal axis to respond normally with an increased production of endogenous corticosteroid, e.g. in times of intercurrent illness. Similarly, patients on steroid therapy who undergo surgery require an increased steroid dosage to enable them to withstand the stress of the operation. Such patients need to carry a steroid card (or bracelet/necklace) so that they can be identified as steroid dependent in the event of an accident/emergency. They should understand the need for uninterrupted treatment and report any problem (vomiting/diarrhoea) immediately. Patients on steroids are now specifically advised to avoid contact with people who have chickenpox or shingles and to see their doctor if such contact occurs. If travelling to remote areas they should be instructed in the self-administration of intramuscular hydrocortisone and given the appropriate equipment and drugs.

Topical therapy

Topically applied steroids are absorbed through the skin and in the case of very potent drugs, such as clobetasol or betamethasone, adrenal suppression and the toxic effects described above can occur. This usually happens only if recommended doses are exceeded, extensive areas of skin are covered or very prolonged administration is used.

Other effects peculiar to topical application are:

1 Worsening of local infections. This is particularly important in the eye, where ulcers caused by herpes simplex (dendritic ulcers) spread dramatically and dangerously following application of steroids.

2 Local thinning of the skin. This slowly resolves on stopping steroids, but some permanent damage may remain.

3 Atrophic striae; these are irreversible.

4 Increased hair growth.

5 The use of high doses of beclometasone by aerosol inhalation can result in hoarseness or candidiasis of the mouth.

Clinical use and dose

Hydrocortisone

Hydrocortisone is used in three different situations:

1 Replacement therapy, when it is given orally in a dose of 20 mg in the morning and 10 mg in the afternoon. Body size needs to be taken into consideration (12–15 mg/m^2 surface area).

2 Shock and status asthmaticus, when it is given intravenously up to 200 mg 6-hourly.

3 Topical application: e.g. 1% cream or ointment in eczema; 100 mg dose as enema or foam in treating ulcerative colitis.

Cortisone acetate

Cortisone acetate is metabolized to cortisol, although some patients may be deficient in the relevant enzyme.

Prednisolone

Prednisolone is used orally in three types of condition:

1 Inflammatory diseases, e.g. severe rheumatoid arthritis, ulcerative colitis, chronic active hepatitis.
2 Allergic diseases, e.g. severe asthma, minimal change glomerulonephritis.
3 Acute lymphoblastic leukaemia and non-Hodgkin lymphoma.

A single dose of up to 60 mg daily is given, depending on disease severity, reducing to a maintenance dose in the range 2.5–15 mg daily.

It is used topically in ulcerative colitis as a 20-mg enema.

Prednisone

Prednisone is a synthetic steroid that is metabolized to prednisolone in much the same way as cortisone acetate is converted to cortisol.

Beclometasone

Beclometasone is a fluorinated, and therefore polar, steroid which passes poorly across membranes. It is used topically in:

1 Asthma, when it is given by metered aerosol doses. About 20% reaches the lungs; the rest is swallowed and destroyed by first-pass metabolism (Chapter 11).
2 Severe eczema, when it is used as 0.025% cream.

Betamethasone

Betamethasone is used for:

1 Cerebral oedema caused by tumours and trauma; given either orally or intramuscularly in doses up to 4 mg 6-hourly. It is ineffective in cerebral oedema resulting from hypoxia.
2 Severe eczema; given topically as 0.1% cream.

Dexamethasone

Dexamethasone is used in cerebral oedema.

Triamcinolone

Triamcinolone is used for:

1 Local inflammation of joints or soft tissue; given by intra-articular injection in doses up to 40 mg depending on joint size.
2 Severe eczema; given topically as 0.1% cream.

Clobetasol

Clobetasol is used topically in severe resistant eczema and discoid lupus erythematosus.

14.2 Mineralocorticoids

Pharmacological effects

These drugs produce retention of salt and water by the same mechanism as aldosterone on the distal renal tubule. Their main adverse effect is excessive fluid retention and hypertension.

Clinical use and dose

Fludrocortisone is a fluorinated hydrocortisone with powerful mineralocorticoid activity and very little anti-inflammatory action. It is used in:

1 Replacement therapy in doses of 50–200 μg daily.
2 Congenital adrenal hyperplasia in doses up to 2 μg/day.
3 Idiopathic postural hypotension 100–200 μg each day.

Comment. Steroids are powerful drugs. Dramatic improvement in certain severe diseases is matched by equally dramatic ill health resulting from adverse effects when these drugs are used in mild inflammatory disorders for which they are not indicated.

Steroids therefore should be used only when other less toxic drugs have failed, or when the severity of the condition justifies aggressive treatment with steroids in high doses. Once control of the clinical state has been achieved, steroid dose should be reduced to the minimum necessary to maintain the desired effect and, if possible, stopped altogether.

CHAPTER 15

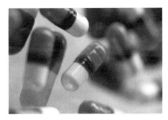

Drugs and the Reproductive System

15.1 Sex steroids

Oral contraceptives

Oral contraceptives have revolutionized the place of women in society. Their efficacy, convenience and overall safety have allowed women to decide if and when they will become pregnant and to plan their domestic and business lives accordingly. They are, however, potent pharmacological agents and under certain circumstances the use of oral contraceptives presents an unacceptable risk.

Composition
The contraceptive pill contains either an oestrogen and progestogen combined or a progestogen alone. Both of the naturally occurring steroids, estradiol (oestradiol) and progesterone, are ineffective orally because of extensive first-pass metabolism; thus synthetic compounds are used. At present, the oestrogen is usually ethinylestradiol (ethinyloestradiol) or its methoxy derivative, mestranol. The term progestogen is misleading, because the progestogens in use as contraceptives are mainly synthetic derivatives of 19-nortestosterone and are often metabolized to oestrogens. Therefore, progestogens can have some androgenic and oestrogenic as well as progestational properties. As a matter of convention, norethynodrel is considered a first-generation,

levonorgestrel and norethisterone are second-generation, and desogestrel, gestodene and norgestimate are third-generation progestogens. The latter combine high progestational potency with low androgenicity.

Mechanism
The combined oestrogen and progestogen pill inhibits ovulation. The oestrogen component inhibits the release of follicle stimulating hormone (FSH) while the progestogen prevents luteinizing hormone (LH) release. The abrupt withdrawal of progestogen at the end of each dosing period assures a prompt onset of withdrawal bleeding similar to normal menstruation. The progestogen-only pill contains less steroid than the combination tablets and probably works by altering cervical mucus so that it becomes thick and progestogenic. In addition, ovulation is prevented in about 40% of women.

Pharmacokinetics
The constituents of contraceptive pills are well absorbed and are eliminated after liver metabolism.

Adverse effects
The most important, but not the most common, adverse reactions involve the effects of *oestrogen* on the cardiovascular system.

Venous thromboembolic disease
1 The risk is increased by:
  (a) Oestrogen content above 50 g/mg.
  (b) Desogestrel or gestodene as the pro-gestagen component.
  Studies in relation to venous thromboembolism have provided reassurance about thromboembolic risks associated with oral contraceptives containing levonorgestrel, norethisterone or etynodiol (ethynodiol) (excess risk around 5–10 cases per 100 000 women per annum). However, the studies indicated that oral contraceptives containing desogestrel and gestodene are associated with around a twofold increase in the risk compared to those containing other progestogens and should not be used by women with risk factors for venous thromboembolism.
  (c) Intercurrent major surgical procedures.
  (d) Factor V Leiden.
2 The increased risk is confined to those actually taking the pill:
  (a) Develops within first month.
  (b) Remains constant during use.
  (c) Returns to normal within 1 month of stopping.
3 Pathogenesis:
  (a) Decreased antithrombin III.
  (b) Decreased plasminogen activator in endothelium.

Myocardial infarction and stroke (including subarachnoid haemorrhage)
1 The risk is increased by:
  (a) Age.
  (b) Cigarette smoking.
  (c) Oestrogen.
  Age and cigarette smoking multiply, rather than add to, the risks of the oral contraceptives with regard to myocardial infarction and stroke. Most cases occur in women aged over 35 years who smoke. It is assumed that the risk is also enhanced by hypertension, diabetes, obesity and hyperlipoproteinaemia but numbers are too small for statistical analysis.
2 The risk is not confined to those currently taking the pill, but persists after stopping.

3 Third-generation pills reduce the risk of arterial disease—users have one-third of the risk of myocardial infarction compared with second-generation pill users.
4 Pathogenesis:
  (a) Acceleration of platelet aggregation.
  (b) Decreased antithrombin III.
  (c) Decreased plasminogen activator.

Hypertension
1 Blood pressure rises by a small amount in all women on the pill. There is a progressive rise with duration of use. In most cases this increase in pressure is small and of little clinical significance. Less frequently there is a rise to levels at which treatment might ordinarily be considered. The best course of action in these cases is to stop the pill and observe for several months. Rarely, malignant hypertension occurs and should be treated as a medical emergency. Blood pressure should be checked at each clinic visit in women receiving an oral contraceptive.
2 Blood pressure usually returns to normal 3–6 months after stopping the contraceptive pill.

Oral contraceptives and cancer
This is a controversial area. Oral contraceptive use appears to protect against endometrial and ovarian carcinoma. Cervical cancer has been identified more frequently in pill users than in women using an intrauterine contraceptive device (IUCD). Interpretation of this finding is difficult because age at first intercourse and number of sexual partners are risk factors for cervical carcinoma and could differ substantially between these two groups. The suggestion that oral contraceptive use at a young age increases the risk of breast cancer remains unproven.

Glucose tolerance and lipid metabolism
There is a small decrease in glucose tolerance. Oestrogens increase, and progestogens decrease, high density lipoproteins. The clinical relevance of these observations is unknown.

Focal migraine and stroke
Oestrogen-containing contraceptives increase the risk of strokes in women with focal migraine.

Other adverse effects
Additional effects of oral contraceptives frequently include:
1 Irregular bleeding during the first few cycles.
2 Headaches.
3 Mood swings.
    Less commonly subjects may present with:
1 Cholestatic jaundice; particularly if a history of jaundice or pruritis in pregnancy.
2 Increased incidence of gallstones.
3 Elevation of thyroid binding globulin (does not affect analysis of free T4).
4 Precipitation of porphyria.
    There is no evidence that oral contraceptives containing low doses of oestrogen either impair established lactation or harm a breast-fed infant.

Drug interactions

Oral contraceptive failure with unwanted pregnancy can be precipitated by enzyme induction (see below) resulting from the coadministration of drugs that induce hepatic microsomal enzymes (Chapter 1, Section 1.3).
    This applies to oestrogen-containing and progestogen-only contraceptives. If long-term treatment with one of these drugs is necessary (e.g. epilepsy) then a higher dose should be used if oral contraception is the method of choice.
    Failure of oestrogen-containing oral contraceptives can be precipitated by reduced absorption resulting from altered bowel flora caused by the coadministration of broad-spectrum antimicrobials. The mechanism depends on the fact that oestrogens undergo conjugation in the liver but hydrolytic enzymes produced by gut bacteria cleave these conjugates and release free hormone, which is then reabsorbed. Broad-spectrum antimicrobials prevent this process by altering gut flora, and hormone absorption is decreased. When an antibiotic such as ampicillin is prescribed for a woman who is also taking an oral contraceptive, she should be advised to use additional contraception during and for 14 days after the course of antibiotic.

Clinical use and dose

The dose of both oestrogen and progestogen should be kept as low as possible.
1 Combination pill: one tablet daily for 21 days starting on day 1 of the menstrual cycle and repeating after 7 pill-free days.
2 Progestogen-only pill: continuous administration of one tablet daily starting on the first day of menstruation and taking the dose at the same time each day. A delay of more than 3 h risks loss of efficacy.
3 Intramuscular medroxyprogesterone acetate: this is a long-acting (3 months) progesterone derivative.
4 Phased formulations (biphasic or triphasic). These provide varying doses of oestrogen and progestogen during the cycle. Deviations from normal metabolism are small and triphasics are recommended for women aged over 35 years. They are taken from day 1 with a 7-day interval.
    The combination oral contraceptive is the most effective form of contraception currently available: the failure rate is around 1/100 woman years. The efficacy of progestogen-only pills is controversial, but is probably equal to that of intrauterine devices, i.e. a

HEPATIC MICROSOMAL ENZYME INDUCERS

Phenytoin	Primidone
Carbamazepine	Rifampicin
Phenobarbital (phenobarbitone)	

failure rate of about 2/100 woman years. They have the advantage of being suitable where the combined pill is contraindicated because of cardiovascular risk, e.g. history of thromboembolism and hypertension.

Contraindications

These are summarized in Table 15.1.

Patients with established diabetes mellitus may use the combined pill with appropriate adjustment of insulin requirements. Ideally, nobody with a relative contraindication should receive an oestrogen-containing oral contraceptive. However, real life is not ideal and pressure of social circumstances sometimes dictates that the risks of an unwanted pregnancy outweigh those accompanying the use of the contraceptive pill; the other forms of contraception are less reliable. The presence of two or more relative contraindications strengthens the case against using an oestrogen-containing contraceptive.

Comment. The widespread use of oral contraceptives is a testament to their popularity. Serious cardiovascular complications are clearly of concern and must be explained to a woman proposing to take the pill. However, they must be explained in the perspective that risk of myocardial infarction and stroke is concentrated largely in older women who smoke and that some, at least, of the morbidity in currently available statistics can still be ascribed to the use of now obsolete high-dose oestrogen preparations.

Hormone replacement therapy

This is used for the alleviation of menopausal vasomotor symptoms and symptoms related to tissue atrophy, for example vaginitis. There is also good evidence that oestrogen administration will reduce postmenopausal osteoporosis. Evidence to show convincingly that hormone replacement therapy (HRT) use is cardioprotective (reduces risk of myocardial infarction) is not available, although some authorities consider that there are cardiovascular benefits from HRT use.

Natural oestrogens (estradiol, estrone (oestrone) and estriol (oestriol)) provide a more physiological effect for HRT than synthetic oestrogens (ethinylestradiol and mestranol). Oestrogen may be administered in various ways, for example, tablet, transdermal patch, cream, gel or implant. Oral oestrogens are subject to first-pass metabolism; therefore, subcutaneous or transdermal administration is more representative of endogenous hormone activity than other preparations. A woman with a uterus requires oestrogen with cyclical progestogen for the last 10–13 days of her cycle in order to prevent endometrial hyperplasia or carcinoma. Some preparations combine both oestrogenic and progestogenic activity. This also means

CONTRAINDICATIONS TO ORAL CONTRACEPTIVE USE	
Absolute	Relative
History of thromboembolism	Diabetes
Moderate/severe hypertension	Cigarette smoking
Focal migraine	Mild hypertension
Active liver disease	Age >35 years
Age >35 years and cigarette smoker	
Porphyria	
Oestrogen-dependent tumour	
Impending major surgery	
History of jaundice in pregnancy	
Major haemoglobinopathy	

Table 15.1 Contraindications to the use of oral contraceptives.

that a post-menopausal woman can take HRT without necessarily having to undergo a cyclical bleed.

Studies indicate that there is an increased risk of breast cancer in women taking HRT. The increased risk is related to duration of use and the excess risk disappears within about 5 years of stopping. For example, for women over 50 years the risk of developing breast cancer increases by 2 per 1000 in those taking HRT. In those women taking HRT for 15 years this figure rises to 12 per 1000.

Progestogens

1 Dysfunctional uterine bleeding. Cyclical gestogens may be used to treat dysfunctional uterine bleeding secondary to anovulation. Side-effects are mild but may include nausea, fluid retention and weight gain.
2 Progestogens are also used in the treatment of endometrial carcinoma.

15.2 Dopamine agonists

Mechanism

These drugs are dopamine receptor agonists that prevent the release of prolactin by stimulating dopamine receptors in the pituitary. They increase growth hormone (GH) release in normal subjects but suppress GH release in acromegaly.

Pharmacokinetics

Bromocriptine is effective orally and eliminated by liver metabolism followed by biliary excretion. Cabergoline has actions and uses similar to bromocriptine, but its duration of action is longer. Other similar drugs are pergolide, lisuride (lysuride) and terguride.

Adverse effects

Bromocriptine
Nausea and vomiting may limit dose increases. Postural hypotension can occur. Constipation is common. High doses (>20 mg/day) can produce a wide range of neuropsychiatric effects,

including confusion, psychosis, dyskinesias and bizarre choreiform movements.

Cabergoline
The pattern of side effects is different to bromocriptine. Therefore, patients intolerant of one drug may tolerate the other.

Clinical use and dose

Bromocriptine
Hyperprolactinaemia: up to 7.5 mg twice a day. Postpartum suppression of lactation: 2.5 mg twice a day for 2 weeks. Acromegaly: 5 mg 6-hourly. Parkinsonism: high doses up to 100 mg daily (Chapter 20, Section 20.2).

Cabergoline
Hyperprolactinaemia: 500 mg weekly. Postpartum suppression of established lactation: 250 mg every 12 h for 2 days.

15.3 Danazol

Mechanism

Danazol inhibits pituitary gonadotrophin release, thereby reducing ovarian function and producing atrophy of the endometrium. It also blocks oestrogen and progesterone receptors and has some androgenic activity.

Adverse effects

Avoid danazol during pregnancy: virilization of female fetus has been reported.

Danazol is not an effective contraceptive and non-hormonal methods should be used during treatment. Acne, hirsutism and voice changes occasionally occur.

Drug interactions

Danazol potentiates the action of carbamazepine and anticoagulants.

Clinical use

Endometriosis, menorrhagia, premenstrual syndrome and hereditary angioedema.

15.4 Gonadotrophin-releasing hormone analogues (GnRH analogues)

Mechanism

Gonadotrophin-releasing hormone (GnRH) is a decapeptide. It was isolated and characterized in 1971. GnRH analogues are produced by altering the amino acids in positions 6 and/ or 10, resulting in compounds with high affinity for the GnRH receptor, and a long half-life as a result of their resistance to cleavage by endopeptidases. After an initial brief stimulation, the GnRH analogues paradoxically result in the suppression of the pituitary and therefore of ovarian activity.

Adverse effects

The main disadvantages of GnRH analogues are secondary to the induced hypo-oestrogenic state, affecting the cardiovascular, skeletal and urogenital systems while producing vasomotor symptoms. Add-back therapy using oestrogens, progestogens or both may be used to negate their harmful effects.

Clinical use

Their short-term use is of proven benefit in assisted reproduction and prior to endometrial resection or ablation. Long-term applications range from shrinking fibroids before surgery, to the management of endometriosis, ovarian hyperandrogenism, the premenstrual syndrome, precocious puberty and dysfunctional uterine bleeding.

15.5 Ovulation induction agents

Anti-oestrogens

Mechanism

Clomifene (clomiphene) and tamoxifen are oestrogen receptor antagonists that prevent negative feed-back of oestrogen at the hypothalamus, leading to increased secretion of FSH and LH.

Clinical use and dose

Female subfertility: clomifene, 50 mg/day for 5 days starting within about 5 days of the onset of menstruation.

An important 'side effect' is the increased risk of multiple pregnancy, i.e. twins or occasionally triplets. There is a 7% chance of twins and a 0.5% chance of triplets. Recently, there has been a suggestion that clomifene may be associated with an increased risk of ovarian cancer. Although this association is far from proven, it has been advised that clomifene should not normally be used for more than six treatment cycles.

Tamoxifen: 20 mg/day starting on the second day of the cycle for 5 days.

Additional use of tamoxifen

Tamoxifen competes with oestrogen at binding sites on oestrogen-dependent breast tumours in pre-menopausal women. Remission occurs in about 40% of patients (Chapter 13, Section 13.1). Dose: 10 mg twice daily. Tamoxifen can cause hot flushes and uterine bleeding secondary to endometrial hyperplasia.

Metformin

Metformin is a biguanide. It exerts its effect mainly by decreasing gluconeogenesis and by increasing peripheral utilization of glucose. Studies of metformin in obese insulin-resistant women with polycystic ovarian syndrome (PCOS) have shown significant improvements in insulin sensitivity and hyperinsulinaemia. Also the ovulatory response to clomifene can be increased in obese women with PCOS by decreasing insulin sensitivity with metformin. It should be noted that metformin is not licensed for this use in the UK.

15.6 Testosterone

Mechanism

Testosterone is the major male sex hormone and is responsible for secondary sexual characteristics.

Pharmacokinetics

Testosterone has an extensive first-pass metabolism: it is given either transdermally or by intramuscular injection.

Drug interactions

Oral anticoagulant requirements are decreased by testosterone.

Clinical effects

Testosterone is used as replacement therapy in hypogonadal or castrated men. In the normal male it inhibits pituitary gonadotrophin secretion and depresses spermatogenesis. Menopausal women are also sometimes given implants of testosterone as an adjunct to hormone replacement therapy.

15.7 Anti-androgens

Cyproterane acetate is a progestagen with antagonist properties at the androgen receptor. It can be used in low dose (2 mg) as part of a combined oral contraceptive (Dianette) in the treatment of hirsutism. Higher doses (50 mg/day) can also be administered where more effective anti-androgen actions are required.

15.8 Drugs adversely affecting sexual function

Several drugs can adversely influence sexual function and the more frequently used are listed in Table 15.2. Remember that patients might not volunteer information about an adverse effect which they consider embarrassing, and which they might not relate to their drug treatment.

15.9 Drug treatment of impotence

Sildenafil

Objective and subjective measures show sildenafil improves rigidity and the number of erections in men with erectile dysfunction. The

DRUGS DECREASING SEXUAL FUNCTION

Drug	Comment
Methyldopa	Impotence; failure of ejaculation; loss of sexual drive
Clonidine	Impotence Difficulty in achieving orgasm (women)
Tricyclic antidepressants	Delayed ejaculation
Phenothiazines	Difficulties in erection and ejaculation
Phenelzine	Delayed ejaculation
Cimetidine	Impaired spermatogenesis (reversible) Impotence
Isoniazid	Menstrual disturbance
Diuretics	Impotence and reduced libido: mechanism unknown
Guanethidine	Impotence, retrograde ejaculation
Sulfasalazine (sulphasalazine)	Impaired spermatogenesis (reversible)

Table 15.2 Drugs which can adversely influence sexual function.

final common pathway for sexual arousal and stimulation leading to erection is the production in cavernosal tissues of cyclic guanosine monophosphate (cGMP) which relaxes the smooth muscle and permits swelling of the corpora with blood. Sildenafil is a potent and specific inhibitor of cGMP-specific phosphodiesterase type 5, the isoenzyme responsible for the breakdown of cGMP in the corpus cavernosum.

The most common side effects are headache, flushing, dyspepsia, nasal congestion and transient disturbance of colour discrimination. A very important drug interaction is the potentially dangerous potentiation of the haemodynamic effect of nitrates, specifically hypotension. This contraindication is important as erectile dysfunction is commonly associated with cardiovascular disease but also because amyl nitrates ('poppers') are drugs of misuse, particularly in the homosexual community.

CHAPTER 16

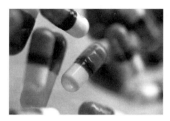

Drugs and Gastrointestinal Disease

16.1 Peptic ulcer

Aims
1 To relieve pain.
2 To heal the ulcer.
3 To prevent ulcer diathesis.

Relevant pathophysiology
It is traditional to regard peptic ulceration as the result of an imbalance between aggressive and protective factors in the upper gastrointestinal tract. The principal aggressive forces are gastric acid and pepsin. The two most important factors disrupting the balance between acid/peptic attack and mucosal resistance are *Helicobacter pylori* infection and non-steroidal anti-inflammatory drugs (NSAIDs). *Helicobacter pylori* stimulates increased gastrin release and thereby increased acid secretion. In addition, it causes direct damage to the mucosa, thus further disrupting the physiological balance. NSAIDs impair mucosal resistance but do not alter acid secretion.

Almost all patients with duodenal ulcer (DU), and most patients with gastric ulcer (GU) have *H. pylori* infection. It is now clear that eradication of *H. pylori* infection is associated with prolonged remission from peptic ulceration, and perhaps with permanent cure. Recognition of the role of *H. pylori* infection in peptic ulcer, and development of effective eradication treatments for it, have had enormous

impact on our approach to the patient with peptic ulceration.

Drugs used in the treatment of peptic ulcer
1 Antacids.
2 Drugs that inhibit gastric acid secretion:
    (a) H_2-receptor antagonists.
    (b) Proton pump inhibitors.
    (c) Synthetic prostaglandin analogues.
3 Drugs that do not directly inhibit gastric acid secretion:
    (a) Chelated salts of bismuth.
    (b) Sucralfate.
4 Drug combinations to eradicate *H. pylori*.

Antacids
Mechanism. These drugs are weak alkalis so they partly neutralize free acid in the stomach. They may also stimulate mucosal repair mechanisms around ulcers, possibly by stimulating local prostaglandin release.

Pharmacokinetics. Most antacids (principally salts of magnesium or aluminium) are not absorbed from the alimentary tract to any appreciable extent. Some, such as sodium bicarbonate, are absorbed.

Adverse effects. Antacids that contain aluminium tend to cause constipation. Those containing magnesium have the opposite effect. Sodium bicarbonate in large quantities may alter acid–base status causing metabolic alkalosis and may promote the formation of phosphate-containing renal calculi. Absorbable antacids should not be administered in the long term. Antacids with a high sodium content should be avoided in patients with impaired cardiac function or chronic liver disease.

Drug interactions. Antacids may reduce the absorption of a number of different drugs from the gut. These include digoxin, phenothiazines and tetracyclines.

Clinical use and dosage. Antacids are mainly used for symptomatic relief in patients with peptic ulcer, gastro-oesophageal reflux disease or non-ulcer dyspepsia 'indigestion'. They can accelerate the healing of peptic ulcers but must be given frequently and in high doses.

Suitable antacids are:

Aluminium hydroxide 5–15 ml 6-hourly.

Magnesium trisilicate 10–20 ml or 1–2 tablets as required.

Drugs that inhibit gastric acid secretion

H_2-receptor antagonists

Currently, there are four such agents available (cimetidine, ranitidine, nizatidine and famotidine). They are all competitive antagonists for histamine at the H_2-receptor found mainly on parietal cells.

Mechanism. By competing with histamine at the H_2-receptor, these drugs reduce acid secretion by the parietal cell, especially at night and in the fasting state. They are less effective in reducing food-stimulated acid secretion.

Pharmacokinetics. They are well absorbed following oral administration. They have relatively short half-lives and are excreted largely unchanged by the kidneys.

Adverse effects. These are rare and are usually of a minor nature. Cimetidine is weakly anti-androgenic in humans. It may cause impotence or gynaecomastia. Either cimetidine or ranitidine may cause reversible mental confusion, particularly in sick elderly patients. Some potentially serious cardiac dysrhythmias have occurred following intravenous injections of H_2-receptor antagonists.

Drug interactions. Cimetidine inhibits oxidative drug metabolism by the liver. It interacts with many drugs but only three are of clinical importance. These are phenytoin, theophylline and warfarin. These three drugs are metabolized in the liver and have narrow therapeutic indices; cimetidine will slow their metabolism and may induce toxicity.

To date, no clinically relevant drug interactions have been reported with the other H_2-receptor antagonists.

Clinical use and dosage. H_2-receptor antagonists can heal duodenal ulcers (DU) and benign gastric ulcers (GU). Patients with GU should have endoscopy and biopsy to exclude gastric carcinoma. Healing of GU should also be documented endoscopically. The H_2-receptor antagonists can be effective in some patients with gastro-oesophageal reflux disease (GORD), especially in milder grades of severity. For patients with erosive or ulcerative oesophagitis complicating GORD, the H_2-receptor antagonists are unlikely to be effective unless higher doses are given (see below).

Seventy-five to 80% of DUs will heal within 4 weeks, increasing to around 90% by 8 weeks. GUs tend to be slower to heal, but over 80% should have healed by 8 weeks. If single evening doses are used, it is important that patients are advised to have nothing further by mouth after the dose. Eating food will stimulate gastric acid secretion through gastrin release and vagal activity and can reduce the pharmacological effect of the H_2-receptor antagonist.

Higher doses are recommended for GORD. Single evening dosage regimens are not appropriate. In GORD, H_2-receptor antagonists should be given at least twice daily. For ranitidine, the dose may go up to 300 mg four times daily.

H$_2$-receptor antagonists are of no proven value in the management of patients with upper gastrointestinal haemorrhage, whether from peptic ulceration or other sources. They may be used prophylactically in some critically ill patients in an effort to prevent stress-related gastric mucosal bleeding. However, this should not be a major problem in countries where high standards of intensive care are available.

Comment. Although H$_2$-receptor antagonists can heal peptic ulcers, relapse is common after stopping treatment. These drugs can be continued as long-term maintenance treatment, typically in half of their initial dose. However, the role of such treatment has become markedly reduced since the importance of eradication of H. pylori has been appreciated (see below).

H$_2$-receptor antagonists are of no proven value in non-ulcer dyspepsia. Their use in patients with undiagnosed upper abdominal pain is not recommended. Some of the H$_2$-receptor antagonists are now available in low doses 'over the counter'. They are likely to be used in this way by patients with mild GORD for relief of heartburn.

Proton pump inhibitors: omeprazole, lansoprazole, pantoprazole and rabeprazole
Mechanism. These drugs are irreversible inhibitors of the proton pump on the parietal cell membrane. The proton pump is an enzyme (H$^+$/K$^+$-ATPase) that actively secretes hydrogen ions into the gastric lumen. It is therefore responsible for the final step in the process of acid secretion. Blocking this enzyme causes a marked, but temporary, suppression of gastric acid secretion to any stimulus, including food.

Pharmacokinetics. Both drugs are administered as capsules of enteric-coated granules. The bioavailability of omeprazole after the first dose is limited, but increases with repeated once daily dosing to reach a plateau by around the fifth day. These drugs have short elimination half-lives (1–2 h) but a prolonged pharmacological effect and are converted in the liver to inactive metabolites.

Adverse effects. These are mild and infrequent. Diarrhoea, skin rash and headache have all been reported. No serious life-threatening adverse effects have been encountered.

Drug interactions. Omeprazole reduces the clearance and prolongs the elimination of diazepam, phenytoin and the R enantiomer of warfarin, through inhibition of their hepatic metabolism. No clinically important drug interactions have been reported with the other proton pump inhibitors.

Clinical use and dosage. Used in the treatment of severe, erosive oesophagitis; in the short-term management of duodenal and gastric ulcers; in treatment and prophylaxis of NSAID induced ulcers; in combination with antibiotics in the eradication of H pylori; and in the treatment of Zollinger–Ellison syndrome.

For DU, omeprazole 20 mg daily, or lansoprazole 30 mg daily will heal around 90% of ulcers within 4 weeks. In patients with GU,

H$_2$-RECEPTOR ANTAGONIST DOSES

Recommended doses for duodenal ulcer and gastric ulcer are:
Cimetidine 400 mg twice daily or 800 mg in the evening.

Ranitidine 150 mg twice daily or 300 mg in the evening.
Nizatidine 300 mg in the evening.
Famotidine 40 mg in the evening.

the same doses are used, but treatment for 8 weeks is recommended.

Synthetic prostaglandins: misoprostol
Mechanism. Prostaglandins are weak inhibitors of gastric acid secretion when given in pharmacological doses. Their mechanism of action is not fully understood. In addition, prostaglandins have a series of properties loosely referred to as 'cytoprotection'. This means that they have been shown in animal studies to prevent or limit experimental damage to the gastric or duodenal mucosa from a variety of noxious stimuli. It is unclear whether or not this is an important property regarding their clinical use. 'Cytoprotection' can be demonstrated at doses below those required for inhibition of gastric acid secretion.

Pharmacokinetics. Misoprostol has a short plasma half-life. It may act on the stomach both locally and systemically.

Adverse effects. There is diarrhoea in up to 40% of patients, but this is usually mild and self-limiting. Misoprostol and other prostaglandins are potentially abortifacient and so should not be given to women of child-bearing age.

Clinical use and dose. The main indication is to prevent gastric mucosal damage and gastric ulcers in patients on NSAIDs. Dose is 200 μg twice to four times daily.

Comment. Misoprostol should be considered for those patients who genuinely require to take NSAIDs and who have a past history of peptic ulcer or upper gastrointestinal bleeding.

For patients already on NSAIDs who are found to have a peptic ulcer, the NSAID should be stopped if possible. However, even if the NSAID has to be continued (in a patient with rheumatoid arthritis, for example) the ulcer can be healed with any type of antiulcer drug. There is no specific indication for misoprostol in this situation.

Drugs that do not directly inhibit gastric acid secretion

Chelated salts of bismuth: tripotassium dicitrato bismuthate
Mechanism. The means whereby bismuth salts heal ulcers are not fully understood. They do not directly inhibit acid secretion. However, they do suppress *H. pylori* infection and thus reduce the hypersecretion of acid induced by the infection. In addition, they may form an insoluble protective layer over the ulcer base, preventing further damage by acid and pepsin. They may also stimulate local prostaglandin production.

Pharmacokinetics. A small quantity of bismuth is absorbed following oral administration. Urinary excretion of bismuth continues for over 2 weeks after stopping a course of treatment.

Adverse effects. The liquid preparation should be avoided because of an unpleasant smell and taste and the fact that it discolours the tongue. The liquid or tablet preparation may colour the faeces black. The long-term consequences of bismuth absorption are unknown, so this drug is not recommended for continuous or repeated administration.

Comment. In the management of patients with peptic ulcer, the main use of a bismuth-containing compound is as part of a drug combination against *H. pylori*. This compound, when combined with metronidazole and another antibiotic, such as tetracycline, can eradicate the infection in 80–90% of patients within 2 weeks. However, frequent doses are necessary and compliance may be a problem.

Sucralfate (sucrose aluminium octasulphate)
Mechanism. The exact mechanism of ulcer healing by sucralfate is unknown. It may act by coating ulcer bases or by stimulating local prostaglandin release. It does not directly

affect acid secretion. However, like the Bismuth salts it suppresses *H. pylori* infection and thus reduces the acid hypersecretion stimulated by the infection. It probably suppresses *H. pylori* by interfering with the ability of the organism to bind to the mucosal epithelial cells.

Clinical use and dosage. Sucralfate is indicated for the treatment of duodenal ulcer and benign gastric ulcer. The usual dose is 1 g four times daily or 2 g twice daily. Healing rates are comparable to those obtained with H_2-receptor antagonists. Sucralfate should not be used in patients with chronic renal failure because of the risk of aluminium absorption and toxicity.

Pharmacokinetics. Sucralfate acts locally; only small amounts of aluminium are absorbed.

Adverse effects. Constipation.

Drug interactions. Sucralfate can reduce the absorption of a number of different drugs, including phenytoin and tetracyclines.

Drug combinations to eradicate Helicobacter pylori

Almost all patients with DU, and many patients with GU, are infected with *H. pylori*. Successful eradication of this bacterium is associated with prolonged remission from ulcer recurrence, and possibly with permanent cure of the ulcer diathesis. Reinfection with *H. pylori* after eradication appears to be rare, at least in developed countries.

Eradication of *H. pylori* requires both acid suppression and antibiotic treatment. The most widely used regimen combines a proton pump inhibitor with clarithromycin and amoxicillin for one week. Metronidazole can replace amoxicillin in allergic patients.

16.2 Gastro-oesophageal reflux disease

Aims
1 To relieve symptoms.
2 To heal lesions of oesophagitis.
3 To prevent complications.

Relevant pathophysiology
Most patients have a functionally incompetent lower oesophageal sphincter that relaxes inappropriately, at times other than during swallowing. This allows excessive reflux of gastric contents, containing acid and pepsin, into the oesophagus. Once refluxed into the oesophagus, acidic material remains in contact with the mucosa for prolonged periods as a result of impairment of physiological clearance mechanisms. This will be further exacerbated by the presence of a hiatus hernia. Gastric acid secretion is usually normal. Some patients have delayed gastric emptying.

Drugs used in the treatment of gastro-oesophageal reflux disease

Antacids and antacid/alginate preparations
Antacids are discussed above. In combination with an alginate, they are thought to provide a protective coating to the lower oesophagus, preventing some contact with refluxed gastric contents.

Drugs that inhibit gastric acid secretion

H_2-receptor antagonists
These are discussed above. They have generally been less successful in the management of gastro-oesophageal reflux disease than in peptic ulcer. To be effective in the treatment of gastro-oesophageal reflux disease, they may have to be given in much higher doses than in peptic ulcer (e.g. ranitidine, 300 mg 6-hourly).

GASTRO-OESOPHAGEAL REFLUX DISEASE

1 Antacids and antacid/alginate combinations.
2 Drugs that inhibit gastric acid secretion:
  (a) H_2-receptor antagonists;
  (b) proton pump inhibitors: omeprazole, lansoprazole.

3 Drugs that act on oesophageal and/or gastric motility:
  (a) metoclopramide, domperidone;
  (b) cisapride.

Proton pump inhibitors
These drugs are discussed above. They are highly effective in treating all grades of gastro-oesophageal reflux disease. They are superior to H_2-receptor antagonists in controlling the symptoms of the condition, and in healing oesophagitis.

Comment. Based on the pathophysiology of the condition, it should be apparent that relapse will be rapid in most patients once treatment is withdrawn. Many patients, particularly those with severe grades of the condition, will require long-term treatment with a proton pump inhibitor. Patients with mild GORD may obtain sufficient symptom relief from an H_2-receptor antagonist taken as required.

Drugs that act on oesophageal and/or gastric motility

Metoclopramide, domperidone
These drugs are discussed in greater detail later in this Chapter. They may be effective in patients with mild grades of gastro-oesophageal reflux disease because of some of their actions on motility of the upper alimentary tract. They have a weak tonic effect on the lower oesophageal sphincter, they may improve oesophageal clearance, and may also improve gastric emptying. They are seldom effective alone. They may be combined with another agent, such as an H_2-receptor antagonist, but this may not be cost-effective. Metoclopramide is not recommended for long-

term use because of its adverse effects on the central nervous system (CNS) (see below).

Cisapride
Mechanism. This drug probably promotes motility in the upper gastrointestinal tract by causing release of acetylcholine from nerve endings in the myenteric plexus. It speeds up gastric emptying and oesophageal clearance and may increase lower oesophageal sphincter tone.

Pharmacokinetics. Cisapride is extensively protein bound and is metabolized extensively in the liver.

Adverse effects. No significant adverse effects have been reported to date.

Drug interactions. No clinically important interactions are known.

Clinical use and dose. In gastro-oesophageal reflux disease, cisapride is about as effective as a conventional dose of an H_2-receptor antagonist. Its use should probably be restricted to patients with mild degrees of severity. Usual dose is 10–20 mg three or four times daily. It can be combined with an H_2-receptor antagonist, but this may not be cost effective.

16.3 Diarrhoea and constipation

Diarrhoea
In all patients presenting with diarrhoea it is important to identify and eliminate a cause

where possible. If the cause is unclear, symptomatic relief may be helpful. The drugs used will depend upon the cause of the diarrhoea and are discussed below under the conditions that cause diarrhoea.

Irritable bowel syndrome

This common condition is the most frequent cause of chronic, recurrent abdominal pain. It may also cause upset of bowel habit, with diarrhoea, constipation or both. The pathophysiology is poorly understood. There are abnormal motility patterns in the bowel and patients may be unduly sensitive to distension or contraction of visceral smooth muscle. Some patients' diets are deficient in fibre. There is a relationship between psychological stress and symptoms in some patients.

Mebeverine is an antispasmodic agent which does not have significant anticholinergic effects. It is useful in relieving symptoms in some patients in a dose of 135 mg three times daily.

Enteric coated capsules of peppermint oil are useful in relieving gut spasm in some patients. The capsules may cause heartburn if bitten into.

Pancreatic insufficiency

A preparation of exogenous pancreatic enzymes containing trypsin, lipase and amylase is given for patients with chronic pancreatic exocrine insufficiency, as in chronic pancreatitis or cystic fibrosis. H_2-receptor antagonists may be given also in order to prevent denaturation of the pancreatic enzymes by gastric acid.

Drugs used in non-specific diarrhoea

Codeine phosphate

This is a useful agent for symptomatic control of diarrhoea. It raises intracolonic pressure and sphincter tone. It should not be given to patients with colonic diverticular disease and should be used only cautiously in patients with inflammatory bowel disease, and only under careful supervision.

Morphine

Kaolin and morphine mixture British Pharmaceutical Codex (BPC) is a time-honoured remedy containing only small quantities of morphine. It is unpalatable so is taken as a liquid.

Diphenoxylate

This is an opiate derivative. It is combined with atropine in the preparation Lomotil. It is more expensive than codeine phosphate and probably no better.

Loperamide

Loperamide is a synthetic opiate with some anticholinergic activity. It may cause dizziness or dryness of the mouth. The usual dose is 2 mg three or four times daily.

Constipation

Drugs used in non-specific constipation

Drugs which increase faecal bulk

These consist of non-absorbable polysaccharides as in bran, ispaghula or sterculia. They are generally effective in simple constipation, particularly where the intake of dietary fibre is poor. They are the agents of choice where treatment is likely to be prolonged.

Stimulant laxatives

These agents stimulate intestinal motility, probably through an effect on the myenteric nerve plexus. Examples are senna and bisacodyl. Prolonged use leads to hypotonicity of the bowel and thereby eventually exacerbates chronic constipation.

Stool softeners

The best known agent in this group is liquid paraffin. It acts by lubricating the faeces, which aids passage along the bowel. It may cause slight perianal irritation. Long-term use can lead to malabsorption of fat-soluble vitamins. It is not indicated for infants as inhalation of the liquid may produce a lipoid pneumonia.

Osmotic laxatives
These agents retain water in the bowel. They increase faecal bulk and moisten faeces. Examples are lactulose and salts of magnesium.

Comment. The commonest cause of constipation is lack of dietary fibre and most cases will respond to a high fibre diet. Both the constipation and diarrhoea associated with diverticular disease may improve with a high-fibre diet.

16.4 Nausea and vomiting

Aims
1 To establish an underlying cause and give specific treatment if possible.
2 To give symptomatic treatment.

Relevant pathophysiology
Vomiting is controlled by two separate brainstem centres: the vomiting centre and the chemoreceptor trigger zone. The trigger zone may be activated endogenously or exogenously by toxins or drugs such as opiates. Activation of the trigger zone stimulates the vomiting centre. The act of vomiting is controlled by the vomiting centre, mainly through vagal action. The vomiting centre has afferent input from the gut, higher cortical centres and the vestibular apparatus. Muscarinic receptors and histamine H_1-receptors are highly concentrated around the area of the vomiting centre.

Drugs used in treatment of vomiting

Anticholinergic drugs: hyoscine
Mechanism. They compete with acetylcholine at muscarinic receptors in the gut and CNS and have antispasmodic action in the gut wall. They may be successful in motion sickness because of their central action.

Adverse effects. Adverse effects are drowsiness plus typical anticholinergic effects of dry mouth, blurred vision and difficulty in micturition.

Clinical use. A 0.3–0.6 mg dose of hyoscine is usually adequate prophylaxis for motion sickness.

Antihistamines: promethazine
Mechanism. Antihistamines are competitive antagonists of histamine at H_1-receptors, acting mainly on the vomiting centre rather than on the chemoreceptor trigger zone. They have weak anticholinergic effects.

Adverse effects. Adverse effects are drowsiness, occasional insomnia and euphoria. Central effects are accentuated by alcohol.

Clinical use. Antihistamines are used in motion sickness or in vestibular disorders. They are widely used in the treatment of allergic rhinitis and other allergic reactions (Chapter 13, Section 13.2).
   Promethazine is given at a dose of 25 mg 8-hourly.

Dopamine antagonists

Phenothiazines: chlorpromazine, prochlorperazine
Mechanism. The general clinical pharmacology of phenothiazines is described in Chapter 19. These drugs act mainly on the chemoreceptor trigger zone. They have dopamine receptor antagonist properties as well as anticholinergic and other actions.

Adverse effects. Prolonged use may produce parkinsonian type tremor or other dyskinesias.

Clinical use and dose. Phenothiazines are effective in a variety of situations, including the vomiting of chronic renal failure and neoplastic disease, and drug-induced vomiting.
   Recommended doses are:

Chlorpromazine 25–50 mg 8-hourly.
Prochlorperazine 5–25 mg orally or 12.5 mg i.m.

Metoclopramide
Mechanism. Metoclopramide is a central dopamine receptor antagonist, effective at blocking stimuli to chemoreceptor trigger zone. It also has effects on upper gastrointestinal tract motility, as described above.

Adverse effects. Metoclopramide may cause acute extrapyramidal reactions, such as opisthotonous, oculogyric crisis or other dystonias. These can be treated with an intravenous anticholinergic agent, such as benzotropine.
   Metoclopramide raises serum prolactin levels and may cause gynaecomastia by virtue of its antidopaminergic effects.

Drug interactions. Metoclopramide potentiates the extrapyramidal side effects of phenothiazines.

Clinical use and dose. Metoclopramide is effective in most causes of vomiting, apart from motion sickness. The usual dose is 10 mg 8-hourly, orally or parenterally.

Domperidone
Mechanism. Domperidone is a dopamine antagonist, effective at the chemoreceptor trigger zone.

Adverse effects. Domperidone is less likely to cause extrapyramidal reactions than metoclopramide. It raises prolactin levels and may produce cardiac dysrhythmias following rapid intravenous injection.

Clinical use and dose. Domperidone is effective in most situations, especially nausea and vomiting related to cytotoxic drug therapy. The usual dose is 10–20 mg 4- to 8-hourly, orally or parenterally.

Cannabinoids: nabilone
Mechanism. Tetrahydrocannabinol is one of the active constituents of marijuana. Nabilone is a synthetic cannabinoid used in the treatment of nausea and vomiting during cytotoxic therapy. Mode of action is unclear.

Adverse effects. Nabilone causes drowsiness, dizziness and dryness of the mouth. Euphoria and hallucinations are rare.

Clinical use and dose. Nabilone at a dose of 1–2 mg twice daily is of value in treating patients receiving cytotoxic agents. Prolonged use may produce toxic effects on CNS.

Serotonin antagonists: ondansetron
Mechanism. Ondansetron is a selective antagonist of serotonin at 5-HT$_3$-receptors. Its exact mode of action in controlling nausea and vomiting is unclear but it has both CNS and peripheral actions.

Adverse effects. Ondansetron causes constipation and headache; flushing may occur.

Clinical use and dose. Ondansetron is indicated for the treatment of nausea and vomiting associated with cytotoxic therapy or radiotherapy. The dose and rate of administration depends on the severity of the problem and on the chemotherapy used.

16.5 Inflammatory bowel disease

Aims
1 To obtain remission in periods of relapse.
2 To prolong periods of remission.

Relevant pathophysiology
Ulcerative colitis and Crohn's disease are chronic inflammatory conditions of unknown aetiology. Both are characterized by episodes of remission and relapse. Drug treatment is aimed at controlling inflammation and bringing about remission. Treatment of these conditions is not only pharmacological but also

depends on psychological support, correction of nutritional deficiencies and possibly surgery.

Drugs used in the treatment of inflammatory bowel disease

Corticosteroids

These agents are discussed in detail in Chapter 14.

Steroids are of proven value in the treatment of acute relapses of ulcerative colitis and Crohn's disease. They may be given rectally, orally or intravenously depending on the extent and severity of the condition.

Steroids are of no value for ulcerative colitis in remission and should be withdrawn once clinical remission is achieved. There is no good evidence that long-term steroids help Crohn's disease.

Aminosalicylates

Mesalazine (a controlled release preparation of 5-aminosalicylic acid (5-ASA)), olsalazine (two molecules of 5-ASA linked by an azo bond that is split by colonic bacteria to release 5-ASA within the colon) and balsalazide (a pro-drug of 5-ASA).

Mechanism. It is thought that 5-ASA exerts a local anti-inflammatory effect.

Adverse effects. Blood dyscrasias, renal damage and (with olsalazine) watery diarrhoea

Clinical use. These drugs are used in the management of mild–moderate ulcerative colitis and in the maintenance of remission.

Azathioprine

Mechanism. This is an immunosuppressive agent which may be useful in improving control in patients with severe inflammatory bowel disease proving difficult to control on steroids and aminosalicylates.

Side effects. It may cause bone marrow suppression. It also reduces the immune response particularly to viral infection.

Clinical use. Patients on azathiprine should be told to report to their doctor immediately if they develop symptoms such as sore throat of a bleeding tendency. In addition, their blood count must be checked regularly.

16.6 Drugs adversely affecting gastrointestinal function

Virtually any drug may cause nausea, vomiting or diarrhoea and a detailed drug history is essential in patients with such complaints. Some specific drug-induced gastrointestinal problems are listed in Table 16.1.

Diarrhoea is common in patients receiving antibiotics. This is usually attributed to an alteration in the intracolonic bacterial flora. In some patients a colitis may result from antibiotic therapy: antibiotic-associated colitis, or pseudomembranous colitis. This is a result of the proliferation of *Clostridium difficile* in the bowel and the secretion of an endotoxin. Treatment of this condition depends on the prescription of an antibiotic, which is poorly absorbed when given orally. Two suitable agents are vancomycin and metronidazole.

DRUGS AFFECTING GASTROINTESTINAL FUNCTION

Drug	Comment
Antacids containing aluminium sucralfate	Constipation
Antacids containing magnesium	Diarrhoea
Oral iron salts	Nausea; constipation or diarrhoea (only nausea is dose-related); darkens stools as does bismuth
Bisphosphonates	Severe oesophagitis, oesophageal ulcers and erosions
Antibiotics	Oral *and/or* oesophageal candidiasis; diarrhoea
Aspirin/NSAIDs	Dyspepsia; gastric erosions (with or without significant bleeding); gastric ulcers; increased risk of perforation or bleeding of existing gastric or duodenal ulcer; NSAIDs may cause ulceration, stricture or perforation of small intestine; NSAIDs may promote relapse of inflammatory bowel disease
Oral potassium supplements	Ulceration or perforation at sites of stasis (e.g. oesophageal or intestinal stricture)

NSAIDs, non-steroidal anti-inflammatory drugs.

Table 16.1 Drugs which may adversely affect gastrointestinal function.

CHAPTER 17

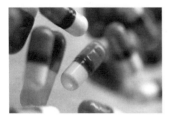

Drugs and the Blood

17.1 Anaemia and haematinics

Aims
1 To relieve symptoms.
2 To correct the underlying disorder.
3 To replace any deficiencies: iron, vitamin B_{12}, folic acid.

Relevant pathophysiology
The cellular constituents of the blood—the red cells, white cells and platelets—exist as a result of the balance between production and destruction. Anaemia occurs when the concentration of haemoglobin in the blood falls below the normal for the age and sex of the patient. The lower limits of normal are:
1 For adult males: 13.0 g/dl.
2 For adult females: 11.5 g/dl.
The balance between production and destruction may be disturbed by:
1 Blood loss.
2 Impaired red cell formation: haematinic deficiency or bone marrow depression.
3 Increased red cell destruction: haemolysis.
Iron, vitamin B_{12} and folic acid are essential for normal marrow function. Deficiency of any or all of these results in defective red cell synthesis and eventual anaemia. As each of the agents plays a different part in cellular production in the marrow, individual deficiencies are manifested in different ways. Accurate diagnosis is therefore essential before any specific agent is given. Lack of iron causes a hypochromic, microcytic anaemia with low serum ferri-tin. Lack of vitamin B_{12} or folic acid causes a macrocytic anaemia with a megaloblastic bone marrow. If the marrow is deprived of either or both vitamin B_{12} and folic acid the blood picture and the marrow look the same, but it is essential to determine which substance is missing. If folic acid is given to a patient who has vitamin B_{12} deficiency neurological damage, subacute combined degeneration of the cord may be provoked or aggravated.

Iron deficiency anaemia

Iron
As iron is usually absorbed from the gut, a satisfactory response is achieved in most patients when iron salts are given orally. Several ferrous salts are available. There is little to choose between them although they vary greatly in cost. The cheaper salts such as ferrous sulphate should be used unless gastrointestinal adverse effects are severe. Slow-release preparations should be avoided because of unreliable absorption. The duration of treatment, and its success, depends on the underlying cause of the anaemia. Haemoglobin should rise by approximately 1 g/week. The achievement of normal haemoglobin levels should then be followed by further treatment for 6 months in an attempt to replenish iron stores throughout the body.

Adverse effects
Some people cannot tolerate oral iron preparations. The main complaints are nausea,

epigastric discomfort, constipation and diarrhoea. A change in the ferrous salt form may help but improvement may be related to a lower content of iron in the alternative preparation.

Dose
Ferrous sulphate is given at a dose of 200 mg three times daily until anaemia is corrected and iron stores are replenished.

Parenteral iron
Oral iron therapy occasionally fails to achieve its objective because of lack of patient cooperation, severe adverse effects or gastrointestinal malabsorption. The total dose of parenteral iron required is calculated for each patient on the basis of body weight and haemoglobin level. Iron sorbitol is given by deep intramuscular injection only; initially 1.5 mg iron/kg to a maximum of 100 mg per injection. Iron dextran is now only available on a named patient basis as an alternative to iron sorbitol. Iron dextran may be given either by deep intramuscular injection or by slow intravenous infusion. In the latter case the patient must be carefully monitored for signs of hypersensitivity.

Megaloblastic anaemia

Vitamin B_{12}
Vitamin B_{12} deficiency demands that vitamin B_{12} should be injected in adequate doses for life. Usually the underlying disease, such as pernicious anaemia, cannot be corrected and a route that bypasses the defective absorption mechanism in the gut therefore must supply the vitamin. Treatment should correct the anaemia and then maintain a normal blood picture. It should arrest, reverse or prevent lesions of the nervous system and replenish depleted stores.

A dramatic response often follows within 2–3 days of the start of vitamin B_{12} therapy. Symptoms improve and the haemoglobin concentration rises progressively to normal. An early index of success is a rise in the reticulocyte count, which reaches a peak after about 1 week and then gradually declines to normal in the next 2 weeks.

Marrow changes reverse rapidly.

Adverse effects
These are rare and probably related to contamination or impurities in the injected solution.

Dose
Hydroxocobalamin is given at a dose of 1 mg daily by intramuscular injection for 1 week, then at 2 monthly intervals for life.

Folic acid
Folic acid deficiency in Western countries is frequently the result of low dietary intake. Less commonly it is the consequence of malabsorption. Pregnancy makes such demands on iron and folic acid stores in the mother that it has been routine for iron and folic acid to be prescribed throughout pregnancy. Recent evidence that periconceptional maternal folic acid deficiency is associated with the birth of infants with neural tube defects has led to the recommendation of the use of supplements of small doses of folic acid by women who are planning pregnancy and until at least 12 weeks gestation.

Dose
An oral dose of 5–15 mg daily is given initially, then 5 mg daily for 3–4 months, depending on the cause. When combined with iron for prophylactic use in pregnancy, 200–500 µg are given daily. A dose of 400 µg daily is recommended for routine periconceptional prophylaxis, but 5 mg daily is recommended for women who have already given birth to an infant with a neural tube defect.

Comment. Whatever the type of anaemia, a cause must always be sought. Anaemia is an observation, not a diagnosis, and there could be an important underlying cause requiring treatment.

17.2 Haemopoietic growth factors

These naturally occurring glycoproteins have a physiological role in the regulation of haemopoiesis. Most are synthesized by bone marrow stromal cells. Some act on pluripotent stem cells, whilst others are lineage specific and act only on committed progenitors. Molecular biological techniques have made possible the production of recombinant forms of some of the haemopoetic growth factors, and these are now in clinical use for a number of specialized indications. All these agents are given parenterally, usually by subcutaneous or sometimes by intravenous injection.

Erythropoietin

Physiologically, erythropoietin is synthesized in the kidney, and its synthesis is regulated by the oxygen tension in renal tissues. It acts on committed erythroid precursors to increase erythropoiesis. In severe renal failure erythropoietin production is defective and this contributes to the anaemia of renal disease. Recombinant human erythropoietin was the first of the growth factors to come into therapeutic use and is indicated for the treatment of anaemia associated with severe renal failure. Patients on dialysis and those not yet being dialysed are suitable. Haematinic deficiency, infections and aluminium accumulation should be ruled out as major contributory causes of anaemia before prescribing erythropoietin to renal patients. Potential adverse effects of erythropoietin include hypertension, clotting of vascular access sites, flu-like symptoms and seizures. It follows that erythropoietin is contraindicated in patients with uncontrolled hypertension.

Granulocyte-colony stimulating factor (G-CSF)

G-CSF is a growth factor that acts at relatively late stages of myelopoiesis in a lineage specific manner to enhance the production and function of neutrophils. Recombinant human G-CSF has been available for therapeutic use in recent years. It is effective in shortening the duration of neutropenia following myelosuppressive chemotherapy, including bone marrow transplantation. Its use should be confined to specialized haematology or oncology units. Its exact role even in these settings is still evolving; many trials are underway, but cost still limits its applications. It has also been used in the treatment of some forms of severe congenital neutropenia.

Granulocyte macrophage-colony stimulating factor (GM-CSF)

GM-CSF acts on committed progenitors of the myeloid lineage, at a stage earlier than G-CSF. These cells are capable of differentiating either into granulocytes or macrophages, and GM-CSF increases the production of both these types of cells. Recombinant human GM-CSF is used therapeutically for indications very similar to those for G-CSF, and again its use should be limited to specialized units (Chapter 13, Section 13.2).

17.3 Drug-induced blood conditions

Drug-induced blood loss

Drugs used to relieve pain and inflammation in rheumatoid and osteoarthritis are often associated with chronic, occult blood loss from the gastrointestinal tract. Aspirin ingestion is a well-recognized cause of this type of anaemia and all other non-steroidal anti-inflammatory drugs, e.g. indometacin, ibuprofen, etc., carry the same risk (Chapter 12, Section 12.2).

Drug-induced megaloblastic anaemia

Two important mechanisms result in drug-induced megaloblastic anaemia:

1 Interference with cellular DNA synthesis by cytotoxic drugs such as cytosine arabinoside, 5-fluorouracil or 6-mercaptopurine.

2 Interference with folate absorption or use of anticonvulsants such as phenytoin and phe-

nobarbital or the cytotoxic drug methotrexate, which inhibits dihydrofolate reductase.

Drug-induced sideroblastic anaemia

Some drugs and chemicals are involved in the aetiology of sideroblastic anaemia (a type of refractory anaemia) in a small proportion of patients. This can occur following administration of the antituberculous drug isoniazid, or following excessive alcohol consumption or exposure to lead.

Drug-induced marrow depression: aplastic anaemia

This occurs when cellular activity in the bone marrow is suppressed and is usually associated with the suppression of white cell and platelet formation (pancytopenia).

Drugs causing aplastic anaemia usually incorporate a benzene ring with closely attached amino groups. The outcome depends on the dose and the length of exposure, and to less well defined factors such as the degree of susceptibility, idiosyncrasy or hypersensitivity exhibited by an individual.

Certain drugs have a high risk of causing aplastic anaemia. These include cytotoxic drugs and gold salts. In other cases this is a rare idiosyncratic adverse effect, e.g. with antimicrobials such as chloramphenicol and the sulphonylureas.

Some drugs have a tendency to suppress white cells, e.g. phenylbutazone, meprobamate and chlorpromazine, while others inhibit platelet production, e.g. gold salts.

Unless the risk is acceptable, as in the treatment of some forms of malignant disease, aplastic anaemia should be prevented at all costs. The risks can be minimized by avoiding known marrow depressants, especially in patients with a history of allergy or idiosyncrasy. If the risk is accepted, then every effort should be made to detect early signs and symptoms of bone marrow depression. The patient should be advised that sore throat, fever, malaise and bruising may be an indication. Regular peripheral blood examination is of limited value but should nevertheless be performed. In many circumstances, where the degree of exposure to the causative agent has not been excessive, withdrawal of the agent leads to recovery within 2–3 weeks. Otherwise, intensive therapy is required, including comprehensive antibiotics, transfusion of blood products, administration of androgens and immunosuppressive agents and, in extreme cases, bone marrow transplantation.

Drug-induced haemolytic anaemia

A haemolytic anaemia occurs when the rate of red cell destruction is increased and red cells survive for a shorter time than the normal 100–200 days. Many drugs can reduce red cell survival:

1 Those that inevitably cause haemolytic anaemia (direct toxins).

2 Those that cause haemolysis because of hereditary defects in red cell metabolism.

3 Drugs that cause haemolysis because of the development of abnormal immune mechanisms.

Direct toxins

Drugs and chemicals that have powerful oxidant properties are likely to cause haemolysis. Damage by these agents results in fragmentation and irregular contraction of red cells, spherocytosis, basophilic stippling, Heinz bodies, methaemoglobinaemia and sulphaemoglobinaemia. In addition to many domestic and industrial agents, haemolytic anaemia may follow the use of sulphones in the treatment of leprosy and sulphonamides, including sulfasalazine and dapsone.

Interaction with hereditary defects in red cells

Glucose-6-phosphate dehydrogenase deficiency in Negroes and Mediterranean races may give some protection against falciparum malaria, but the red cells in these individuals are abnormally sensitive to oxidizing agents, resulting in haemolysis.

A large number of compounds may cause this haemolytic reaction, notably:

1 Antimalarial drugs, e.g. primaquine and pamaquin.

2 The sulphones used in leprosy, e.g. dapsone.

3 Some sulphonamides including cotrimoxazole.

4 Quinolone antibiotics including ciprofloxacin and nalidixic acid.

5 Water-soluble vitamin K analogues.

Immune mechanisms

Drugs can be associated with two immune haemolytic mechanisms.

Immune haemolytic anaemia

Antibodies may be formed against the drug or its metabolites. Antibodies can only be demonstrated *in vitro* in the presence of the drug. They may be stimulated by the drug binding directly to red cells forming a drug–red cell complex (the hapten cell mechanism, e.g. penicillin and cephalothin) or by the drug itself with subsequent adsorption on to the red cell surface. Activation of complement then causes lysis (immune complex mechanism, e.g. quinidine, *p*-aminosalicylic acid and rifampicin).

Autoimmune haemolytic anaemia

Antibodies are formed against the red cells. They can be demonstrated *in vitro* in the absence of the drug. This not uncommon form of haemolytic anaemia has been associated most often with the antihypertensive drug methyldopa. While at least 15% of patients on methyldopa develop a positive direct antiglobulin test, less than 0.1% develop overt haemolytic anaemia. If the drug is withdrawn, the haemoglobin level recovers but it may take many months for the antiglobulin test to become negative. Other drugs occasionally causing this kind of haemolytic anaemia are levodopa and mefenamic acid.

Drug-induced neutropenia

The most common adverse effect of drugs on the white cell system is a reduction in the number of neutrophils below the lower limit of normal (neutropenia).

Drugs causing this do so either as part of aplastic anaemia (pancytopenia) or as a selective neutropenia which does not involve the red cells or platelets. Drugs causing pancytopenia have been discussed in relation to aplastic anaemia.

Drugs may also cause selective neutropenia. This may occur either because of selective myeloid suppression, or because of an immune mechanism that may affect mature neutrophils only, or may also involve late myeloid precursors in the bone marrow (agranulocytosis). A large number of agents have been documented as causes of neutropenia, and a careful drug history should be taken in patients presenting with neutropenia. In most cases individual patient susceptibility to a particular drug underlies the problem. The following have a particular association with neutropenia:

Treatment of drug-induced neutropenia calls for:

1 Withdrawal of the drug.

2 Bone marrow examination.

3 In severe cases expert supportive care for the prevention and treatment of infection.

4 In selected cases treatment with myeloid growth factors, e.g. G-CSF, may be worthwhile.

DRUGS AND NEUTROPENIA

1 Antibiotics: chloramphenicol, cotrimoxazole.

2 Anti-inflammatory drugs: phenylbutazone.

3 Oral hypoglycaemics.

4 Psychotropic drugs: including phenothiazines and the antipsychotic agent clozapine which may cause agranulocytosis in 1 in 300 patients and which requires patient registration for use.

5 Anticonvulsants: carbamazepine.

6 Antithyroid drugs.

17.4 Drug-induced thrombocytopenia

Platelets may be reduced in number (thrombocytopenia) or function by drugs and chemicals. This may be part of aplastic anaemia or selective thrombocytopenia. The latter is a rare effect of various drugs, including thiazides, sulphonamides and sulphonylureas, and sodium valproate.

Drug-induced thrombocytopenia may occur as a result of suppression of platelet production or may involve an immune mechanism, akin to drug-induced immune haemolysis. A further mechanism is drug-induced platelet aggregation, for example, heparin-induced thrombocytopenia which is a consequence of antibody-dependent platelet aggregation (see Chapter 9, Section 9.3). Rarely, drugs may be involved in the aetiology of microangiopathic syndromes associated with thrombocytopenia (thrombotic thrombocytopenic purpura and haemolytic uraemic syndrome). Oral contraceptive agents and ciclosporin have occasionally been implicated in such cases.

Drug-induced thrombocytopenia should be treated according to haematological advice. The offending agent should be withdrawn and a bone marrow examination is usually indicated. If an immune mechanism is implicated, intravenous immunoglobulin treatment may be helpful. In others, particularly if platelet production is suppressed and the thrombocytopenia is severe or the patient is haemorrhagic, platelet transfusion may be indicated. Platelet transfusion should *not* be given in suspected cases of heparin-induced thrombocytopenia. Heparin should be stopped and advice regarding alternative anticoagulation sought from a haematologist. Platelet transfusions are also contraindicated in microangiopathic syndromes.

Comment. Whenever a disorder of blood cell formation is observed and an adverse drug effect suspected, take a careful drug history and consult reference books describing adverse effects.

CHAPTER 18

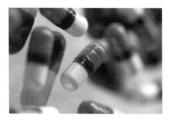

Anaesthesia and the Relief of Pain

18.1 Relevant pathophysiology

Sensory receptors for pain are found in all tissues of the body. A variety of noxious stimuli (thermal, chemical, mechanical or electrical) causes them to respond and lead to the subjective experience of pain.

1 The first-order afferent neurones transmitting pain impulses are of two types:

(a) The rapidly conducting (12–30 m/s) small-diameter myelinated fibres of the A group (delta).

(b) The slow (0.5–2 m/s) non-myelinated C fibres.

Both rapid and slow conducting fibres terminate in the dorsal horns of the spinal cord.

2 Second-order neurones carry the pain stimuli to the thalamus in the lateral spinothalamic tracts. Branches from both A and C fibres form synapses with cells in the dorsal horns of the spinal cord. A network of cells in this area, which includes the substantia gelatinosa, regulates transmission between the nociceptive neurones and those in the spinothalamic tract. Descending fibres from higher centres act to inhibit transmission.

3 From the thalamus, third-order neurones convey pain impulses to the postcentral gyri of the cerebral cortex. The thalamus is the main region responsible for the integration of pain input but the cortical area is concerned with the exact and meaningful subjective interpretation of pain.

The transducing qualities of free nerve endings are affected by chemical changes in the immediate vicinity, e.g. changes in the concentrations of hydrogen ions, substance P, 5-hydroxytryptamine (5-HT), histamine, bradykinin and eicosanoids. Bradykinin and related substances are formed in extracellular fluid whenever there is tissue damage and account for the vascular and exudative changes of inflammation. Bradykinin sensitizes and stimulates nerve endings and causes pain. The analgesic effects of aspirin and other non-steroidal anti-inflammatory drugs result from the impaired release of mediator by mechanisms including inhibition of prostaglandin synthesis (Chapter 12).

Within the central nervous system (CNS), opiate receptors are localized in the substantia gelatinosa of the spinal cord and the central grey matter of the brain stem. There are several subgroups. Mu and kappa receptors are responsible for analgesia and respiratory depression, while delta receptors bind endogenous enkephalins. Endogenous opiates (such as the enkephalins, endorphins and dynorphins) are released as neurotransmitters from specific opiate-containing neurones and act on receptors in these sites to modify pain sensation. These substances provide a rational basis for the use and actions of morphine-like drugs.

Transmitters in the pain pathway include substance P and other opioid peptides, biogenic amines like 5-HT and excitatory amino acids.

Principles of drug treatment

From a practical point of view, there are two types of pain:

1 Visceral pain, which is a dull, poorly localized pain, e.g. peritoneal pain.

2 Somatic pain, which is sharply defined, e.g. pain of a fractured femur.

Pain is a valuable symptom of underlying pathology and may be vital in the diagnosis of disease, e.g. in management of the acute abdomen. However, inadequate administration of relief to a patient in distress while steps are taken to confirm the diagnosis should be avoided.

There is a pronounced placebo effect in the treatment of pain. Thirty per cent of patients in pain experience some relief from a doctor taking an interest in their pain and prescribing any drug.

18.2 Opioid analgesics

Morphine

Mechanism of action

Morphine produces a range of depressant effects by a central action on mu opiate receptors within the CNS and in peripheral tissues.

The CNS effects include analgesia, euphoria and sedation; depression of respiration; depression of the vasomotor centre resulting in hypotension; cough suppression; release of antidiuretic hormone; miosis and nausea and vomiting. Peripheral effects include smooth muscle contraction with reduced motility of the gastrointestinal tract; reduced secretion of gastrointestinal tract; biliary spasm; urinary retention; constriction of bronchi partly as a result of histamine release; vasodilatation and itching.

Pharmacokinetics

Morphine is unreliably absorbed after oral administration and subject to high first-pass metabolism. However, there is a slow-release oral preparation that results in delayed but sustained therapeutic plasma morphine concentrations. The drug can be given intravenously, intramuscularly or subcutaneously. After intramuscular injection, peak brain concentrations occur between 30 and 45 min but relatively little of the administered drug crosses the blood–brain barrier.

The major route of elimination is conjugation with glucuronic acid to form morphine-3-monoglucuronide, which is excreted in the urine. Only a very small amount of free morphine appears in the urine, bile or faeces. About 90% of the administered dose is eliminated within the first 24 h.

Adverse effects

Many of the adverse effects of morphine represent an extension of its pharmacological effects as a result of relative overdosage (see below).

Drug interactions

Morphine delays the absorption of other drugs when they are given orally. In addition, its depressant effects are potentiated by other drugs such as phenothiazines and tricyclic antidepressants. Morphine will, in turn, potentiate the effect of most hypnotics and all volatile anaesthetic agents.

ADVERSE EFFECTS OF MORPHINE

1 Respiratory depression, periodic breathing or apnoea.
2 Hypotension.
3 Nausea and vomiting.
4 Constipation.
5 Tremor.
6 Urticaria and itch.
7 Tolerance and addiction to the drug.
These are rare when morphine is given during anaesthesia or for the relief of pain after surgery.

Clinical use and dose

1 The relief of visceral and traumatic pain.

2 The relief of anxiety and pain after myocardial infarction.

3 In acute left ventricular failure (pulmonary oedema) to reduce preload by venodilation (Chapter 7).

4 Before, during and after anaesthesia, as part of a balanced anaesthetic technique.

The usual dose for relief of severe pain is 10–15 mg i.m. every 2–3 h. For postoperative pain morphine is increasingly given intravenously using syringe drivers activated by the patient (patient-controlled analgesia).

5 Opiates, particularly codeine derivatives, are used as antitussives (Chapter 11) and anti-diarrhoeal agents (Chapter 16).

Other opioid analgesics

Many opioid drugs are available and the properties of some are summarized in Table 18.1. Others such as pentazocine, butorphanol, dextromoramide, levorphanol and dipipanone have very limited use.

Papaveretum

This is a solution containing the pure alkaloids of opium. It has the same uses as morphine.

Diamorphine or heroin

This is more potent and more lipid soluble than morphine. It is metabolized to mono-acetylmorphine and then morphine. It is claimed to be less emetic than morphine but there is little evidence for this. Its physical properties make it particularly suitable for administration into the epidural space to relieve postoperative pain in patients undergoing major surgery. It is otherwise rarely used.

Codeine or methylmorphine

The actions of codeine are similar to those of morphine but it is a less potent analgesic. It is used as a cough suppressant, and also to con-

OPIOID ANALGESIC DRUGS

	Dose (mg)	Route	Duration of action (h)	Notes
Natural opiates				
Morphine	10–15	i.m., s.c.	4	
	10–30	oral as sustained release	8	Slow onset, needs regular dosage to be useful
Papaveretum	20	i.m., s.c.	4	
Semi-synthetic				
Diamorphine	5	i.m., s.c.	4	
Oxycodone	10	i.m.	4–6	Used in chronic pain
	30	Rectal	4–8	
Dihydrocodeine	50	i.m., s.c.	4	
	30–60	Oral	4	
Synthetic				
Pethidine	100–150	i.m., s.c.	2–3	
Buprenorphine	0.3	i.m., s.c.	8	Partial agonist
	0.3	Sublingual	8	Slow onset
Methadone	5–10	Oral/ i.m.	5–6	Used in chronic pain
Tramadol	50–100	Oral	5–6	Used in chronic pain
	100	i.m.	5–6	Used in postoperative pain

Table 18.1 Comparison of opioid analgesic drugs.

trol diarrhoea, and in combination with aspirin or paracetamol as a mild analgesic. It is metabolized to morphine.

Pethidine

This is a synthetic narcotic analgesic that has a more rapid onset than morphine and a shorter duration of action. Smooth muscle contraction is less prominent and therefore it is used in biliary and ureteric colic. Constipation does not occur to the same extent. One of its metabolites, norpethidine, is active and may accumulate and cause convulsions in patients with hepatic or renal impairment. The risk of toxicity may be increased in patients taking other drugs which induce hepatic enzymes.

Fentanyl, alfentanil and remifentanil

These are opioids used intravenously during anaesthesia. They have a very short duration of action (20–30 min for fentanyl). Fentanyl is lipophilic and can be absorbed transdermally and by inhalation. Remifentanil was designed to be metabolized rapidly by tissue esterases. Its effects dissipate promptly even after prolonged infusion and so it is useful as part of a total intravenous anaesthetic technique.

Partial agonists and opiate antagonists

Buprenorphine

This is a partial agonist at mu opiate receptors. It is a potent long-lasting analgesic drug that can be absorbed sublingually. Dependence or addiction potential is claimed to be low. Respiratory depression is not reversed by the opiate antagonist naloxone except in very high dose (15 mg or more). Hallucinations can occur. Note that it is not advisable to give buprenorphine to augment inadequate analgesia from morphine and more potent agents.

Tramadol

This synthetic opioid acts via partial agonism at mu receptors and via activation of monoaminergic (5–HT and noradrenaline) pathways responsible for spinal inhibition of pain. Advantages include a low incidence of respiratory depression and a low potential for abuse. The main disadvantages are nausea and vomiting.

Nalbuphine and meptazinol

These are synthetic opioids used parenterally in the treatment of surgical and chronic pain.

Naloxone

This is a specific opioid antagonist without agonist activity. It is used to antagonize all of the actions of opioid analgesic drugs. It precipitates withdrawal symptoms if given to addicts or the neonate born to a mother addicted to narcotics. Naloxone may be given intravenously or intramuscularly in a dose of 0.4–1.2 mg. When given intravenously, the onset of action occurs within 1–2 min and it lasts 20–30 min. Thus, if it is used to reverse an opioid that has a longer duration of action it may have to be given repeatedly, preferably by intravenous infusion.

18.3 Local (regional) anaesthesia

Transmission of impulses in peripheral nerves is associated with depolarization of the nerve cell membrane, which is the result of an increased membrane permeability to sodium ions. Local anaesthetic agents produce a localized, reversible block to nerve conduction by reducing the permeability of the membrane to sodium. Most of the clinically useful local anaesthetic agents act by reversibly blocking the sodium channel through a direct interaction between the anaesthetic molecule and a few amino acids of the receptor protein. These agents may exist in the charged and uncharged form in solution. The uncharged form diffuses more readily through the neural sheath while the charged form attaches to the receptor. The relative proportion of the charged and uncharged form depends upon the pK_a of the drug, the pH of the solution and the pH at the injection site. The smaller the nerve fibre, the more sensitive it is to local anaesthetic block. Thus it is possible, but practically difficult, to block pain and autonomic fibres and leave proprioception, i.e. touch and movement, intact.

Local anaesthetics are administered locally and do not rely on the circulation to take them to their site of action. However, uptake into the systemic circulation terminates their effects. The rate of systemic absorption is determined by the factors listed below.

A vasoconstrictor, such as adrenaline, may be used in solution with the local anaesthetic to delay systemic absorption, prolong the local block and limit toxicity.

Local anaesthetics are weak bases with pK_a values between 7.5 (mepivacaine) and 8.9 (procaine). Marked changes in the ratio of ionized to non-ionized drug occur with changes in acid–base balance. They are extensively bound to plasma proteins. Differences in binding between agents may influence the intensity and duration of effect and placental transfer.

Local anaesthetic drugs are of two types:
1 *Esters*, e.g. procaine, which are metabolized in the plasma by esterases.
2 *Amides*, e.g. lidocaine (lignocaine), which are extensively metabolized in the liver, the clearance being dependent on liver blood flow. In the liver, *N*-dealkylation of the tertiary amine produces a more soluble secondary amine that may be active and is in turn dealkylated. Very little of an injected dose of local anaesthetic is excreted unchanged in the urine.

The physicochemical and pharmacokinetic properties of several local anaesthetics are shown in Table 18.2.

Lidocaine

Lidocaine (lignocaine) has both local and systemic effects. Local effects include loss of pain and other sensations, vasodilatation and loss of motor power. Systemic effects occur following absorption from the site of local administration or following systemic administration and result from generalized membrane stabilization. Myocardial excitability is

SYSTEMIC ABSORPTION OF LOCAL ANAESTHETICS

1 Pharmacokinetic properties of the drug.
2 Vascularity of the injection site.
3 Concentration of the solution used.
4 Rate of injection.

LOCAL ANAESTHETIC DRUGS

Agent	Relative dosage	pK_a	$t_{1/2}$ (h)	Onset	Duration
Amides					
Lidocaine	1.0	7.9	1.6	Rapid	Medium
Bupivacaine	0.25	8.1	2.7	Slow	Long
Prilocaine	1.0	7.9	–	Slow	Medium
Ropivacaine	0.33	8.1	3.3	Slow	Long
Esters					
Cocaine	1.0	–	*	Slow	Medium
Procaine	2.0	8.9	*	Slow	Short
Tetracaine (amethocaine)	0.25	8.5	*	Slow	Long
Chloroprocaine	3.0	8.7	*	–	–

* $t_{1/2}$ is very short owing to hydrolysis in plasma.

Table 18.2 Comparison of local anaesthetic drugs.

depressed. Adverse effects are a consequence of overdosage and include anxiety and excitement progressing to sedation, disorientation, lingular and circumoral anaesthesia, restlessness, twitching, tremors, convulsions and unconsciousness. Coma may be accompanied by apnoea and cardiovascular collapse.

A 1 or 2% solution of lidocaine is used for local infiltration, intravenous regional or extradural analgesia. The maximum safe dose for a 70 kg man is 200 mg without adrenaline and 400 mg with adrenaline. The first effects are noted 5–10 min after administration, and the duration of action is of the order of 2–3 h. Lidocaine is also used in the treatment of ventricular tachyarrhythmias (Chapter 6) as it possesses class I antiarrhythmic activity.

Other local anaesthetics

Prilocaine

This is equipotent with lidocaine and can be used for all types of local analgesia. It is less toxic than lidocaine because of its greater degree of tissue uptake. Large doses may produce methaemoglobinaemia, which is caused by a metabolite, O-toluidine. The maximum dose is 300–400 mg. The drug is widely used for intravenous regional anaesthesia. Reformulated in a mixture of prilocaine and lidocaine crystals (eutectic mixture of local anaesthetic—EMLA), it is absorbed transdermally and gives good surface analgesia for procedures such as venepuncture in children.

Bupivacaine

This is an amide that is four times as potent as lidocaine and considerably longer lasting. It is available as a 0.25, 0.5 or 0.75% solution and the maximum dose is 100–150 mg. This agent must not be used for intravenous regional anaesthesia as it is cardiotoxic in high doses.

Ropivacaine

Ropivacaine was developed in an attempt to reduce cardiotoxicity. It is similar to bupivacaine but may cause less motor block and cardiotoxicity, although this may simply relate to reduced potency.

Cocaine

This is an ester and is unique in that as well as local anaesthetic properties it is a CNS stimulant. It is used clinically for topical analgesia and for its central euphoriant effects in the management of terminal malignant disease, often together with opiate analgesics.

18.4 General anaesthesia

Modern anaesthesia is characterized by the balanced technique in which drugs are used specifically to produce analgesia, sleep, muscle relaxation and abolition of reflexes. Nowadays, a single drug is rarely used to produce all the components of surgical anaesthesia.

Intravenous anaesthetic agents

These drugs are used to produce a rapid and pleasant induction of sleep. In most cases, anaesthesia will be maintained by other agents and thus it is rapidity of onset and not brevity of action that is the most desirable property. The mechanism of action of these agents remains unclear. They are all highly lipid-soluble agents and cross the blood–brain barrier rapidly. Their rapid onset of action is a result of this rapid transfer into the brain and high cerebral blood flow. Action is terminated by distribution of the drugs away from the brain to less well perfused tissues.

Non-barbiturate anaesthetics

Propofol

Propofol is the most widely used intravenous anaesthetic. It is a phenolic derivative emulsified with soybean oil and egg phosphatide. After administration of 2–2.5 mg/kg, sleep occurs in one arm–brain circulation time (15–20 s) but this may be delayed in patients with cardiac disease or shock. Loss of consciousness is pleasant and lasts for 2–5 min. Recovery is rapid following redistribution of propofol from the brain to other tissues. Elimination is faster than with other intravenous anaesthetics because of glucuronide conjugation in the liver. There is thus no pronounced after-effect. Similarly, infusion of the drug does not produce significant cumulation, making it suitable for total intravenous anaesthesia. Advantages include depression of upper airway reflexes and an antiemetic effect; disadvantages are hypotension, respiratory depression and pain on injection.

Etomidate

This is an imidazole derivative with a very short duration of action owing to rapid redistribution. It has minimal effect on myocardial contractility and is preferred in very sick patients. It is metabolized in the liver and has a half-life of 4.6 h. Injection may be painful and causes muscle twitching with involuntary movements. Infusion of the drug blocks 11-β-hydroxylation in the adrenal cortex, inhibiting cortisol synthesis.

Ketamine

This is a derivative of phencyclidine. It may be administered intravenously or intramuscularly and has both analgesic and anaesthetic properties. It is now used infrequently in the UK but is given extensively in underdeveloped countries. It produces full surgical anaesthesia but the form of this anaesthesia is different from other agents like barbiturates. Adverse effects include hypertension, hallucinations and confusion.

Barbiturates

Thiopental (thiopentone)

Thiopental, the sulphur analogue of pentobarbitone, was once the most widely used intravenous anaesthetic. After administration, the initial decay of plasma concentration is very rapid and the half-life of the initial distribution phase is 2.5 min. Elimination is by hepatic metabolism and the terminal half-life is 6.2 h (Table 18.3).

The adverse effects of thiopental include respiratory depression, myocardial depression and vasodilatation. Laryngeal reflexes are not depressed and laryngospasm may occur. The drug has no analgesic properties. Thiopental, like all barbiturates, may exacerbate porphyria.

Methohexitone

This is an oxybarbiturate that is three times as potent as thiopental. The initial decline in plasma concentrations because of distribution is similar to that seen after thiopental but the elimination phase is more rapid. Adverse effects include muscle twitching and involuntary movements.

Inhalation anaesthetic agents

These agents, usually with others, such as intravenous analgesics, are used to maintain a state of general anaesthesia after induction. The depth of anaesthesia produced by these drugs is related to the tension or the partial pressure of the agent in the arterial blood.

ANAESTHETIC INDUCTION AGENTS

Drug	Distribution volume (l/kg)	Clearance (ml/min)	Plasma half-life $t_{1/2}$ (h)
Propofol	5.0	1500	2.0
Etomidate	4.5	740	4.6
Ketamine	3.3	1296	3.4
Thiopental (thiopentone)	1.6	144	6.2
Methohexitone	1.1	825	1.6

Table 18.3 Comparison of intravenous anaesthetic agents.

Because the alveolar epithelium of the lung presents virtually no barrier to their diffusion, the alveolar concentration or partial pressure of the drug in the alveoli determines the depth of anaesthesia. This alveolar concentration is influenced by the factors listed below:

As a general rule, drugs with low blood-gas solubility, such as nitrous oxide and sevoflurane, act rapidly and drugs with a high blood-gas solubility, such as ether, act slowly.

The potency of these agents is related to, but is not dependent on, fat solubility. The minimum alveolar concentration (MAC) is the alveolar concentration that produces a state of surgical anaesthesia in 50% of patients. Put another way, it is the dose that abolishes movement in response to incision in 50% of patients. MAC is a population median that varies with age and other factors.

In practice, clinical signs are used to monitor anaesthetic administration. Depth of anaesthesia monitors continue to be research tools rather than practical theatre devices.

Nitrous oxide

This is a gas at room temperature. It cannot produce surgical anaesthesia when administered alone as its MAC is over 100%. It is used in a concentration of 50% to produce analgesia. Prolonged exposure to nitrous oxide may result in bone marrow depression.

Isoflurane

This is the most commonly administered inhalational anaesthetic agent. It is a halogenated ether that is a liquid at room temperature and must be vaporized before use. Over 99% of an administered dose is excreted unchanged by the lungs and the remainder is metabolized. In common with other volatile anaesthetics, it depresses the respiratory and cardiovascular systems but causes less myocardial depression and arrhythmias than other agents.

The MAC is 1.2% and it is normally given as a 0.5–2% concentration in a mixture of oxygen and nitrous oxide.

Desflurane

This differs from isoflurane by the substitution of a fluorine for a chlorine atom. It boils at room temperature and so requires a heated, pressurized vapouriser. Its solubility is similar to that of nitrous oxide allowing rapid uptake and, more importantly, rapid elimination of the drug. Its properties are otherwise similar to those of isoflurane.

Sevoflurane

Like desflurane this is an ether completely halogenated with fluorine atoms. Its low solubility allows rapid emergence from anaesthesia and its low level of airway irritation make it very suited for inhalational induction of anaesthesia, e.g. in children.

Halothane

This is a halogenated hydrocarbon. The liver metabolizes 20%; hepatic damage very rarely occurs 7–10 days after halothane anaesthesia, especially following repeated exposures, because of an immunological response to one of its metabolites. This has virtually abolished the use of halothane in adults. Arrhythmias, bradycardia and myocardial depression are more troublesome than with other volatile agents.

Enflurane

An halogenated ether, its properties are similar to those of halothane. As the liver

---

FACTORS AFFECTING ALVEOLAR CONCENTRATION OF ANAESTHETICS

1 The concentration of the drug in the inspired gas.
2 Alveolar ventilation.
3 Cardiac output.
4 The solubility of the drug in the blood.

metabolizes much less enflurane than halothane the risk of hepatitis is reduced.

18.5 Neuromuscular blocking drugs

When an electrical impulse in a motor nerve reaches the nerve ending it releases acetylcholine at the neuromuscular junction. Acetylcholine acts on nicotinic cholinergic receptors on the muscle membrane, resulting in a wave of depolarization. The acetylcholine is then destroyed rapidly by a specific cholinesterase.

Neuromuscular blocking drugs may interfere with neurotransmission in one of two ways:

1 Prolongation of the normal depolarization, e.g. suxamethonium.

2 Competitive inhibition of acetylcholine at the receptors, e.g. vecuronium, atracurium.

These drugs are used during anaesthesia to:

1 Produce muscle paralysis for any operation which will be assisted by neuromuscular blockade, but particularly for abdominal surgery.

2 Facilitate tracheal intubation.

After administration, the anaesthetist must always ventilate the patient's lungs because paralysis includes all voluntary muscle, notably the respiratory muscles. The use of these drugs is an integral part of a balanced anaesthetic technique, but great care must be taken to ensure that the patient is unconscious and anaesthetized and not just paralysed.

Factors that influence the action of neuromuscular blocking drugs are listed below.

Suxamethonium

This is a very short-acting depolarizing neuromuscular blocking drug. A dose of 1 mg/kg produces muscle fasciculations within 1 min followed by complete paralysis for 5–10 min.

Respiration must be maintained artificially. The drug is broken down very rapidly by plasma cholinesterase. In patients with the genetically determined abnormality and atypical enzyme, paralysis is prolonged for 6–24 h and artificial ventilation of the lungs must be continued throughout this period. Adverse effects of suxamethonium include bradycardia, muscle pains and raised intraocular pressure.

Non-depolarizing muscle relaxants

Vecuronium

This is an aminosteroid that produces competitive neuromuscular paralysis. It has replaced the traditional relaxants tubocurarine, a benzylisoquinolinium compound, and pancuronium, also an aminosteroid. Its advantages are its lack of effects on the heart and an intermediate duration of action (20–40 min). Rocuronium is structurally similar. Duration of action is the same as vecuronium but its onset is more rapid.

Neuromuscular blockade may be reversed at the end of surgery by administering an anticholinesterase such as neostigmine. This drug

FACTORS AFFECTING NEUROMUSCULAR BLOCKADE

1 Muscle blood flow (the most important factor). Muscles with high blood flow have the earliest onset and shortest duration of action.

2 Changes in temperature.

3 pH.

4 Potassium concentrations influence the degree of paralysis.

5 Aminoglycoside antibiotics prolong competitive blockade by reducing acetylcholine release.

6 Drugs that produce central muscle relaxation, e.g. benzodiazepines or isoflurane, prolong the muscle paralysis.

7 Renal disease, as most competitive blockers are excreted unchanged in the kidney to a greater or lesser extent. Atracurium is, however, metabolized in the blood.

8 Hereditary atypical cholinesterase markedly prolongs the effect of suxamethonium.

is always given with atropine or glycopyrrolate, which prevent the muscarinic effects of acetylcholine and allow the nicotinic effects to be manifest.

Atracurium

This is a benzylisoquinolinium compound with few cardiovascular side effects. It has an intermediate duration of action because of rapid non-enzymatic degradation in plasma and is particularly favoured in patients with renal or hepatic disease. The principal disadvantage is histamine release. This can be avoided by using cisatracurium, an isomer of atracurium, which does not provoke histamine release.

Mivacurium

Mivacurium is also a benzylisoquinolinium compound. It is hydrolysed rapidly by plasma cholinesterase and has a shorter duration of action than atracurium or vecuronium, making it suitable for shorter procedures.

CHAPTER 19

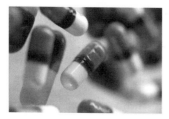

Drugs and Psychiatry

The last 50 years have seen major changes in psychiatric practice, with the advent of effective psychotropic drugs and the trend away from custodial to community care. The introduction of the phenothiazines in the 1950s transformed the lives of many patients with schizophrenia by abolishing troublesome symptoms and permitting a return to more normal behaviour. Next came the antidepressants, a welcome alternative to the effective but to some, controversial, electroconvulsive therapy. Since the 1960s lithium has been used effectively in acute mania, as prophylaxis in bipolar affective illness and more recently as adjunctive therapy for refractory depression. The 1960s also saw the introduction of chlordiazepoxide, the first clinical use of benzodiazepines. These sedative and anxiolytic agents were a welcome improvement upon the more dangerous barbiturates they replaced but their widespread use has led to concerns over dependency. A relatively quiescent couple of decades then gave way to an explosion of new pharmacotherapies. Antidepressant treatments expanded, first with the introduction of selective serotonin reuptake inhibitors followed by a range of other novel agents. Lithium now shares a stage with several anticonvulsant drugs shown to be effective as mood stabilisers. The management of schizophrenia and related psychoses has benefited from a new generation of antipsychotics with improved side effect profile and, particularly in the case of clozapine, evidence of improved efficacy. Most recently, pharmacotherapy for substance use disorders and dementia has also been the focus of renewed interest.

The classification of psychiatric disorders remains heavily dependent upon the identification of clusters of symptoms, and as a result diagnostic categories have a disconcerting tendency to merge. In general, where a particular illness does not fall clearly into a diagnostic category, treatment is best directed at relief of the predominating symptoms. Table 19.1 presents a working outline of the major categories in which drug treatment is likely to be required.

Comment. Elucidation of the cause of psychiatric symptoms is frequently difficult. It is important to try to characterize the principal underlying abnormality, as specific drug treatment is available for most of these categories. Misdiagnosis may exacerbate psychiatric symptoms; for example, sedative benzodiazepines given to a depressed patient may lead to further impairment of function and even increased risk of suicide. Tricyclic antidepressants may precipitate or aggravate psychotic symptoms in a patient with schizophrenia.

PSYCHIATRIC DISORDERS IN WHICH DRUG TREATMENTS ARE COMMONLY USED

Acute and chronic organic brain syndromes (including delirium, dementia and drug-related psychoses)
Bipolar affective (manic-depressive) disorder
Unipolar depression (psychotic and non-psychotic)
Schizophrenia and delusional disorders (paranoid psychoses)
Generalized anxiety and panic disorders
Phobias
Obsessive compulsive disorder
Less commonly, complications of drug dependence, alcohol misuse and personality disorder may require drug treatment

Table 19.1 Psychiatric disorders in which drug treatments are commonly used.

19.1 Neuroleptic drugs (antipsychotics, major tranquillizers)

Aims

The main aims are to inhibit the most florid subjective and behavioural disturbances of psychosis, and to restore the patient to as near normal a life in society as possible. Some novel antipsychotics also aim to diminish 'negative symptoms' of schizophrenia such as amotivation, flattened affect and social withdrawal.

Relevant pathophysiology

The neuroleptics are used in acute schizophrenia to diminish disturbance as a consequence of delusional thinking, hallucinations, inappropriate behaviour and anxiety. In chronic schizophrenia maintenance neuroleptic therapy reduces risk of relapse. Novel agents may also reduce negative symptoms more resistant to conventional neuroleptics. In affective disorders neuroleptics are used to control manic symptoms, and in depression where delusions, or anxiety and agitation are prominent. They are also used to treat drug-related psychoses.

The pathophysiology of the psychoses is still unclear and the mechanisms by which drugs exert their effect are still largely hypothetical. The 'dopamine hypothesis', which proposes an over-activity of the brain dopamine system in

schizophrenia, is the most favoured explanation for the antipsychotic effects of neuroleptics. The finding of increased dopamine concentrations in the brains of both treated and untreated patients with schizophrenia, together with the dopamine receptor antagonistic effects of neuroleptics, are in keeping with this hypothesis. On the other hand, 'atypical' neuroleptics such as clozapine, which have additional pharmacological properties, may be effective where typical neuroleptics have failed. Furthermore, traditional neuroleptic agents have little effect upon the 'negative' symptoms of schizophrenia. Thus it is important to recognize that although the 'dopamine hypothesis' might help to explain some of the therapeutic effects of neuroleptics, it does not in itself explain the pathophysiology of schizophrenia.

Conventional neuroleptics

Mechanism

Neuroleptic antipsychotics act as competitive antagonists of dopamine (particularly D_2) receptors in the central nervous system and compete for dopamine binding sites *in vitro*. Although all have similar efficacy, they show a range of other pharmacological properties that might contribute to their therapeutic effects and which are also of importance in determining the profile of adverse effects for any individual drug.

1 Muscarinic blockade causing anticholinergic activity is considerable with thioridazine and much less with fluphenazine and haloperidol.

2 Alpha$_1$-adrenoceptor blockade is prominent with chlorpromazine and thioridazine and less so with fluphenazine.

3 Histaminergic (H$_1$) blockade results in sedation most commonly with chlorpromazine and thioridazine.

4 Dopaminergic blockade is greater with 'high-potency' drugs such as haloperidal. This is also closely linked to propensity for adverse extrapyramidal (parkinsonian) side effects (EPS).

EPS may need to be controlled by reduction in the dose of neuroleptic or temporary co-administration of anticholinergic drugs such as procylidine, trihexyphenidyl (benzhexol), orphenadrine or benzatropine (benztropine) (Chapter 20, Section 20.9).

Pharmacokinetics

Chlorpromazine, the prototype neuroleptic, is absorbed orally and metabolized by the liver to many active and inactive metabolites. It has a plasma half-life of over 16h that, together with the long-lived active metabolites, makes once-daily dosing practical although rarely used. No clear-cut therapeutic range can be defined because of the presence of unmeasured active metabolites and a wide range of individual responses in patients. Plasma or urine drug levels are only of help in assessing compliance. First-pass metabolism is immense, of the order of 80%, making intramuscular administration considerably more potent than the oral alternative.

Adverse reactions

Dose-related adverse reactions from known pharmacological properties include those listed below.

Clinical use and dose

Chlorpromazine: orally 75–300 mg daily, increasing up to 1 g gradually if required. Chlorpromazine: intramuscular injection, 25–50 mg 6- to 8-hourly as required to control acute symptoms. Haloperidol: orally 1.5–

ADVERSE EFFECTS OF CONVENTIONAL NEUROLEPTICS

Dose-related adverse reactions from known pharmacological properties.

1 Extrapyramidal side effects (EPS), caused by dopamine receptor blockade, including: (i) acute dystonia; (ii) parkinsonism; (iii) akathisia; and (iv) tardive dyskinesia—involuntary choreoathetoid movements which, unlike other EPS, may persist even after withdrawal of the neuroleptic drug. Tardive dyskinesia may be aggravated by anticholinergic drugs and treatment is generally unsatisfactory. Benzodiazepines, diazepam and clonazepam may be helpful.

2 Increased prolactin (also resulting from dopaminergic blockade), e.g. galactorrhoea, infertility and impotence.

Hypersensitivity reactions not related to dose.

1 Cholestatic jaundice with portal infiltration occurs in 2–4% of patients, usually early in treatment. It presents the biochemical features of cholestasis and resolves slowly on drug withdrawal.

3 Anticholinergic effects, e.g. blurred vision, constipation, urinary hesitancy, dry mouth, tachycardia or arrhythmias.

4 Alpha$_1$–adrenoceptor blockade, e.g. postural hypotension.

5 Histamine$_1$–receptor blockade, e.g. sedation.

6 Neuroleptic malignant syndrome (potentially fatal hyperthermia, muscle rigidity and autonomic dysfunction).

7 Hypothermia in the elderly.

8 Other adverse effects such as confusion, nightmares and insomnia and weight gain.

2 Agranulocytosis occurs rarely.

3 Skin rashes, including photosensitivity dermatitis and urticaria, may be seen.

3 mg, 2–3 times daily with doses of up to 120 mg daily in treatment resistant cases.

Neuroleptics administered in lower doses are used in nausea and vomiting (Chapter 16, Section 16.4), hiccough, vertigo and labyrinthine disturbances, and during drug withdrawal reactions. They are also widely used as premedication in anaesthesia (Chapter 18, Section 18.4). Other psychiatric indications are mentioned above.

Novel (atypical) neuroleptics

These include clozapine, risperidone, olanzapine, quetiapine, zotepine and amisulpride. They differ from conventional neuroleptics (and from each other) in their pattern of receptor binding, e.g. clozapine has affinity for 5-hydroxytryptamine (5-HT) and D$_4$ receptors in addition to the more conventional sites listed above. All atypicals share a reduced propensity to cause EPS (most importantly tardive dyskinesia). Claims have been made for their effectiveness in treating negative symptoms but only clozapine has been demonstrated clearly to be superior to conventional neuroleptics in treatment-resistant patients.

Other adverse effects of atypicals include weight gain (most commonly with clozapine, olanzapine and quetiapine) and sedation. Clozapine may cause agranulocytosis and prescription is restricted initially to hospital patients who can be provided with weekly blood monitoring.

Depot neuroleptics

Long acting depot neuroleptic preparations play an important part in the community maintenance of more disabled and therefore poorly compliant psychiatric patients. A number of different neuroleptics are used in this way. Commonly used examples are fluphenazine and flupentixol (flupenthixol). Fluphenazine is a phenothiazine derivative. As the decanoate or enanthate ester it can be given as a depot by intramuscular injection at intervals of 14–40 days. Adverse effects of fluphenazine are similar to those of chlorpromazine but sedation and anticholinergic adverse effects are less common. EPS are correspondingly more common, particularly dystonia and akathisia or restlessness. Liver and bone marrow toxicity and skin rashes have been reported, as with most other phenothiazines. Flupentixol is a thioxanthine, and as such is somewhat less sedating than other classes of neuroleptic. It is more likely to cause EPS.

Dose

Fluphenazine decanoate: 25–100 mg by injection into the gluteal muscles every 15–40 days determined by response and side effects. A test dose (12.5 mg) should be given when treatment is begun, to assess possible extrapyramidal reactions.

Flupentixol decanoate: 40–400 mg (test dose 20 mg) similarly administered.

Comment. Neuroleptic antipsychotic drugs play a central role in the initial treatment and long-term management of psychoses. The dose should be determined individually from response and adverse effects. Novel drugs (with the exception of clozapine) are increasingly prescribed now as first-choice interventions. Ineffectiveness after a minimum of six weeks treatment on any one drug should result in a trial of a second drug of a different class. Clozapine should be considered if there is lack of response to two neuroleptics. Depot intramuscular preparations are useful for long-term outpatient management. Adverse effects are common and may be disabling or even dangerous. Patients on long-term antipsychotic medication should remain under close medical supervision.

Neuroleptics should not be used in the management of simple anxiety as an alternative to anxiolytics, minor tranquillizers or other forms of treatment.

19.2 Antidepressants

Aims

The main aims are to relieve symptoms of depression, restore normal social behaviour and prevent further episodes.

Relevant pathophysiology

Depression is common in all populations. Pathological feelings of sadness and despair may be associated with physical and emotional withdrawal. Depressive illnesses are a common factor in suicide.

Major depression is characterized by despair with physical symptoms, e.g. anorexia, sleep disturbance, weight loss. Psychotic symptoms, such as delusions of unworthiness, may also occur. Episodes may be recurrent (unipolar depression) or alternate with mania (bipolar affective disorder).

A range of drugs, including sedatives, steroids, opiates and the antihypertensive methyldopa may cause depressive symptoms. The causative drug should be withdrawn if possible.

The neurochemical basis of depression is thought to involve underactivity of central neuronal pathways where noradrenaline or serotonin act as transmitters. This amine hypothesis is supported by biochemical measurement of these transmitters and their metabolites *in vivo* in cerebrospinal fluid and in brain tissue at postmortem, and from neuroendocrine evidence of abnormal aminergic neurotransmission in depressed patients. There is further support from the therapeutic actions of drugs that modify amine turnover.

Monoamine oxidase inhibitors (MAOIs) block the intrasynaptic breakdown of noradrenaline and serotonin and thus increase transmitter activity.

Tricyclic antidepressants block neuronal reuptake (uptake 1) of noradrenaline and/or serotonin into noradrenergic/serotonergic neurones, altering transmitter levels in the synaptic cleft.

The selective serotonin reuptake inhibitors (SSRIs) selectively inhibit the reuptake of serotonin.

Other 'atypical' antidepressants influence noradrenergic and/or serotonergic neurotransmission in a variety of other ways.

Comment. The diagnosis of depression is complicated by frequent non-specific somatic symptoms of anorexia, malaise, weight loss and constipation. Conversely, the symptoms of depression often accompany non-psychiatric physical illness and understandably depressing adjustments such as bereavement. Nevertheless, pathological depression is common, responsive to drug treatment and therefore important to identify and treat appropriately. Suicide is a serious and well-recognized complication of depression.

Tricyclic antidepressants

Mechanism

This group of drugs includes the closely related agents amitriptyline, nortriptyline, imipramine and clomipramine. They competitively block neuronal uptake of noradrenaline and serotonin into nerve endings and in the short term increase transmitter levels in the synaptic cleft. In the long term these agents lead to down-regulation of pre- and post-synaptic adrenoceptors and serotonin receptors in the brain.

All tricyclics have a range of other pharmacological properties that may contribute to their therapeutic actions and adverse effects:
1 Alpha$_1$–adrenoceptor blockade.
2 Anticholinergic effects.
3 Antihistaminergic effects.
4 Other non-specific sedative actions.

The therapeutic response to tricyclics develops over 3–4 weeks. Suicide by overdose of antidepressant is a risk during this lag period during treatment. There is some evidence that long-term tricyclic treatment is superior to placebo in reducing the frequency of recurrent depressive symptoms. Amitriptyline, which has more sedative properties, may be useful in agitated depression or where insomnia is troublesome. Imipramine, with less sedative properties, is indicated in those who have marked motor retardation.

Pharmacokinetics

Tricyclics are extensively metabolized by the liver. The half-life of amitriptyline is > 24 h and the formation of metabolites with antidepressant activity further extends the duration of

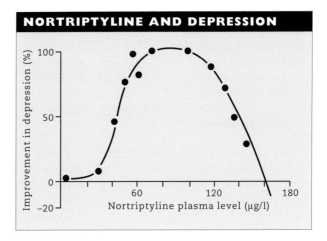

NORTRIPTYLINE AND DEPRESSION

Fig. 19.1 Relationship between drug plasma level and effect with nortriptyline.

drug activity. Once-daily dosing, ideally at night, is indicated for most tricyclics.

Hepatic metabolism of tricyclics is determined by genetic and environmental factors. There are wide differences in plasma level when the same dose is given to a group of individuals. Thus the dose of tricyclic should be titrated individually, with therapeutic response or adverse effects as end points.

Studies with nortriptyline have shown an unusual relationship between drug plasma level and effect (Fig. 19.1). At low drug levels and also at high drug levels there is little effect, while optimal effect is seen within a very narrow concentration range (50–150 µg/l) or therapeutic window. This has led some to propose drug level monitoring as a guide to antidepressant therapy, but this is not routine clinical practice.

Adverse effects (see p. 202)

Clinical use and dose
As the many side effects can limit compliance, it is often prudent to begin with a relatively low dose and titrate upwards to a therapeutic dose over a period of 1–2 weeks: 25–75 mg orally, titrated to 100–200 mg daily. Imipramine may also be useful in nocturnal enuresis and hyperactivity syndrome in childhood. Ami-

triptyline is also used in some forms of neurogenic pain.

Other related antidepressants
Monocyclic, bicyclic and tetracyclic drugs have been developed with similar therapeutic properties to the tricyclics.

Selective serotonin reuptake inhibitors (SSRIs)
Drugs in this group include fluoxetine, fluvoxamine, paroxetine, sertraline and citalopram.

Mechanism
These drugs inhibit the reuptake of serotinin 5-HT into neurones in the central nervous system.

Pharmacokinetics
SSRIs have good oral bioavailability and are eliminated by liver metabolism. They have long half-lives (e.g. fluoxetine 2 days) and can be given once daily.

Adverse effects
SSRIs have the same *incidence* of adverse effects as the tricyclics but the nature of these effects is different: nausea, diarrhoea, headache, insomnia and agitation are the main problems. They are less sedative than

tricyclics and safer in overdose. Those with shorter half-lives should be withdrawn slowly—a discontinuance syndrome is recognized. SSRIs increase the levels of carbamazepine, phenytoin, MAOIs (2 weeks should elapse between treatments and five weeks in the case of fluoxetine) benzodiazepines, lithium and possibly warfarin.

Comment. Tricyclic antidepressants and SSRIs have similar efficacy but a different range of side effects. The main significance of SSRIs is that they have much reduced toxicity in overdose.

Monoamine oxidase inhibitors

Mechanism
Phenelzine, tranylcypromine and iproniazid are non-competitive irreversible antagonists of monoamine oxidase (MAO). They block MAO type A, in contrast to selegiline, which is described in Chapter 20. The enzyme is blocked not only in brain monoamine neurones but also in peripheral neurones, enterocytes in the gut wall and platelets. Inhibition of MAO leads to increases in serotonin, noradrenaline and dopamine in the brain.

The problems with MAOIs result from widespread enzyme inhibition, and as a result other drug treatments for depression have been favoured. There are now reversible MAOIs, such as moclobemide, which promise a safer alternative. Apart from therapeutic failure with other antidepressants, indication for the use of MAOIs include phobic states and 'agitated' depression.

When used, the response may be delayed for 2–3 weeks. After the use of irreversible MAOIs the enzyme recovers slowly (2–3 weeks) after the drug is stopped, as it requires re-synthesis. This problem does not accompany the use of reversible MAOIs.

Adverse effects
1 Postural hypotension.

2 Headache.
3 Anticholinergic side effects.
4 Drug-induced liver damage (phenelzine and isocarboxazid).
5 Hypertensive crisis.

The most important adverse effect is hypertensive crisis following amine-containing foods, beverages or drugs. Inhibition of MAO in the gut wall allows absorption of tyramine and other sympathomimetic substances in food or drink. MAO usually metabolizes these to inactive products during absorption. The amines are taken up from the circulation by peripheral sympathetic nerve endings. They displace endogenous noradrenaline from storage sites (indirect sympathomimetic action) leading to hypertension, tachycardia and headache.

Severe paroxysmal hypertension may cause a cerebrovascular accident. Foods rich in tyramine, particularly cheese, meat, yeast extract and red wine, should be avoided.

Comment. The dangers of hypertension, the limitations on food intake and the availability of alternatives have greatly reduced the role of monoamine oxidase inhibitors in depression. They are rarely used as first-line agents.

Other antidepressants

Mianserin
A tetracyclic compound with sedative properties and low cardiotoxicity. Blood dyscrasias can occur in patients (particularly the elderly) treated with this drug. A 30–60 mg daily dose is given at bedtime, increasing if necessary and if tolerated to 200 mg daily.

Nefazodone
Causes 5-HT reuptake inhibition and 5-HT_2 blockade. The commonest side effects of nausea and restlessness can be minimized by building up the dose gradually to an optimal range of 300–600 mg daily. There is a beneficial effect on sleep.

Venlafaxine

A combined serotonin and noradrenaline reuptake inhibitor (SNRI) but without the anticholinergic and sedative effects commonly seen with the tricyclics. Dosage should be 75 mg daily or greater and a once daily slow-release form is available. The most frequent side effect is nausea, usually resolving after a week, but blood-pressure elevation may occur at higher doses.

Mirtazepine

Termed a NaSSA (noradrenergic and specific serotonergic antidepressant) this drug has a novel action in enhancing noradrenaline and (indirectly) serotonin transmission by blocking presynaptic $alpha_2$ adrenergic receptors. It also causes $5-HT_2$ and $5-HT_3$ receptor blockade, minimizing serotonergic side effects. Dose range is 15–45 mg with sedation more prominent at lower doses.

Reboxetine

Specifically causing noradrenaline reuptake inhibition (NARI), reboxetine is administered in a dose range 4–12 mg daily. Claims have been made for its greater effect on social functioning. Dry mouth is the commonest side effect.

19.3 Mood stabilizing agents

Relevant pathophysiology

Mania and hypomania are characterized by a pathologically elevated mood and disinhibited behaviour. They usually occur as part of a bipolar affective (manic depressive) disorder. Mania is characterized by expansive mood with motor over-activity, non-stop talk, flight of ideas, grandiosity and a progressive lack of contact with reality.

Treatment of an acute manic episode includes sedation with haloperidol or other major tranquillizers, together with general supportive measures. Specific therapy with lithium salts is used both in the acute attack (the main disadvantage to its use as sole agent

being its delayed onset of effect) and for prophylaxis between attacks. Lithium is also now recognized to have a place in the prophylaxis against recurring depressive disorder and as adjunctive therapy in antidepressant-resistant depression. The anticonvulsants carbamazepine and sodium valproate are also used as prophylactic agents in bipolar disorder.

Lithium carbonate

Mechanism

The monovalent lithium cation, given as the carbonate salt, modifies the effect in mania. The mechanism of action of lithium is not clear. It appears to substitute for sodium and potassium cations in cellular transport processes. It has effects on the release of monoamine neurotransmitters and alters intracellular and extracellular ion concentrations, fluxes across excitable membranes and the concentrations of 'second messengers' such as inositol phosphate. Lithium may take several days to achieve its effect.

Pharmacokinetics

Lithium is rapidly and completely absorbed after oral dosing. It is not metabolized and is excreted unchanged by the kidney with a half-life of 12 h. Lithium is distributed in total body water, slowly enters cells and reaches steady state levels after dosing for 5 days. There is a narrow therapeutic range for lithium (0.5–1.0 mmol/l, with higher levels sometimes used in acute mania), with severe adverse effects occurring at higher levels. Monitoring of drug levels in plasma is essential for optimal control of therapy (Chapter 2). Change in renal function is the most important factor modifying elimination and thus plasma levels. Lithium clearance is 0.2 times the creatinine clearance, and the dose must be modified in the presence of renal impairment and in the elderly. The sodium and potassium status of the patient also influences lithium levels and response. Thus dehydration, salt depletion or diuretic

ADVERSE EFFECTS OF TRICYCLICS

1 Sedation and confusional states, especially with amitriptyline.
2 Anticholinergic effects, e.g. dry mouth, constipation, urinary symptoms, sexual dysfunction and precipitation of glaucoma.
3 Postural hypotension, especially in the very young and old.
4 Cardiac tachyarrhythmias (seen in overdose) and conduction defects that are quinidine/
procainamide-like. May occur more frequently in patients treated with long-term tricyclics.
5 Self-poisoning by tricyclic overdose is common and its management is discussed further in Chapter 23, Section 23.2.
6 Fits may occur on withdrawal of tricyclics.

therapy all tend to increase the plasma drug concentration.

Adverse effects (see p.204)
These are more common and severe when the plasma lithium level exceeds 1.2 mmol/l or in the presence of salt depletion or diuretic therapy.

Drug interactions
Lithium levels rise following the introduction of diuretics. Other drugs altering sodium balance (e.g. steroids, ACE inhibitors) may have the same effect. Lithium potentiates the neurotoxicity of haloperidol and flupentixol. Owing to the wide range of further possible interactions, always check carefully before administering another drug with lithium.

Dose
Lithium carbonate: 0.4–2.0 g daily in divided doses, depending on renal function and drug plasma levels achieved.

Other mood stabilizers

Carbamazepine
This commonly used anticonvulsant is an effective treatment both for acute mania and as prophylaxis in bipolar disorder. Trials suggest that its prophylactic effect is less marked than lithium and so should be reserved for those where lithium is contraindicated or has proven ineffective. There is an uncertain relationship between blood levels and treatment response.

A dose of 600–800 mg should be aimed for depending on response and side effects.

Sodium valproate
While there is not as much evidence available for valproate, what there is suggests effectiveness in treatment of acute mania and prophylaxis of bipolar disorder. Blood levels above 45 mg/l are associated with response but side effects prominent at levels above 100 mg/l.

Neuroleptic drugs
Haloperidol and other antipsychotic major tranquillizers have long been used in the management of acute mania. Symptoms are controlled, but it is not clear whether the duration of the manic episode is reduced. These drugs are useful in the treatment of acute attacks.

Haloperidol or chlorpromazine have been used successfully and may be used either alone or in combination with lithium carbonate so long as the dose of haloperidol does not exceed 15 mg/day and the plasma lithium concentration does not exceed 0.8 mmol/l. For adverse effects see Chapter 20, Section 20.1.

Comment. Lithium carbonate is used for long-term prophylaxis in bipolar affective disorder and recurring depressive illness, and it is used together with phenothiazines for control of symptoms in acute attacks. The daily dose of lithium depends on renal function and should be determined individually. Monitoring of lithium plasma levels is essential for optimal treatment without unacceptable adverse effects.

Carbamazepine and valproate may be more effective in lithium-resistant cases (e.g. rapid-cycling affective disorder, mania with depressive symptoms) and combinations of any two of the three mood stabilizers may be more effective than monotherapy.

19.4 Anxiolytics

Aim
The aim is to control symptoms of anxiety without interfering with normal physical or mental function.

Relevant pathophysiology
The experience of anxiety, with physical and psychological symptoms, is a universal phenomenon. Furthermore, better defined and clearly morbid anxiety disorders such as agoraphobia are amongst mankind's commonest seriously disabling conditions. As a result there has always been widespread and excessive use of whatever anxiolytic agents are available. Since the introduction of chlordiazepoxide in 1960, the anxiolytic benzodiazepines have become the most widely prescribed group of drugs in UK and in the USA (15–20% of the population at any one time). Medical practitioners, conditioned to 'treat', often find it extremely difficult to resist demands for a pill to relieve anxiety even though such problems invariably require other forms of intervention.

The principal groups of drugs used in the management of anxiety are the benzodiazepines, the beta-receptor blockers and recently developed agents affecting 5–HT systems. There is also growing interest in the use of imipramine and selective serotonin reuptake inhibitors in the treatment of patients with panic attacks, the use of serotonergic agents in the treatment of patients with obsessional or compulsive disorders and the use of MAOIs in the treatment of certain phobic conditions.

Comment. Anxiety in appropriate circumstances is a normal response. If anxiety symptoms are frequent or persist in a severe form, they may interfere with normal function. Such pathological anxiety is an indication for assessment and appropriate treatment, which might include a pharmacological agent.

Benzodiazepines

Mechanism
Benzodiazepines have a relatively selective action on the limbic system, cerebral cortex and the ascending amine systems that govern arousal. They potentiate gamma-aminobutyric acid (GABA) transmission. The identification of specific binding sites for benzodiazepines has led to speculation that these 'receptors' are normally present to be activated by an, as yet, unidentified 'endogenous benzodiazepine', deficient in anxiety states. Clear proof of this has yet to emerge.

The amnesic action of benzodiazepines is useful in addition to sedation for use as pre-medication for minor investigative procedures like gastroscopy and bronchoscopy.

The benzodiazepines currently available range from very short-acting drugs such as flurazepam or temazepam, which are used as hypnotics, to longer-acting agents such as diazepam, chlordiazepoxide and oxazepam, which are most useful as anxiolytics. Variations in pharmacokinetics and metabolism are responsible for these differences.

Pharmacokinetics
Diazepam is rapidly absorbed from the gastrointestinal tract and extensively metabolized by oxidation in the liver. It forms several active metabolites, including oxazepam, which is used therapeutically in its own right. The plasma half-life is long (24 h) and its duration of effect even longer, as the active metabolites have half-lives of several days. The half-life may be increased in the elderly, who may also be more sensitive to the drug.

Oxazepam is an active metabolite of diazepam. It is cleared by conjugation in the liver and has a half-life of 10–20 h.

Chlordiazepoxide was one of the earlier benzodiazepines. It is still used as an anxiolytic, and is the drug of choice in serious alcohol withdrawal states.

Adverse effects

Benzodiazepines are drugs of dependence. The risk of physical dependence is apparently greater with short-acting agents. Prescriptions should be limited to short-term use (no longer than 6 weeks) and in the case of anxiety only if the condition is severely disabling.

Other adverse effects are listed on p. 206.

Drug interactions

Benzodiazepines have additive or synergistic effects with other centrally acting drugs—antihistamines, alcohol, barbiturates. This may increase the impairment of motor or intellectual function or worsen respiratory depression.

Diazepam and chlordiazepoxide do not interfere with the metabolism of other drugs and do not interact with warfarin.

Clinical use and dose

Benzodiazepines are appropriate in the short-term management (2–4 weeks) of severe disabling anxiety. Chlordiazepoxide is the treatment of choice in severe alcohol withdrawal states including delirium tremens.

Diazepam: orally, 4–30 mg daily in divided doses titrated to control symptoms and continued only as long as is necessary; intramuscularly or slow intravenous injection, 10 mg repeated after 4–6 h if required. Diazepam is used as a sedative in acutely agitated hospitalized patients or as premedication before minor procedures.

Comparable doses of the benzodiazepines are shown in Table 19.2.

Comment. Use the lowest possible dose.

The use of benzodiazepines to treat mild anxiety is unjustifiable. Long-term use is to be avoided. If a patient has taken a benzodiazepine for a long time, the drug should be

ADVERSE EFFECTS OF LITHIUM CARBONATE

1 Nausea and vomiting.
2 Drowsiness, confusion and fits.
3 Ataxia, nystagmus and dysarthria.
4 Hypothyroidism by interference with iodination; rarely hyperthyroidism.

5 Oedema and weight gain.
6 Nephrogenic diabetes insipidus.

ANXIOLYTIC DRUGS AND DOSES

Drug	Group	Dose (mg)
Chlordiazepoxide		75–100
Diazepam		4–30
Lorazepam	Benzodiazepines	1–10
Medazepam		10–30
Oxazepam		30–120
Propranolol	Beta-blocker	40 (when need anticipated)
Buspirone	$5HT_{1a}$ receptor agonist	15–30

Table 19.2 Anxiolytic drugs and dose range used.

withdrawn slowly, at a rate determined by the severity of the withdrawal syndrome.

Other drug treatment of anxiety

Beta-receptor blockers

Beta-receptor blockers reduce cardiovascular and other beta-receptor mediated effects of increased sympathetic activity. Most experience has been acquired with propranolol, a non-selective beta-blocker. Their value in the treatment of morbid anxiety is limited but occasional use in patients disabled by performance anxiety can be of value. The clinical pharmacology and adverse effects of beta-blockers are discussed in Chapter 8. Beta-blockers should be used with caution in patients with a past history of asthma, peripheral vascular disease, cardiac failure or bradyarrhythmias.

Dose

Propranolol: 40 mg before a predictably anxiety-provoking situation.

Serotonergic agents

Buspirone is a 5-HT_{1a} receptor agonist for which reasonable evidence of clinical efficacy exists. It does not appear to interact with the same receptors as the benzodiazepines, but early claims of freedom from physical dependence should be treated with caution.

Clomethiazole

Clomethiazole has few advantages over benzodiazepines, and prolonged use may lead to dependence and severe respiratory depression can occur.

Tricyclic antidepressants, SSRIs and MAOIs

Imipramine and SSRIs have a part to play in the treatment of patients disabled by recurrent panic attacks. SSRIs and clomipramine are used in the treatment of obsessive-compulsive disorder, and MAOIs used in the treatment of certain phobic disorders. Their effects are probably a result of long-term changes in central noradrenergic and/or serotonergic activity. Optimal treatment of such patients also involves an appropriate psychological intervention. Use of these agents depends upon careful assessment of the clinical problem and requires specialized advice.

Comment. Anxiety symptoms should only be treated with drugs if they are severe and interfere with the patient's lifestyle or if alternative social or psychotherapy is not possible or appropriate. Treatment should be regularly revised and stopped as soon as possible. Benzodiazepines are effective but beta-blockers may be an alternative, with fewer dependence problems and less abuse potential. The treatment of more severely disabled patients with anxiety disorder may benefit from one of the various noradrenergic or serotonergic agents traditionally used in the treatment of depression, but such use should be restricted to specialized services.

19.5 Hypnotic drugs and the treatment of insomnia

Aim

By short-term use the aim is to restore normal restful sleep without a residual hangover the next day and to aid a return to normal sleep without drugs.

Relevant pathophysiology

Insomnia is an interference with the quality or quantity of sleep and is a very common complaint. Insomnia is a subjective symptom and reflects what the patient considers to be the 'normal' length and quality of sleep. Individuals vary in their expectation of sleep. Requirements for sleep may vary and diminish with advancing age. A reduced duration of total sleep is common in the elderly and may not be pathological.

The treatment of sleep disorders requires:
1 Assessment of the type of sleep disorder.
2 Assessment of accompanying symptoms of anxiety or depression and their treatment.

3 Diagnosis and treatment of other physical symptoms interfering with sleep, e.g. pain, nocturnal dyspnoea or urinary frequency.

4 Consideration of non-pharmacological strategies, including changes in lifestyle. Simple measures like bathing, exercising or enriched milk drinks at bedtime may help.

Drug treatment should be offered only when the alternatives given above have been excluded, and where there is evidence of frequent and marked sleep impairment. Hypnotics should ideally be used for short periods of days or weeks when required, and not given for regular long-term use.

Comment. A successful hypnotic should act rapidly, allow the subject to wake if necessary without severe sedation and be free from residual hangover effects in the morning. Unfortunately, few of the available agents meet these criteria.

Benzodiazepines

Mechanism

Benzodiazepines exert hypnotic effects by similar mechanisms to their anxiolytic actions but at higher doses. At the peak of drug action, in addition to the anxiolytic effect, the drugs affect brain arousal systems by potentiating the inhibitory effects of GABA.

Nitrazepam, flurazepam and temazepam are widely used (Table 19.3). They induce sleep within 20–40 min of dosing and produce sleep with a reduction in deep sleep (stage 4) and a reduction in rapid eye movement (REM) sleep.

Residual hangover effects with cumulative adverse reactions in chronic dosing may occur with nitrazepam and flurazepam, which have a long half-life and an active metabolite, respectively.

Temazepam appears to have the advantage of a short half-life and no active metabolites. Residual impairment is less with temazepam than with other benzodiazepines.

Adverse effects

Benzodiazepines are drugs of dependence. Particular problems relevant to their use as hypnotics include oversedation (especially in the elderly), 'hangover' effect, paradoxical agitation, and withdrawal phenomena including rebound insomnia, vivid dreams and fits.

ADVERSE EFFECTS OF BENZODIAZEPINES

1 Drowsiness, agitation, ataxia and lightheadedness, especially in the elderly.
2 Incontinence, nightmares and confusion.
3 Excessive salivation.
4 Changes in libido.
5 Respiratory depression, hypotension.
6 Impaired alertness with motor and intellectual dysfunction, e.g. driving, operating machinery.
7 Paradoxical stimulant effects in some violent patients.
8 Disinhibition can lead to suicidal behaviour.
9 Withdrawal can be associated with rebound increased agitation, hallucinations and epileptic seizures.
10 Thrombophlebitis may follow intravenous diazepam.
11 Psychological adjustment to bereavement may be inhibited by benzodiazepines.

BENZODIAZEPINE HYPNOTICS

Drug	Plasma half-life (h)	Active metabolite
Nitrazepam	20+	None
Flurazepam	2–4	Yes, with long half-life
Temazepam	5–6	None

Table 19.3 Benzodiazepine hypnotic drugs.

Clinical use and dose

Benzodiazepines are indicated in the short-term management of severe, disabling insomnia.

Temazepam: 10–30 mg ⎫ 30 min
Nitrazepam: 5–10 mg ⎬ before
Flurazepam: 15–30 mg ⎭ bedtime

Comment. Hypnotic drugs should only be used for short periods of time. They should certainly not be prescribed without very careful thought. Other physical, psychiatric and social factors may well require attention.

19.6 Drug-induced psychiatric disorder

Central nervous system adverse effects of drugs are common, especially in the case of lipid-soluble drugs with specific effects on:
1 Receptors.
2 Transmitter synthesis.
3 Degradation of transmitters.
4 Electrophysiological effects on excitable membranes.

A careful history of recent drug ingestion is an essential feature of the evaluation of a patient with psychiatric illness and, where possible, the first step in the management of drug-induced psychiatric symptoms should be withdrawal of the offending drug.

There are many well documented examples of drugs causing behavioural adverse effects, and these are summarized in Table 19.4.

19.7 Abuse of psychoactive drugs

Abuse of drugs and related agents is a major social problem amongst young people, especially in urban communities. Therapeutic drug use may also lead to dependence, e.g. benzodiazepines used for anxiety or insomnia, or opiate analgesic abuse in patients first treated for chronic severe pain. However, the concept of drug misuse or abuse must be judged in a cultural and historical context. Attitudes to the non-therapeutic use of cannabis and even opiates differ greatly throughout the world.

The problems of drug abuse are:
1 The direct specific toxic effects, e.g. respiratory depression with opiates.
2 Generalized actions on mood, disinhibition of social behaviour and impaired level of consciousness.
3 Short-term consequences of drug withdrawal, e.g. psychological and physical symptoms of dependence.
4 Long-term medical complications of the contemporary drug 'subculture', e.g. hepatitis, septicaemia, acquired immunodeficiency syndrome (AIDS) and bacterial endocarditis.

Psychoactive drugs, like analgesics or sedatives, have a high potential for abuse because of:
1 *Central effects.* They modify mood or behaviour, leading to either pleasurable experiences, depersonalization or intoxication and amnesia.
2 *Tolerance.* If there is tolerance to the effect with regular use, and thus a need to increase the dose to get the same effect, then not only is the drug-taking habit reinforced but there is a greater risk of chemical toxicity or adverse effects at the higher doses.
3 *Withdrawal symptoms.* Symptoms on withdrawal of the abused drug further reinforce the need for continued drug use (or abuse). While these withdrawal symptoms may often be psychological, in the case of benzodiazepines, opiates and barbiturates, physical symptoms on withdrawal create further dependence or 'addiction'.

Drugs with a high abuse potential can be divided into:
1 Therapeutic agents:
(a) Benzodiazepines.
(b) Barbiturates.
(c) Other hypnotics and sedatives.
(d) Opiate analgesics and analogues, including dextropropoxyphene.
2 Non-therapeutic agents ('street' drugs):
(a) Cannabis.

DRUG-INDUCED PSYCHIATRIC DISORDER

Depression

Antihypertensives	*Steroids*
Methyldopa	Corticosteroids
Clonidine	Oral contraceptive pill
Reserpine	
Propranolol	*Analgesics*
Guanethidine	Opiates
	Non-steroidal anti-inflammatory drugs

Sedatives

Benzodiazepines	*Others*	
Alcohol	Levodopa	Cimetidine
Barbiturates	Tetrabenazine	Triamcinolone
	Methysergide	Mefloquine

Neuroleptics
Phenothiazines and other antipsychotics

Psychotic states

Sympathomimetics (amfetamine (amphetamine)) and the amfetamine-derived 'designer' drug Ecstasy
Anticholinergic drugs (atropine, trihexyphenidyl (benzhexol))
Levodopa and dopamine agonists (bromocriptine, apomorphine)
Steroids (prednisolone, dexamethasone)
Phencyclidine (PCP: 'angel dust')
Cannabis

Anxiety and anxiety symptoms

Sympathomimetics (amfetamine, ephedrine, phenylpropanolamine, etc.)
Beta$_2$-adrenoceptor agonists (isoprenaline, salbutamol, terbutaline)

Drug-withdrawal states

Benzodiazepines, clonidine, barbiturates, opiates and alcohol

Table 19.4 Drug-induced psychiatric disorder.

(b) Cocaine.

(c) Opiates.

(d) Amfetamines (amphetamines); their therapeutic use now is very limited.

(e) LSD, psylocybin, phencyclidine and other hallucinogens.

(f) Solvents.

(g) Alcohol.

The following agents are used in the management of psychoactive substance misuse:

Benzodiazepines

Their primary use is in the management of severe alcohol withdrawal states, which may present with autonomic overarousal and fits, and delirium tremens. Long-acting compounds such as chlordiazepoxide are preferred and prescribed on a reducing dose regime over 5–7 days. Initial doses are judged on symptom severity and may range from 60 to 160 mg/d. Vitamin supplementation (B1) ought to also be given to minimize risk of amnesic (Wernicke–

Korsakoff) syndrome. Vitamin deficiency and malabsorption require high doses to be used.

Disulfiram

The metabolism of ethanol is blocked by disulfiram, which causes inhibition of ALDH leading to accumulation of acetaldehyde. Symptoms of the alcohol–disulfiram reaction include flushing, tachycardia, headache, nausea, vomiting and hypotension. Rarely, significant medical complications can arise. The practice of patients receiving a test challenge has now been abandoned and disulfiram therefore acts as a deterrent to drinking in patients who are motivated toward abstinence. Enzyme inhibition (and thus potential for reaction) lasts up to seven days and patients must be warned of potential interactions with alcohol in foods and over-the-counter medications.

Acamprosate

Acamprosate enhances GABA inhibitory neurotransmission and antagonizes glutamate excitation. This is thought to be the mechanism by which it reduces craving for alcohol. It is prescribed in a usual dose of 666 mg three times daily. It should be commenced while abstinent but can be maintained during brief relapses.

Opiate dependence

May be treated by use of substitute prescribing (methadone) or by drugs that abolish the euphoric effects of opiates (naltrexone). Drugs such as lofexidine are used to minimize symptoms of opiate withdrawal.

Comment. The management of drug abuse is not easy and involves:
1 Management of acute pharmacological toxicity.
2 Treatment of any acute medical complications, e.g. septicaemia, endocarditis.
3 Psychiatric assessment and treatment of any underlying psychopathology, e.g. depression.

4 Controlled planned withdrawal of the drug, if necessary, with temporary substitution, e.g. methadone for heroin.
5 Long-term measures such as family or community support (Alcoholics Anonymous), psychotherapy or drug therapy (disulfiram for alcoholics).

19.8 Treatment of dementia

Aim

Traditionally, drugs have been used to minimize behavioural disturbance in dementia. New agents, such as donepezil, stabilize or reverse cognitive decline, albeit temporarily.

Relevant pathophysiology

Dementia is a chronic, progressive organic brain disorder resulting in memory decline and eventual loss of all aspects of cognitive functioning. A small number of cases are reversible where certain specific aetiologies can be found (e.g. vitamin B_{12} deficiency, normal pressure hydrocephalus, hypothyroidism). The majority however, are irreversible, the commonest being Alzheimer's disease (and its variant, Lewy Body dementia) and multi-infarct dementia.

Alzheimer's disease is characterized by postmortem findings of senile plaques, neurofibrillary tangles and reduced neurotransmitter levels, particularly of acetylcholine, the severity of which correlates with neuronal loss. Acetylcholinesterase inhibitors have recently been introduced in the management of mild to moderate Alzheimer's disease. Compounds currently available include donepezil and rivastigmine. They may slow the rate of cognitive and non-cognitive decline in 40% of patients.

Donepezil

This is prescribed in an initial dose of 5 mg daily, rising to 10 mg/day after one month. Side effects, which include nausea, vomiting and diarrhoea, are minimized by careful dose titration.

Rivastigmine

Similar side effects to donepezil are seen. Rivastigmine is prescribed twice daily in doses of 6–12 mg/day, titrated weekly to maximum tolerated dose.

Comment. While drugs may slow cognitive decline, they do not alter ultimate disease progression and, on withdrawal, rapid deterioration may occur, even when no clear response has been seen. This should be explained to patients and their relatives. Baseline assessment of cognitive functioning should precede treatment and patients should be reassessed again at three months. If no clear improvement has occurred the drug should be stopped. Other drugs, including antidepressants and antipsychotics are often used to control behavioural disturbance. However, antipsychotics should be avoided if at all possible in patients with Lewy Body dementia, where they may cause severe EPS.

CHAPTER 20

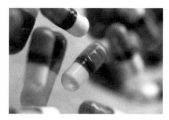

Drugs and Neurological Disease

20.1 Epilepsy

Pathophysiology

Epilepsy is recurrent unprovoked seizures. A seizure is a paroxysmal event resulting from abnormal, hypersynchronous discharges of cortical neurones. Convulsions refer to a seizure where motor manifestations predominate. Two major categories of seizures are recognized: generalized seizures and partial seizures. Generalized seizures lead to loss of consciousness and are bilaterally symmetric. In a partial seizure, symptoms begin locally that may progress to a secondary generalized seizure. Common types of primary generalized seizures are grand mal (tonic–clonic), tonic, myoclonic, petit mal (absence) and atonic (akinetic). There are two main types of partial seizures: simple, with no impairment of consciousness and complex, where consciousness may be altered and patients may have automatism (lip-smacking or aimless walking). An aura is the subjective onset of a minor partial seizure and may appear as olfactory, visual or psychic symptoms. Seizures that occur as the consequence of an identifiable brain pathology (trauma, tumour or infarction) are called secondary or symptomatic epilepsy; all other types of epilepsy are primary. *Status epilepticus* is continuous seizures (generalized or partial) lasting for 30 min. Convulsive (tonic–clonic) status epilepticus is defined as two or more discrete convulsive seizures with incomplete recovery of consciousness in between. It is a medical emergency.

Aim and principles of therapy

In treating epilepsy, the drug chosen needs to be matched to the individual patient and the type of epileptic seizures. A wide range of treatments is currently available and 70–80% of epileptic patients will become seizure-free with appropriate drug therapy.

Sodium valproate is the first choice for generalized seizures; carbamazepine and phenytoin are alternatives. Valproate is also the treatment of choice for juvenile myoclonic epilepsy. For partial seizures, carbamazepine is the first choice; lamotrigine, valproate and phenytoin are the alternatives in the decreasing order of preference. Ethosuximide is the only available alternative to valproate for petit mal (absence seizures); phenytoin or carbamazepine are ineffective. Clonazepam is usually an adjunct to valproate for treating myoclonic seizures and clobazam is particularly useful for seizures occurring in clusters (e.g. during menstrual periods). Phenobarbital is a cheap and effective treatment for generalized seizures but is currently used only when other treatments fail. Phenobarbital is also the active ingredient in primidone, effective in all types of epilepsy except absence seizures. It is rarely used now.

The therapeutic goal in epilepsy treatment is complete remission of seizures without side effects, using a single drug (monotherapy). Table 20.1 is a list of anti-epileptic drugs with their doses, common side effects and interactions. Most anticonvulsants have important interactions with other drugs, especially those that are highly protein bound or are metabolized by the liver, including other anticonvulsants and oral contraceptives. Interactions between anti-epileptic drugs are complex and may enhance toxicity without a corresponding increase in the anti-epileptic effect. There is good correlation between therapeutic effect and drug level only with phenytoin and to some extent with phenobarbital and carbamazepine; valproate and newer anti-epileptic drugs do not require monitoring of plasma levels. If ineffective, medications should be increased to the maximum tolerated dose on clinical grounds rather than serum levels. Approximately one-third of patients will require polytherapy with two or more drugs.

Newer anti-epileptic drugs

These are expensive and with the exception of lamotrigine, all current new drugs for epilepsy (vigabatrin, gabapentin, topiramate and tiagabine) are primarily indicated as add-on therapy for seizures poorly controlled with optimal doses of the conventional first-line therapy. Vigabatrin has been recommended as monotherapy only for infantile spasms (West's syndrome). Experience with oxcarbamazine, felbamate, zonisamide and flunarizine has been largely restricted to trials. Levetiracetam is currently being evaluated as a potential anti-epileptic drug. Patients with certain epilepsy syndromes (e.g. temporal lobe epilepsy) refractory to medical therapy will benefit from surgical excision of the seizure focus and could achieve significant reduction or permanent discontinuation of their anti-epileptic drug therapy.

Anti-epileptic drugs in common use

Carbamazepine

A tricyclic derivative, it is likely that carbamazepine acts by blocking the neuronal calcium and sodium channels. It is also effective in neuralgia and certain forms of dystonia. It is metabolized in the liver and is a powerful enzyme inducer, inducing its own metabolism so that its elimination half-life falls from an initial 24–48 h following a single dose to 8–12 h on chronic therapy. For this reason, carbamazepine must be started at a low dose (e.g. 100–200 mg once daily in an adult) and then the dose is gradually titrated upwards over several weeks. It is contraindicated in patients with cardiac conduction defects, a history of bone marrow depression, porphyria and in combination with monoamine oxidase inhibitors. A measles-like skin rash is the commonest side effect (5–15%) that may occasionally proceed to erythema multiforme. Patients must be cautioned about the rare idiosyncratic risk of bone marrow suppression (leukopenia and thrombocytopenia) and liver disorders. Other side effects include vestibulo-cerebellar symptoms as a manifestation of acute toxicity, hyponatremia as a consequence of the syndrome of inappropriate antidiuretic hormone (ADH) secretion and a 1% risk of spina bifida in babies exposed in utero. Cognitive and behavioural effects are also recognized. Paradoxic seizures may occur with carbamazepine toxicity. Carbamazepine is available as a suppository for use in small children.

Valproate

Sodium valproate acts by increasing the level of the inhibitory neurotransmitter gamma-aminobutyric acid (GABA) by a combination of mechanisms that may involve its accelerated synthesis (induction of glutamic acid decarboxylase) and reduced breakdown (inhibition of GABA-transaminase). It can be used in all forms of epilepsy and also for migraine prophylaxis, neuralgia, chorea and cerebellar tremors. It is well absorbed, extensively protein

ANTI-EPILEPTIC DRUGS

Generic name	Principal uses	Typical dosage and dosing intervals	Half-life	Therapeutic range	Adverse effects		Drug interactions
					Neurologic	Systemic	
Valproic acid	Tonic–clonic absence Atypical absence Myoclonic Focal-onset	750–2000 mg/day (920–60 mg/kg) b.i.d.-q.i.d.	9–20 h	50–150 mg/l (400–700 μmol/l)	Ataxia, sedation, tremor	Hepatotoxicity, thrombocytopenia, gastrointestinal irritation, weight gain, transient alopecia, hyperammonaemia	Level decreased by carbamazepine, phenobarbital (phenobarbitone), phenytoin
Carbamazepine	Tonic–clonic Focal onset	600–1800 mg/day (15–35 mg/kg, child) b.i.d.-q.i.d.	12–17 h	4–12 mg/l (17–42 μmol/l)	Ataxia, dizziness, diplopia, vertigo	Aplastic anaemia, leukopenia, gastrointestinal irritation, hepatotoxicity	Level decreased by erythromycin, propoxyphene Isoniazid, cimetidine
Phenytoin (diphenylhydantoin)	Tonic–clonic (grand mal), Focal-onset	300–400 mg/day (3–6 mg/kg, adult; 4–8 mg/kg, child) q.i.d.-b.i.d.	22 h (wide variation, dose-dependent)	10–20 mg/l (40–80 μmol/l)	Ataxia, incoordination, confusion, cerebellar	Gum, hyperplasia, lymphadenopathy, hirsutism, osteomalacia, facial coarsening, skin rash	Level increased by isoniazid, sulphonamides; level decreased by carbamazepine, phenobarbital; altered folate metabolism
Topiramate	Adjunctive for focal-onset, primary and secondary generalized seizures	50 mg daily initially (25 mg in children), then slowly increased to 200–400 mg/day b.i.d.	18–30 h	Not established	Impaired memory and concentration, impaired speech, mood disorder and depression; paresthesia, dizziness, ataxia	Renal calculi, leukopenia, taste disturbance, weight loss, fatigue, asthenia	Accelerated metabolism of contraceptives

continued on p. 214

ANTI-EPILEPTIC DRUGS

Generic name	Principal uses	Typical dosage and dosing intervals	Half-life	Therapeutic range	Adverse effects		Drug interactions
					Neurologic	Systemic	
Phenobarbital	Tonic–clonic Focal-onset	60–180 mg/day (1–4 mg/kg, adult; 3–6 mg/kg, child) q.d.	90 h (70 h in children)	10–40 mg/l (50–170 μmol/l)	Sedation, ataxia, confusion, dizziness, decreased libido, depression	Skin rash	Level increased by valproic acid, phenytoin. Enhances metabolism of other drugs via liver enzyme induction
Primidone	Tonic–clonic Focal onset	750–1000 mg/day (10–25 mg/kg) b.i.d.-t.i.d.	Primidone 8–15 h, Phenobarbital 90 h	Primidone 4–12 mg/l Phenobarbital 10–40 mg/l	Same as phenobarbital		Same as phenobarbital
Ethosuximide	Absence (petit mal)	750–1250 mg/day (20–40 mg/kg) q.d.-b.i.d.	60 h, adult; 30 h, child	40–100 mg/l (283–708 μmol/l)	Ataxia, lethargy, headache	Gastrointestinal irritation, skin rash, bone marrow suppression	No known significant interactions
Gabapentin	Focal-onset	900–2400 mg/day t.i.d.-q.i.d.	5–9 h	Not established	Sedation, dizziness, ataxia, fatigue	Gastrointestinal irritation	No known significant interactions
Clonazepam	Absence, Atypical absence, Myoclonic	1–12 mg/day (0.1–0.2 mg/kg) q.d.-t.i.d.	18–48 h	10–70 pg/l	Ataxia, sedation, lethargy	Anorexia	Increased sedation with hypnotics

Lamotrigine	Focal-onset, Lennox-Gestaut syndrome	150–500 mg/day b.i.d. (with enzyme-inducers); 59 h (with valproic acid)	25 h, 15 h	Not established	Dizziness, diplopia, sedation, ataxia, headache	Skin rash, Stevens–Johnson syndrome	Level decreased by carbamazepine, phenobarbital, phenytoin; Level increased by valproic acid
Vigabatrin	Monotherapy for infantile spasms (West's syndrome); add-on for focal and secondary generalized seizures	0.5 g (40 mg/kg in child) starting dose; increased to 2–4 g (100 mg/kg in children and up to 150 mg/kg in West's syndrome) b.i.d.	12–18 h	Not established	Visual field defects, nystagmus, ataxia, irritability, depression, memory loss, psychoses; excitation in children; rarely photophobia and retinal disorders	Weight gain, oedema, alopecia, gastrointestinal	Level decreased by carbamazepine, phenobarbital irritation
Felbamate	Focal-onset, Lennox-Gestaut syndrome	2400–3600 mg/day, (45 mg/kg, child) t.i.d.-q.i.d.	16–22 h	Not established	Insomnia, dizziness, sedation, headache	Aplastic anaemia, hepatic failure, weight loss, gastrointestinal irritation	Increases phenytoin, valproic acid, active carbamazepine metabolite
Tiagabine	Add-on for focal-onset seizures with or without generalization	5 mg initially, increased to 30–45 mg/day, NOT in children	7–9 h	Not established	Dizziness, tremor, depression, drowsiness, speech and memory problems	Fatigue, leukopenia	No significant interaction

Table 20.1 Anti-epileptic drugs.

bound and metabolized in the liver, and thus contraindicated in active liver disease and porphyria. Fatal hepatic failure has occurred especially in children under 3 years of age and those with metabolic or degenerative disorder and those on multiple anti-epileptic drugs for severe seizure disorder, usually in the first 6 months of therapy. Monitoring of liver function tests is recommended before and during the first 6 months of therapy, especially in patients most at risk. Common adverse effects include weight gain, gastric irritation, ataxia, tremors, polycystic ovary-like symptoms in women, rarely pancreatitis, leukopenia and bone marrow depression. An interesting side effect is loss of hair followed by regrowth of curly hair. The risk of spina bifida in babies exposed *in utero* is 2–3%. A parenteral therapy has recently become available for continuation or initiation of valproate treatment when oral therapy is not possible.

Phenytoin

It acts by neuronal membrane stabilization and blockade of sodium channels. Despite its proven efficacy in tonic–clonic and partial seizures, phenytoin is no longer a first-line therapy because of its narrow therapeutic window. The relationship between dose and plasma concentration is non-linear; small dosage increases in some patients may produce large rises in plasma concentration at saturation (zero-order) kinetics. Monitoring of plasma concentration is extremely useful with phenytoin. It is also an enzyme inducer and is commonly implicated in drug interaction. Phenytoin is also effective in neuralgia and myotonia. It is unsuitable in adolescent patients as a result of its cosmetic side effects (coarse facies, acne, hirsutism and gingival hyperplasia). It is to be avoided in porphyria and in second degree or complete heart block. Phenytoin is the cause of a common drug-induced systemic lupus erythematosus. Concentration-dependent side effects include anorexia, insomnia, nausea, cerebellar symptoms (nystagmus and ataxia), peripheral neuropathy, chorea, obtundation and seizures.

Long-term use can cause osteomalacia (vitamin D malabsorbtion), megaloblastic anaemia (folate malabsorbtion), Dupuytren's contracture and generalized lymphadenopathy that may appear indistinguishable from Hodgkin's lymphoma on histology. Rarely, blood dyscrasias (agranulocytosis), hepatitis, skin rash and erythema multiforme are reported.

The parenteral preparation of phenytoin is the first-line therapy in patients with status epilepticus. The injection must only be given intravenously. The injection solution is strongly alkaline and if extravasated, can cause intense irritation of tissues and in the hands, swelling and discoloration ('purple glove' syndrome). Because of its alkaline pH, phenytoin should not be mixed with solutions with acidic pH, e.g. 5% dextrose in water, which will precipitate the salt (dihydantoin sodium). Rapid intravenous injections may also cause cardiovascular and central nervous system (CNS) depression, heart block, hypotension and respiratory arrest; patients over the age of 50 years are more susceptible. The rate of infusion should not exceed 50 mg/min; resuscitation facilities and a cardiac rhythm monitor must be available.

Fosphenytoin

Fosphenytoin is a new, water-soluble prodrug of phenytoin that is suitable for intramuscular or intravenous injections. It is more neutral in solution and is better tolerated at infusion sites. It is converted to phenytoin (half-life: 15 min) by non-specific phosphatases. Doses of fosphenytoin are expressed as phenytoin equivalents (PE), which are the amount of phenytoin released by the prodrug in the presence of phosphatases. Unlike parenteral phenytoin, fosphenytoin is not formulated with propylene glycol that has been implicated in the cardiovascular side effects of intravenous phenytoin. It can be also administered more rapidly at PE doses up to 150 mg/min. Although cardiovascular complications are less likely, cardiac monitoring is still recommended during intravenous infusion.

Lamotrigine

It acts by blocking the neuronal sodium channels and is effective as monotherapy in partial seizures. It is well absorbed, fully bioavailable and is metabolized largely as a glucuronide conjugate in the liver. It is contraindicated in hepatic impairment. Elimination half-life of lamotrigine is reduced to around 15 h by the enzyme inducing anti-epileptic drugs (carbamazepine and phenytoin), whereas sodium valproate inhibits its metabolism and doubles the half-life to nearly 60 h. It must be given at a very low dose (12.5 mg daily or 25 mg every alternate day) with slow weekly dose increment in patients on concomitant valproate therapy. A pharmacodynamic interaction is common when lamotrigine is co-prescribed in patients taking carbamazepine and the symptoms of neurotoxicity (headache, nausea, dizziness, diplopia and ataxia) can be avoided or ameliorated by reducing the carbamazepine dose. The commonest side effect of lamotrigine is skin rash (3–5%) and there is good evidence that starting with a high dose increases the risk of rash with lamotrigine. Other side effects that are concentration dependent include dizziness, nausea, diplopia and ataxia. Increased toxicity and paradoxic deterioration of seizure control may occur when lamotrigine is used in combination with other anti-epileptic drugs.

Anti-epileptic drug therapy in pregnancy

There is an increased risk of teratogenicity associated with the use of anti-epileptic drugs in pregnancy that may be less with monotherapy. In view of the increased risk of neural tube and other defects associated, in particular, with valproate, carbamazepine and phenytoin ('foetal hydantoin' syndrome), women taking anti-epileptic drugs who may become pregnant should be informed of the risks and must be screened antenatally (alpha-fetoprotein measurement and a second trimester ultrasound scan) if they become pregnant. All women on anti-epileptic drug therapy should take folic acid before and during pregnancy; a dose of 5 mg daily is appropriate for women receiving established anti-epileptic drugs. In view of the increased bleeding associated with carbamazepine, phenobarbital and phenytoin, prophylactic Vitamin K1 should be given to the mother on any of these drugs before delivery. Breast feeding is acceptable with most anti-epileptic drugs with the exception of barbiturates, ethosuximide and some of the more recently introduced drugs.

Status epilepticus

The treatment protocol for convulsive (tonic–clonic) status epilepticus is outlined in Table 20.2.

20.2 Migraine, other headaches and neuralgic pain

Pathophysiology

Migraine (corrupted from hemicrania) may be classical (headache with aura) or common (headache without aura). Family history is often positive and migraine is more common in women. The triad of a classical migraine is visual scotomata or scintillations, unilateral throbbing headache and nausea or vomiting. Headache may be bilateral or generalized in common migraine with a more gradual onset. An attack usually lasts for 2–6 h and may be provoked by wine, cheese, chocolate, contraceptives, stress, exercise or travel. Cluster headache is characterized by recurrent, unilateral throbbing headache that is typically nocturnal, commoner in males, provoked by alcohol and accompanied by retro-orbital searing pain, conjunctival and nasal congestion. Headache as a result of temporal arteritis affects elderly people (two thirds are women) and may lead to blindness if untreated.

Aim and principles of treatment

The principles of treatment in migraine consist of three steps: (i) elimination of known precipitant or trigger; (ii) pharmacological treatment of acute attacks; and (iii) prophylaxis.

DRUGS FOR CONVULSIVE STATUS EPILEPTICUS

Time frame (min)	Intervention
(continuing seizures) 0–5	*In all*: monitor vital signs, administer O_2, establish i.v. access, collect blood for biochemistry, blood gases and toxic screen; drug levels (phenytoin, carbamazepine) if on treatment. Put patient in recovery position. 50 ml of 50% dextrose i.v. (+100 mg thiamine i.m./i.v. if known alcoholic). **Lorazepam** 0.1 mg/kg i.v. at 2 mg/min (maximum dose: children 2 mg and adults 8 mg)
5–25	**Phenytoin** 15–20 mg/kg i.v. at 50 mg/min (typically 1 g in an adult) *or* **Fosphenytoin** 15–20 mg/kg PE i.v. at 150 mg/min. If on oral phenytoin, use 50% of calculated dose. *If seizures persist, then*
25–35	Additional phenytoin (5–10 mg/kg) or fosphenytoin (5–10 mg/kg PE) i.v.
35–50	**Phenobarbital** (phenobarbitone) 10–15 mg/kg at 50 mg/min i.v.; facilities for intubation must be readily at hand
50–60	Additional phenobarbital 5–10 mg/kg (not exceeding a cumulative total dose of 20 mg/kg or 1 g) *Alternatively* **Paraldehyde** by deep intramuscular injections (5 ml in each buttock, max 10 ml using all glass equipment with a steel needle
>60	Patient must be ventilated and monitored in the ICU. *Use one of the following infusions:* **midazolam** (loading dose 0.1–0.2 mg/kg slow i.v., then maintained at a dose of 0.75–10 μg/kg/min) **clomethiazole** (chlormethiazole) as an 0.8% solution intravenously 40–120 mg/min up to a maximum of 800 mg (80 μg/kg in children), then maintained at a rate of 4–8 mg/min **propofol** (loading dose 1–2 mg/kg i.v., followed by 2–10 mg/kg/h) *If this fails, only then use* **Thiopental** (thiopentone) (2.5% solution), given i.v. 100–150 mg in adults over 10–15 s (2–7 mg/kg in children), then maintained at 0.5–1 mg/kg/h If EEG facilities are available, then the dose may be adjusted on the basis of EEG monitoring, the end point is suppression of spikes. If blood pressure is stable, secondary end point is burst-suppression pattern in the EEG with intervals of <1 s between bursts

Notes: 1. Maintenance doses of phenytoin (5–6 mg/kg) and phenobarbital (3–5 mg/kg) must be continued; measure plasma concentrations for optimal doses. 2. Taper infusions of midazolam, clomethiazole or thiopentone after 12 h; if seizures recur, reinstate infusion for at least 12 h. 3. There is a risk of convulsions with propofol. 4. EEG monitoring, though not mandatory, may be useful when available; an ictal EEG also helps to exclude pseudo-status epilepticus. 5. Use i.v. fluids and low-dose dopamine ± dobutamine to treat hypotension.

Table 20.2 Anti-epileptic drug therapy for convulsive status epilepticus.

Treatment of acute attack

This should begin at the very onset of headache. Any standard non-steroidal anti-inflammatory drug (NSAID), e.g. aspirin, paracetamol, naproxen or ibuprofen, often with an anti-emetic in combination (metoclopramide, domperidone or a phenothiazine), is the first choice. Tolfenamic acid is a new NSAID that has been indicated specifically for migraine attacks. Because serotonin (5-hydroxy tryptamine or 5-HT), plays a key role in the neurovascular inflammation that is characteristic of migraine, 5-HT$_1$ agonists ('triptans') are of considerable value in the treatment of an acute attack, especially in those who fail to respond to simple analgesics. The first-generation triptans consist of sumatriptan, naratriptan and zolmitriptan. The second-generation triptans (rizatriptan and eletriptan) cross the blood–brain barrier and have better bioavailability on oral administration. It should be noted that triptans do not abolish nausea or vomiting and require the additional use of an anti-emetic. Unremitting attacks of severe migraine lasting for days ('status migrainosus') require the short-term use of corticosteroids in an anti-inflammatory dose, although this diagnosis should always be made with caution and after exclusion of all other possibilities even in a patient known to be a migraine sufferer. Corticosteroids are also indicated as first-line therapy in the treatment of the headache of temporal arteritis and in severe cluster headache.

Great care should be exercised when prescribing analgesics to patients with headache, because with frequent use, a large proportion will develop chronic daily headaches resulting from the drugs ('analgesic headache') in addition to their primary headache type. Opioid-containing preparations are particularly likely to produce this effect but it does occur with simple analgesics and NSAIDs. Prolonged use of triptans can also give rise to 'rebound headache'.

Treatment for migraine prophylaxis

In patients with two or more attacks in a month, use of prophylactic agents for prevention of migraine is justified. Amitriptyline and propranalol are the two main prophylactic agents that are often used in combination. Other prophylactic agents that may be used in migraine are pizotifen, valproate, carbamazepine, methysergide or selected calcium channel blockers (flunarizine or verapamil). Lithium (1500–2400 mg/day) and verapamil (160–240 mg/day) are used for prophylaxis in cluster headache.

Antimigraine drugs in common use

Sumatriptan

A 5-HT$_{1D}$ agonist, sumatriptan is used for acute attacks of migraine (oral preparation, intranasal spray or subcutaneous injections) and cluster headache (subcutaneous injections only). It should not be taken until 24 h after stopping any preparation containing ergotamine. It has poor bioavailability and less than half of the orally administered dose is absorbed. Further reduction may occur in patients with migraine-induced gastroparesis and vomiting. The dose by mouth is 50 mg (some patients may require 100 mg) and patients not responding should not take a second dose for the same attack. In responders, the dose may be repeated if migraine recurs (max. 300 mg in 24 h). It is available as an intranasal spray and subcutaneous injection for prompt relief. The dose by subcutaneous injection using an auto-injector is 6 mg (max. 24 mg in 24 h) and 1 spray (20 mg) intranasally (max. 40 mg in 24 h). Sumatriptan is also effective in cluster headache. None of the 5-HT agonists should be used for prophylaxis and all are contraindicated in ischaemic heart disease, previous myocardial infarction, coronary vasospasm, uncontrolled hypertension and in attacks of migraine with brain stem dysfunction ('basilar migraine'). Side effects of triptans include sensations of tingling, heat, heaviness, pressure or tightness in the chest, flushing, dizziness, weakness, vomiting and fatigue.

Ergotamine

It is used in rare cases of acute attacks of migraine and cluster headache. Ergotamine has a high affinity for 5-HT$_1$ receptors, which probably explains its mode of action in this condition. Ergot alkaloids are alpha-receptor blockers and also have a direct vascular effect causing vasoconstriction. This may lead to peripheral vasoconstriction with Raynaud's phenomenon, ischaemia and digital gangrene ('ergotism') in patients with coexisting vascular disease and in chronic users who take it habitually to counteract the symptoms of headache caused by vasodilation when the drug is withdrawn. It is contraindicated in patients with known coronary artery disease. The dose of ergotamine (as tartarate) is 1–2 mg sublingually to a total dose of 6–8 mg per attack or max. 12 mg/week; rectally the dose is 2 mg repeated after 1 h to the same total dose; and by aerosol, 360 μg inhalation repeated up to six inhalations daily or 15 per week.

Beta-blockers

Propranolol, a non-selective beta-blocker, is effective in reducing the frequency of migraine attacks in daily doses of 40–120 mg (this may be increased up to 480 mg according to effectiveness) given orally. Only beta-blockers with intrinsic sympathomimetic activity are effective in migraine; those with partial agonist activity have no action. Their mechanism of action in migraine prophylaxis is unknown.

Amitriptyline

A tricyclic antidepressant, its antimigraine effect is not a result of its antidepressant property and small doses are often effective (20–50 mg/day). Sedation and dry mouth are two common side effects. The detailed pharmacology of amitriptyline is given elsewhere in this book.

Pizotifen

It is an antihistamine and serotonin antagonist structurally related to the tricyclic antidepressants. It affords good prophylaxis for migraine but may cause weight gain and drowsiness. The treatment may be started at 500 μg at night; maximum dose is 3 mg/day.

Methysergide

A 5-HT$_2$ antagonist, methysergide is a very effective drug for prophylaxis of migraine and cluster headache but carries serious long-term side effects (retroperitoneal, pleural and cardiac valvar fibrosis, arterial and coronary vasospasm) that widely limit its use now. These risks can be minimized by taking periodic 'drug holidays' (5 months on the drug and 1 month off in a 6-month cycle). The usual dose is 1–2 mg 2–3 times daily. Methysergide is also used in 'serotonin syndrome' and to treat diarrhoea caused by carcinoid tumour in higher doses.

Facial pain and neuralgias

The most common cause of facial pain is dental, triggered by hot, cold or sweet foods. Facial neuralgias (trigeminal and glossopharyngeal) consist of paroxysmal, fleeting, pain akin to electric shock. Most cases are idiopathic although structural disease (e.g. multiple sclerosis) are likely in younger patients. Carbamazepine (400–1200 mg/day) is usually effective; gabapentin, phenytoin, valproate and baclofen are other options.

20.3 Cerebrovascular disease

Pathophysiology

A stroke is the sudden onset of neurological deficit from a vascular mechanism. Eighty percent of strokes are a consequence of ischaemia; a transient ischaemic attack (TIA) is an ischaemic neurodeficit that rapidly resolves. The accepted boundary between a TIA and a completed stroke is 24 h. The remaining 20% of strokes are primary haemorrhages, including subarachnoid, lobar and hypertensive deep cerebral haemorrhages. Multiple factors, both non-modifiable (age and sex) and modifiable (e.g. hypertension and diabetes), influence the risk of cerebrovascular disease. Prolonged hypertension and diabetes are specific risk factors for small vessel cerebral stroke (lacunar infarcts); smoking is a risk factor for all vascular mechanisms causing stroke. Cerebral venous thrombosis may be spontaneous (as seen during pregnancy) or may be secondary to a hypercoagulable state, focal intracranial or ear infections.

Aim and principles of treatment

Intracranial haemorrhage

The specific treatment is often surgical and pharmacological interventions are directed to the reduction of raised intracranial pressure. Nimodipine, a calcium channel blocker that crosses the blood–brain barrier, may be effective in minimizing symptomatic vasospasm following subarachnoid haemorrhage if begun early (by day 4). Cerebral vasospasm after aneurysm surgery is best treated by improving cerebral perfusion with vasopressor agents.

Acute treatment of ischaemic stroke

Patients with TIA or an established ischaemic stroke should receive aspirin (75–300 mg/day) as soon as the diagnosis is confirmed. If fever and/or hyperglycemia are present, these should be treated promptly. Anticoagulation is strictly reserved for patients with high risk of venous thromboembolism, cerebral venous thrombosis without major haemorrhage, recurrent thromboembolic arterial stroke from a known source (e.g. cardiogenic emboli with atrial fibrillation) and progressive stroke in the basilar artery territory (stroke-in-evolution). Systemic or selective intra-arterial thrombolytic therapy with recombinant tissue plasminogen activator (rtPA) cannot yet be recommended for general use. However, it may be offered in selective centres with expertise in patients seen within the first 3 h of the ischaemic event in the absence of any major ischaemia or haemorrhage in the computerized tomography (CT) scan. Despite a higher risk of cerebral haemorrhage as a consequence of thrombolytic therapy in ischaemic stroke, both short-term outcome and long-term disabilities may significantly improve in such patients.

Secondary prevention of stroke

Lifestyle and risk factor modifications will remain the cornerstone of secondary stroke prevention. All patients with ischaemic stroke or TIA should receive life-long aspirin (75–300 mg daily). Higher doses of aspirin have little advantage and only worsen gastrotoxicity. Identical doses of aspirin are given to patients after carotid endarterectomy. Dipyridamole (200 mg twice daily) is recommended for patients intolerant of aspirin or for those with recurrent ischaemic events despite aspirin. Clopidogrel (75 mg/day) is an alternative for patients intolerant of aspirin. Warfarin is indicated for patients with atrial fibrillation or cardioembolic stroke. The combination of aspirin and warfarin carries a high risk of cerebral haemorrrhage, especially in the elderly.

Drugs used in cerebrovascular diseases

(For aspirin and warfarin, see Chapter 9.)

20.4 Raised intracranial pressure (ICP)

Acute rises in ICP can occur as a result of intracerebral or subarachnoid haemorrhage, cerebral infarction, tumours, Reye's syndrome and after head injury. The aim of medical therapy is to maintain cerebral perfusion and prevent global cerebral ischaemia. General treatment of acutely raised ICP (best carried out in an intensive care unit) involves: (i) head elevation to 45 degrees; (ii) restriction of free water by the use of intravenous normal (0.9%) saline to 1000 ml/day; (iii) aggressive treatment of fever; (iv) careful intubation (without causing gagging or coughing) in comatose patients; (v) avoiding a drop in systemic blood pressure; and (vi) stool softeners to prevent straining. Specific treatment depends on the cause of raised ICP. Mannitol, an osmolar diuretic, lowers ICP by decreasing interstitial brain fluid and is given as intravenous boluses of 0.5–1 g/ kg every 4–6 h, maintaining plasma osmolality above 295 mOsm/kg. Furosemide (frusemide) is less effective. Longer periods of treatment with mannitol may not be effective and mannitol should not be given in raised ICP resulting from extracerebral (subdural or extradural) haemorrhage. Dexamethasone is the treatment of choice for raised ICP resulting from vasogenic oedema, as in cerebral tumours or metastases. It is given as an initial dose of 8–12 mg intravenously, followed by 4–6 mg every 6 h. Mechanical hyperventilation in intubated patients to reduce arterial Pco_2 to 3.5 kPa is sometimes helpful.

Cases of chronically raised ICP without any focal cerebral pathology (idiopathic or benign intracranial hypertension) is treated with oral acetazolamide (750–1000 mg/day).

Acetazolamide is an inhibitor of the carbonic anhydrase enzyme that is present in the choroid plexus where cerebrospinal fluid (CSF) is formed. It probably reduces the synthesis of CSF and is the most effective treatment for idiopathic intracranial hypertension (and open-angle glaucoma). It is also used in neurology with remarkable success to prevent attacks of periodic paralysis and episodic ataxia and it is occasionally helpful as an adjuvant therapy in atypical absence, atonic and tonic seizures especially in children. Its use to reduce hydrocephalus caused by choroid plexus papilloma is only of historical interest. The main side effects are nausea, taste disturbance, loss of appetite, paraesthesia, fatigue, metabolic acidosis and electrolyte disturbances; rarely renal calculi, abnormal liver function, blood disorders including agranulocytosis and thrombocytopenia and erythema multiforme are reported.

20.5 Infections of the nervous system

Infections of the CNS may be acute or chronic. The pathogens involved may be bacterial, viral, protozoal or parasitic. Brain abscess and subdural empyema are focal suppurative infections of the brain and require surgical drainage in addition to antibiotics. Treatment for acute bacterial meningitis and herpes simplex encephalitis must begin as soon as possible on clinical suspicion alone, with

intravenous benzylpenicillin and aciclovir, respectively. In tropical countries, cerebral malaria (caused by choloroquine-resistant forms of *Plasmodium falciparum*) and tuberculous meningitis are important causes of mortality and morbidity. HIV infections can involve any part of the nervous system and should be treated with standard antiretroviral combination therapy. Leprosy is the commonest infection of the peripheral nerves in the world. The pharmacology of antimicrobial chemotherapy is given elsewhere in this book (Chapter 10).

20.6 Disorders of sleep

Excessive daytime sleepiness (EDS) causes impaired alertness leading to accidents and is associated with increased cardiovascular morbidity and mortality. Many disorders of EDS are consequences of neurological diseases, e.g. narcolepsy and periodic limb movements during sleep (PLMS). EDS in narcolepsy is often associated with cataplexy (sudden loss of muscle tone, provoked by an emotional stimulus like laughter). Narcoleptic EDS is usually treated with stimulants (methylphenidate, pemoline, dextroamfetamine, methamfetamine, mazindol), all of which carry the risk of dependence with long-term use. Modafinil is a recent addition to this list that has been claimed to act differently with less risk of dependence. Cataplexy and other sleep-related phenomena in narcolepsy frequently respond to tricyclic or SSRI antidepressants. The most effective treatment for the restless leg syndrome and PLMS depends on dopaminergic agents (levodopa, bromocriptine and pergolide) taken before retiring to bed. Tricyclic antidepressants paradoxically aggravate these movements.

20.7 Neuroimmunology

Pathophysiology
Immunological mechanisms are recognized to play an important role in a number of diseases affecting different parts of the nervous system

IMMUNOLOGICAL MECHANISMS	
Central nervous system (CNS)	
Acute	Disseminated encephalomyelitis
	Haemorrhagic leukoencephalitis
	Demyelinating optic neuritis
	Transverse myelitis
	CNS vasculitis (isolated angitis of CNS)
Subacute	Neuro-systemic lupus erythematosus (SLE)
	Subacute cerebellar degeneration and limbic encephalitis (usually paraneoplastic)
Chronic	Multiple sclerosis (MS)
	Stiff-person syndrome
Peripheral nervous system	
Acute	AIDP (Guillain–Barré syndrome)
	Vasculitis of peripheral nerves
Chronic	CIDP, MMN
	Acquired neuromyotonia
Neuromuscular junction	
	Myasthenia gravis
	LEMS
Skeletal muscles	
	Polymyositis and dermatomyositis

Table 20.3 Neurological disorders with a proven or presumed immunological mechanism.

(Table 20.3). One of three treatments may be selected to treat an acute attack following neuroimmunological injury: (i) high doses of corticosteroids (e.g. intravenous methylprednisolone); (ii) human immunoglobulin (IVIg); or (iii) plasma exchange (plasmapheresis). However, one particular treatment may be more specific for one disease than the other. In diseases with an established autoimmune mechanism (e.g. myasthenia gravis or vasculitic neuropathy), long-term immunosuppression is required as well. Azathioprine is the neurologists' most preferred immunosuppressive drug.

Methylprednisolone

Methylprednisolone is usually used for rapid suppression of inflammatory and allergic disorders; its side effect profile is similar to prednisolone except that rapid intravenous administration of large doses has been associated with cardiovascular collapse. Patients often experience a metallic taste at the time of infusion, and psychosis and restlessness are reported occasionally. It is usually given in short courses (1 g daily for 3 days or 500 mg daily for 5 days) When oral prednisolone is used for long-term immunosuppression, care must be taken to avoid long-term complications like osteopenia and prophylactic use of biphosphonates may be desirable in high-risk cases (e.g. post-menopausal women). For the pharmacokinetics and adverse effects of corticosteroids and immunosuppressive drugs, please refer to the relevant sections in this book.

Interferons

Interferons are naturally occurring recombinant proteins with complex effects on immunity and cell function. Three classes of interferons are available for treatment: alpha, beta and gamma. Interferon-alpha is used in selected cancer treatment and chronic viral hepatitis (B and C); interferon gamma-1b is indicated in chronic granulomatous disease to reduce the frequency of infections; only interferon-beta can be effective in patients with multiple sclerosis.

Human immunoglobulin (IVIg)

The mechanism of action of IVIg in acute and chronic inflammatory demyelinating poly-neuropathies (AIDP and CIDP) and in other neuroimmunological disorders is unclear; exogenous IVIg may neutralize putative auto-antibodies as a result of the presence of anti-idiotype antibodies in the healthy donor pool contributing the human IVIg. Another explan-ation is that administered IVIg increases the catabolism of endogenous IVIg that may carry the circulating autoantibody fraction. The usual dose is 2 g/kg given i.v. over 3–5 days; a dose of 1 g/kg may be adequate for maintenance. IVIg is also used for replacement therapy in patients with congenital agamma or hypo-gamma globulinemia, for the treatment of idiopathic thrombocytopenic purpura, Kawasaki syn-drome and for the prophylaxis of infection following bone marrow transplantation. Com-mon side effects are allergic reaction, urticaria, hypotension, venous thrombosis and increased blood viscosity. In patients who are IgA-deficient, oliguric renal failure may occur.

20.8 Specific diseases

Multiple sclerosis

In multiple slerosis (MS), there is destruction of myelin in the CNS. An acute attack causes oedema around the area of demyelination, called a plaque. Recurrent attacks cause destruction of axons that contribute to per-manent disability. Relapsing-remitting MS is the commonest clinical form. Treatment is aimed at the alleviation of acute relapses with new neurological symptoms or an exacerbation of old symptoms that produce functional impair-ment present for at least 48 h or longer. Short courses of intravenous methylprednisolone followed by tapering courses of oral predniso-lone over 2–3 weeks are usually given to most patients. Attacks of demyelinating optic neur-itis, transverse myelitis or disseminated ence-phalomyelitis are treated similarly. Currently three treatments are available as disease modi-fying therapy for slowing the progression in MS: Interferon IFN)b-1b, IFNb-1a and copoly-mer 1 (glatiramer). Each of these three thera-pies reduce annual relapse rates by about one-third but are expensive and should be given regularly (subcutaneous or intramuscu-lar injections) on a long-term basis. Both intramuscular (IFNb-1a, Avonex) and subcuta-neous injections (IFNb-1a, Rebif and IFNb-1b, 'Betaseron') are used. Most frequently reported side effects include irritation at injec-tion sites (including skin necrosis), influenza-like symptoms and fatigue; rarely raised liver enzymes, hypersensitivity reactions, blood dis-orders, mood and personality changes, confu-sion, convulsion and suicide attempts have been reported. For chronic progressive MS, the role for immunosuppression (azathioprine and cyclophosphamide) or IFNb-1b therapy is debatable. Table 20.4 lists the symptomatic therapy available for patients with chronic neu-rological disability as seen in MS. These treat-ments can be delivered in any chronic neurological disorder where similar symptoms emerge.

Peripheral neuropathy

Acute and chronic inflammatory demyelinating polyneuropathies (AIDP, also termed Guillain-Barré syndrome, and CIDP) are rare disorders. They are treated with high doses (2 g/kg) of intravenous human immunoglobulin (IVIg) or therapeutic plasma exchange. Oral corticoster-oids (prednisolone) are also effective in CIDP but not in AIDP. Patients with CIDP usually require maintenance treatment with steroids or with pulses of IVIg or plasma exchange repeated at 1–6 monthly intervals. Some cases of CIDP may require additional immuno-suppression (azathioprine or ciclosporin). Vas-culitic peripheral neuropathy usually presents with multiple painful mononeuropathies. Often responsive to steroids (pulse methylpredniso-lone followed by oral prednisolone 1 mg/kg) alone, some cases may require the addition of cyclophosphamide, e.g. those with an underly-ing systemic vasculitis. After maximal recovery of neurological deficit, steroids are tapered off and cyclophosphamide is continued, usually orally (2 mg/kg daily), for a period of one year.

Muscle diseases

Polymyositis is a condition of presumed auto-immune aetiology in which the skeletal muscle is damaged by a lymphocytic inflammatory process. The term dermatomyositis is used when polymyositis is accompanied by characteristic skin changes. Both are treated with prednisolone (1–1.5 mg/kg/day), tapered after muscle strength improves and muscle enzymes (serum creatine kinase) decline. Approximately 75% of patients will have a good clinical response to steroids alone. The onset of steroid-induced myopathy may complicate therapy. Cytotoxic therapy should be considered for severe disease, inadequate response to steroids, relapsing disease and for steroid-induced complications. One of the three agents is used orally: methotrexate (7.5–15 mg/week), azathioprine (2–2.5 mg/kg/day) and cyclophosphamide (1–2 mg/kg/day).

Diseases of neuromuscular junction

In myasthenia gravis, there is an autoimmune attack by the complement system and antibodies are targeted to the nicotinic acetylcholine receptors in the post-synaptic neuromuscular junction. Typically, patients experience fluctuating symptoms of muscle weakness and fatigue provoked by exertion. Most forms of myasthenia are generalized and only 10% will have weakness restricted only to the extraocular muscles (ocular myasthenia). Administration of drugs with neuromuscular blocking effects can dangerously exacerbate myasthenic symptoms. The thymus, which is abnormal in 75% of patients, plays a central role in sensitizing lymphocytes to the acetylcholine receptors. Thymectomy offers the only possibility of a cure in this condition. Anticholinesterase drugs assist patients with short-term symptomatic improvement but overdose with cholinesterases can lead to weakness resulting from depolarizing neuromuscular blockade ('cholinergic crisis').

DRUGS FOR CHRONIC NEUROLOGICAL DISABILITY

Nature of symptoms	Drugs available
Spasticity	Oral and intrathecal baclofen (GABA agonist) Diazepam (GABA agonist) Dantrolene (direct effect on skeletal muscles) Tizanidine (alpha$_2$ adrenoreceptor agonist) Botulinum toxin (local injections to spastic muscles)
Muscle spasms	Clonazepam Baclofen
Bladder symptoms	Antimuscarinics: flavoxate and oxybutinin for increased frequency tolterodine, propiverine may also be effecive in urge incontinence: *all may cause retention and precipitate angle-closure glaucoma* cholinergics (carbachol, bethanecol) for retention *in the absence of urinary obstruction* adrenergic blockers (prazosin, doxazosin) improve urinary flow by reducing the tone of external uretheral sphincter
Nocturnal enuresis	Adults: desmopressin or propantheline Children: tricyclics (imipramine, amitriptyline)
Dysesthesia	Carbamazepine, lamotrigine
Pain	Tricyclics (amitriptyline, imipramine) Anti-epileptics (carbamazepine, gabapentin)
Fatigue	Amantadine
Depression	SSRI (sertraline, citalopram)
Impotence	Sildenafil

Table 20.4 Symptomatic treatment of chronic neurological disability.

Plasma exchange is probably superior to IVIg for rapid improvement in seriously weak patients with myasthenia ('myasthenic crisis') and to stabilize neuromuscular function prior to thymectomy or other major surgery.

Long-term treatment of acquired auto-immune myasthenia gravis requires immuno-suppression, often started with a combinaton of corticosteroids and azathioprine. Low doses of corticosteroids are generally preferred (prednisolone 15 mg/day, then increased by 5 mg every 3rd or 4th day until a dose of 1 mg/kg is reached). Larger doses of steroids can transiently worsen myasthenic symptoms, particularly bulbar weakness. Initial large doses of steroids (prednisolone 0.75–1 mg/kg) are only given to hospitalized patients, who can be closely monitored, or to the rare patient requiring ventilatory support as a result of myasthenic crisis. Azathioprine is usually introduced at a daily dose of 1.5 mg/kg and then increased to a maintenance dose of 2–2.5 mg/kg/day. Patients with ocular myasthenia are best maintained on low doses of steroids (prednisolone 5–10 mg) alone.

The principle of drug therapy in Lambert–Eaton myasthenic syndrome (LEMS) is broadly similar. In this condition, antibodies directed to the voltage-gated calcium channels in the presynaptic vesicles of the motor end plate affect acetylcholine release. LEMS may be associated with an underlying malignancy (small cell lung cancer) as a paraneoplastic syndrome. As compared to myasthenia gravis, response to treatment is far less satisfactory. 3,4 Di-aminopyridine, a potassium channel blocker, partially improves presynaptic transmission failure in LEMS.

Drugs used for neuromuscular junction disorder

Cholinesterase inhibitors

This class of drugs enhances neuromuscular transmission both in voluntary and involuntary muscles by increasing the intrasynaptic acetyl-choline level as a result of the inhibition of cholinesterases, which normally terminate its action as a chemical transmitter. Muscarinic side effects (sweating, increased salivation, bradycardia, gastro-intestinal and uterine motility) are common to all members of this class. These parasympathomimetic effects are effectively antagonized by atropine. Edrophonium is extremely short-acting and is useful mainly for the diagnosis of myasthenia gravis or to determine whether or not a patient with myasthenia is receiving inadequate or excessive treatment with cholinergic drugs. It has to be given parenterally (i.v.). Neostigmine produces a therapeutic effect for 2–4 h and is available as 15 mg tablets (usual daily dose 120–180 mg). Pyridostigmine is less powerful than neostigmine but has a longer duration of action (3–6 h) and has relatively less gastrointestinal side effects. It is available as 60 mg tablets (usual daily dose 360–720 mg). Propantheline bromide (Pro-Banthine) is usually used as an antimuscarinic to minimize the side effects of cholinesterase inhibitors at a dose of 15 mg two or three times daily.

Cholinesterase inhibitors that cross the blood–brain barrier (donepezil, rivastigmine and galantamine) have been claimed recently to delay progression of dementia in Alzheimer's disease. They are not used for peripheral neuromuscular disorders.

20.9 Movement disorders

Pathophysiology

The movement disorders can be broadly classified as: (i) hypo- or bradykinetic, causing poverty of movement and rigidity (parkinsonism); (ii) dystonic, focal or generalized, which are produced by involuntary spasm of the involved muscles; and (iii) hyperkinetic, such as chorea and various dyskinesias. Parkinsonism is caused by many disorders and may be drug induced. Parkinson's disease (PD) is idiopathic parkinsonism that is characterized by bradykinesia, rigidity, tremor and gait disorder. PD is caused by loss of striatal dopaminergic projections from the substantia nigra pars compacta. The cause of neuronal death in PD is unknown but may result from the generation of free radicals and oxidative stress, perhaps by oxidation of dopamine itself. Levodopa, the aminoacid precursor of dopamine, acts mainly by replenishing striatal dopamine in PD. Parkinsonism caused by more diffuse degenerative brain disease (e.g. multiple system atrophy) does not normally respond to levodopa.

Aim and principles of therapy
The goal of treatment in PD is to restore motor function. Levodopa improves bradykinesia and rigidity more than tremor. It is always given in combination with an extracerebral decarboxylase inhibitor (carbidopa or benserazide), which prevents peripheral degradation of levodopa to dopamine but, unlike levodopa, does not cross the blood–brain barrier. The advantages of using a decarboxylase inhibitor with levodopa are: (i) effective brain concentrations of dopamine can be achieved with lower doses of levodopa; (ii) reduced peripheral conversion to dopamine decreases cardiovascular side effects (hypotension and arrhythmia) and nausea; (iii) there is rapid onset of therapeutic effect; and (iv) a smoother clinical response. A disadvantage is an increased incidence of abnormal involuntary movements on long-term therapy (>5 years). It is currently accepted that levodopa therapy (with carbidopa or benserazide) is best given as modified or controlled release preparations that may also prevent 'end of dose' deterioration and nocturnal immobility and rigidity.

Drugs used for parkinsonism (Table 20.5)

Levodopa
It is always given in combination with one of the two extracerebral dopa-decarboxylase inhibitors: carbidopa (cocareldopa or 'Sinemet') and benserazide (cobeneldopa or Madopar) as fixed drug formulations. Sinemet is

available in two formulations of levodopa : carbidopa (10 : 1 or 4 : 1); 1 part of benserazide is always combined with 4 parts of levodopa. When cocareldopa 100/10 is used, the dose of carbidopa may be insufficient to achieve full inhibition of the extracerebral decarboxylase system that usually requires a daily dose of carbidopa 75 mg. Treatment must be initiated with low doses (typical dose: 'Sinemet CR' 100/25 twice daily) and increased gradually. The final dose is usually balanced between the efficacy and side effects of treatment and the interval between doses may need to be individualized. Treatment should be taken before meals. As the patient ages, the maintenance dose may need to be reduced. Domperidone is useful in controlling nausea and vomiting if present. Other side effects, often dose related, include postural hypotension (rarely labile hypertension), arrhythmias, neuropsychiatric symptoms (insomnia, agitation, hallucinations) and dyskinesias.

Dopamine agonists
Bromocriptine, cabergoline, pergolide and lisuride are ergot derivatives and act as direct agonists of dopaminergic receptors. Ropinirole is a D_2 agonist with comparable efficacy. Pramipexole is a recently introduced, nonergot dopamine agonist with preferential effect only on the D_2 receptor family. The role of dopamine agonists as initial therapy, as opposed to levodopa/dopa decarboxylase inhibitors, in early stages of PD remains controversial and a trial (ELLDOPA trial) is underway to answer this question. Dopamine agonists offer no advantages over levodopa but it is claimed that their use in the early stages of PD can defer the eventual introduction of levodopa by up to 12–18 months, thereby delaying the onset of dopa-induced dyskinesia. These agonists are useful in the advanced stages of PD as add-on therapy and also when response to levodopa therapy becomes less predictable and shows fluctuations with individual dosages ('on–off' phenomenon). Apomorphine is a potent

ANTI-PARKINSONIAN DRUG THERAPY

Drug	Dose	Side effects
Levodopa		
Levodopa/carbidopa		
Regular dose	100/10 to 250/25 Increase slowly to t.i.d. or q.i.d.	Orthostatic hypotension, GI complaints, hallucinations, confusion, chorea, dyskinesias
Slow-release dose	100/25 to 200/50 b.i.d. or t.i.d.	
Dopamine agonists		
Bromocriptine	7.5–30 mg daily in divided doses	Postural hypotension, nausea, vomiting hallucinations, psychosis, dyskinesias
Pergolide	0.05–3 mg daily in divided doses	Nausea, dizziness, hallucinations, confusion, constipation, postural hypotension, dyskinesias
Ropinirole	0.5–3 mg daily in divided doses	Nausea, somnolence, leg oedema, abdominal pain, vomiting, syncope, dyskinesia, hallucinations
Amantadine (acts by NMDA-receptor blockade)	100–200 mg	Livido reticularis, diarrhoea, depression
Apomorphine (subcutaneous injections)	3–30 mg daily in divided doses	Nausea, vomiting, confusion, hallucination, postural hypotension, dyskinesias, local reaction to injections (nodule and ulcers)
Enzyme inhibitors		
Selegeline (inhibits MAO-B)	5 mg b.i.d.	Nausea, dizziness, insomnia, hallucination
Entcapone (inhibits COMT)	200 mg with each dose of levodopa; max 2 g	Nausea, vomiting, abdominal pain, dizziness
Antimuscarinics		
Trihexiphenidyl	2–5 mg t.i.d.	Dry mouth, blurred vision, confusion
Benzatropine (benztropine)	0.5–2 mg t.i.d.	Dry mouth, confusion

Table 20.5 Commonly used anti-parkinsonian drug therapy.

stimulator of dopamine receptors that is sometimes useful in stabilizing PD patients experiencing frequent, unpredictable 'off' periods on levodopa treatment. It is essential to hospitalize such patients and commence domperidone three days before starting apomorphine (given by subcutaneous injections). Selegeline is a monoamine-oxidase B inhibitor used in the treatment of PD for its presumed neuroprotective effect and in conjunction with levodopa to reduce 'end of dose' deterioration. Entcapone, a catechol-*o*-methyl-transferase inhibitor, has also been introduced recently for the latter indication. Amantadine (first introduced for its antiviral activity) has modest anti-parkinsonian effects and improves mild bradykinetic disabilities, rigidity and tremors. Although initially believed to be a dopamine agonist, its anti-parkinsonian effect is probably a result of NMDA-receptor blockade.

Anticholinergics

The role for antimuscarinic drugs (less appropriately called anticholinergics) in the treatment of PD is probably restricted to patients with predominant tremors or mild symptoms. They are believed to exert their anti-parkinsonian effect (mainly on tremor and rigidity with no effect on bradykinesia) by correcting the relative cholinergic excess that occurs in the striatal network as a result of dopamine deficiency. Antimuscarinics are also useful in reducing sialorrhoea and are indicated as the first-line therapy in drug-induced parkinsonism. However, tardive dyskinesia does not respond to antimuscarinics and may actually be made worse. No important differences exist in the efficacy or side effects between the many synthetic antimuscarinics that are available. Those most commonly used are orphenadrine, trihexyphenidyl, benzatropine and procyclidine.

A summary of the sites of action of anti-parkinsonian drugs is given in Fig. 20.1.

Dystonia and other movement disorders

Drug therapy for generalized dystonia is often empirical. Because some forms of generalized dystonia are levodopa responsive, it is mandatory to offer a trial of levodopa in all cases. Non-responders are treated with antimuscarinics, carbamazepine or tetrabenazine, which acts by depleting nerve endings of dopamine. Tetrabanazine is also effective in Huntington's chorea and related disorders. Haloperidol, pimozide and clozapine are used to treat complex motor tics and symptoms of Gilles de la Tourette syndrome. Small doses of haloperidol alone are remarkably effective in Sydenham's chorea; valproate is an alternative. Essential tremors are treated with propranolol or primidone. Focal dystonias (blepharospasm and torticollis) are best treated with botulinum toxin injected periodically in small amounts locally to the involved muscles.

Wilson's disease

This is an autosomal recessive disease of brain and liver that presents between 10 and 30 years of age with a syndrome of tremor, extrapyramidal rigidity, dystonia, dysarthria and cerebellar ataxia. The fundamental defect is probably hepatic failure to incorporate copper into ceuloplasmin, the copper-binding protein

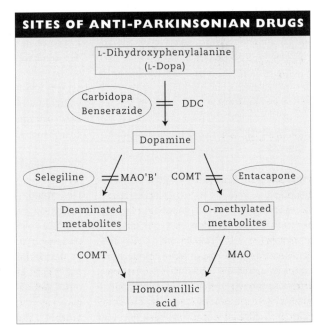

Fig. 20.1 Sites of action of anti-parkinsonian drugs. COMT, catechol-o-methyl transferase; DDC, dopa carboxylase; MAO, monoamine oxidase.

in serum. There are deposits of excess copper in liver that may cause cirrhosis; the presence of rings of copper pigment in the cornea (Kayser–Fleischer or KF rings) is diagnostic. Treatment consists of reducing dietary copper, taking oral zinc to reduce copper absorption in the gut and eliminating tissue-bound copper by using a specific chelator, D-penicillamine. Penicillamine is used for copper and lead poisoning, in the treatment of cystinuria and as disease-modifying therapy in rheumatoid arthritis and in chronic active hepatitis (anti-inflammatory effect). In Wilson's disease, penicillamine is started at a small dose (250 mg twice daily) and then slowly increased to a maximum daily dose of 1.5–2 g in adults (20 mg/kg in children). The serious side effects are hypersensitivity, pemphigus, erythema multiforme, drug-induced lupus erythematosus, myasthenia gravis (with positive autoantibodies), polymyositis, dermatomyositis, nephrotic syndrome, Goodpasture's syndrome, agranulocytosis, aplastic and haemolytic anaemia. Patients on penicillamine must have periodic blood counts, urine tests and renal clearance estimated. Appearance of any of the above side effects must lead to permanent discontinuation of the therapy. A proportion of patients with Wilson's disease may actually deteriorate on penicillamine therapy that may be irreversible in some cases, even on drug withdrawal. Trientine is an alternative to D-penicillamine but it acts differently.

20.10 Drug-induced neurological disorders (Table 20.6)

Neuroleptic malignant syndrome (NMS)

A small percentage (1–2%) of patients exposed to neuroleptics develop this serious and potentially fatal (mortality rate up to 25%) condition. Hyperpyrexia, muscle rigidity, agitation and autonomic hyperactivity, that may progress to mental obtundation, raised muscle enzymes (serum creatine kinase) and leukocytosis are characteristic. Treatment includes

immediate discontinuation of neuroleptics, supportive care and use of dantrolene and bromocriptine. A similar condition may be reproduced by abrupt discontinuation of levodopa in PD patients.

Malignant hyperthermia (MH)

This syndrome is distinct from NMS but shares similar features with it. In susceptible individuals (those with genetic disorder of calcium channels or neuromuscular diseases such as central core disease and other myopathies), fever, muscle rigidity (with raised serum creatine kinase), metabolic and respiratory acidosis occur soon after exposure to halogenated inhaled anaesthetics and/or depolarizing muscle relaxants such as succinylcholine.

Vulnerability to this syndrome can be evaluated by *in vitro* testing of biopsied muscle for a hypercontractile response to caffeine and/or halothane.

Serotonin syndrome

This syndrome consists of altered mental status, autonomic dysfunction and disordered motor function that typically occur within minutes to hours of initiating or increasing the dose of a serotoninergic agent or combining a serotoninergic agent with monoamine oxidase inhibitors. Hyperstimulation of brainstem and spinal cord $5-HT_{1A}$ receptors is the presumed mechanism. Treatment consists of withdrawal of the offending agent, supportive care and use of a serotonin antagonist like cyproheptadine or methylsergide.

Drug used in NMS and MH

Dantrolene

It acts on the skeletal muscle by interfering with the calcium influx in the muscle cell and stopping the contractile process. Because of its muscle relaxant effect, dantrolene is used commonly as an antispasticity agent (initial oral dose 25 mg daily, slowly increased to a maximum of 100 mg 3–4 times daily). It is the drug of choice for NMS and malignant

DRUG-INDUCED COMMON NEUROLOGICAL DISORDERS

Exacerbation of myasthenia
Aminoglycosides
Erythromycin
Phenytoin
Polymyxin

Extrapyramidal effects
Butyrophenones, e.g. haloperidol
Methyldopa
Metoclopramide
Phenothiazines

Myopathy
Colchicine
Corticosteroids
Penicillamine
Quinine

Headache
Ergotamine (withdrawal)
Nitrites
Vasodilators (e.g. hydralazine)
Drugs causing benign intracranial
    hypertension (hypervitaminosis A,
    corticosteroids,
    tetracycline)

Seizures
Amfetamines (amphetamines)
Ciclosporin (cyclosporin)
Isoniazid
Lidocaine
Lithium

Peripheral neuropathy
Amiodarone
Chlorpropamide
Clofibrate
Ethambutol
Ethionamide
DDC and DDI
Isoniazid
Metronidazole
Nalidixic acid
Nitrofurantoin
Vincristine

Optic neuritis
Aminoquinolenes
Ethambutol
Isoniazid
Phenothiazines

Sleep disturbances
Dopamine agonists/levodopa
Monoamine oxidase (MAO) inhibitors

Stroke
Oral contraceptives

Table 20.6 Drug-induced common neurological disorders.

hyperthermia, and dantrolene in these emergent circumstances must be given as rapid i.v. injection, 1 mg/kg, repeated as required to a cumulative maximum of 10 mg/kg. Side effects are drowsiness, fatigue, weakness, liver enzyme rises (occasionally fatal dose-related hepatotoxicity), diarrhoea, urinary symptoms, seizures, pleurisy and pericarditis.

CHAPTER 21

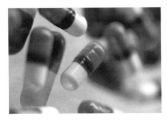

Drugs and Endocrine Disease

21.1 Diabetes mellitus

Pathophysiology

Diabetes mellitus comprises two separate disorders:

1 Non-insulin dependent diabetes mellitus (NIDDM, type 2 diabetes), is a disorder of middle-aged and elderly patients and has a strong genetic basis. Resistance to the action of insulin and hyperinsulinaemia characterizes the early stages. With time, insulin secretion declines and pancreatic failure occurs as a late event. The underlying cause of the disorder remains obscure: there are strong associations with essential hypertension and obesity, and subjects have a very high risk of arterial disease.

Weight reduction improves the metabolic abnormalities, including the insulin resistance; drugs to increase insulin secretion from the pancreas or the peripheral action of insulin are given, but in later stages of the disease when insulin deficiency occurs insulin therapy may become necessary.

2 Insulin dependent diabetes mellitus (IDDM, type 1 diabetes) is the result of autoimmune destruction of pancreatic islet cells, possibly occurring as a late consequence of occult viral pancreatitis. The disease is characterized by absolute insulin deficiency and subjects require insulin therapy from the outset. There is a tendency to develop ketoacidosis owing to unrestrained lipolysis, fatty acid degradation and formation of ketone bodies.

Insulin deficiency (either absolute or relative) results in profound metabolic abnormalities, including altered carbohydrate, fat and protein metabolism. Both types of diabetes mellitus are associated with the long-term complications of nephropathy, retinopathy and neuropathy. In addition, both are associated with a high risk of atherosclerosis.

Aims of treatment

The purpose of treatment is to restore metabolism, including glucose homeostasis, to normal. In type 1 diabetes, strict glycaemic control has been shown to reduce the risk of development of nephropathy and neuropathy. In type 2 diabetes mellitus, the UK Prospective Study in Diabetes (UKPDS) showed that improved glycaemic control reduces the risk of progression of diabetic retinopathy. The risk of cardiovascular (macrovascular) disease is greatly increased in patients with diabetes and an aggressive approach to treat high blood pressure has been shown to be effective in both primary and secondary prevention of macrovascular complications in patients with diabetes. There also is some evidence to suggest that this might delay or prevent the development of the long-term consequences of diabetes mellitus. Other cardiovascular risk factors (e.g. dyslipidaemia) should also be actively treated.

Insulin

Insulin is synthesized as a prohormone in the pancreatic beta cells and secreted into the

ACTIONS OF INSULIN

1 Glucose transport into muscle and fat cells.
2 Increased glycogen synthesis.
3 Inhibition of gluconeogenesis.
4 Inhibition of lipolysis and increased formation of triglycerides.

5 Stimulation of membrane-bound energy-dependent ion transporters (e.g. sodium/potassium ATPase).
6 Stimulation of cell growth.

circulation as a mature dimer composed of two peptides linked by disulphide bridges. The main actions of insulin are shown above.

Pharmacokinetics

Insulin is destroyed in the gut and must be given parenterally. It is degraded in the liver and kidney and has a half-life (either endogenous or exogenous) of approximately 9 min. It should be recognized that insulin is normally secreted into the portal circulation and there is a high level of extraction by the liver. Insulin administration (either subcutaneous or intravenous) will always result in an unphysiological relationship between the amount of insulin systemically and the amount of insulin in the portal circulation. Efforts to develop systems to deliver insulin in a more physiological manner (for example, pancreatic transplant or alternative technological developments) are likely to develop further in the next few years.

Adverse effects

1 Local effects following subcutaneous injection of insulin can lead to either loss of fat (lipo-atrophy) or hypertrophy of fat (lipo-hypertrophy). These reactions are unusual since the advent of human or highly purified animal insulins.
2 Antibodies may develop to insulin (this is not usually seen with human insulin) and binding of insulin to antibody may result in prolongation and attenuation of the action of insulin.
3 Hypoglycaemia is the most frequent and potentially most serious adverse effect. This is normally a consequence of decreased carbohydrate intake, unaccustomed exercise, administration of too much insulin or ingestion of alcohol. Symptoms and signs are those of adrenergic activation (sweating, tachycardia, systolic hypertension and hunger) and of neuroglycopenia (visual disturbance, drowsiness, seizures and coma).

Insulin formulation

Insulin may be made from animal (porcine or bovine) pancreas, although these formulations are very infrequently used. Porcine insulin can be modified biochemically to make it identical to the human amino acid sequence. More commonly, howevever, insulin is synthesized using genetic engineering. Recently, a modified form of human insulin (insulin analogue, Lispro) has become available. In this formulation, a single amino acid change is made in the insulin sequence, which results in more rapid absorption following subcutaneous injection. This allows the timing of insulin administration to be much closer to food ingestion, and this can have some advantages in patients with type I diabetes mellitus. In particular, greater flexibility of lifestyle is offered by this approach. However, this type of insulin does have a slightly greater risk of causing hypoglycaemic episodes.

In order to prolong its biological action, insulin is given by subcutaneous injection, thereby slowing its rate of delivery to the circulation. Absorption can be slowed further by combining the insulin with protamine (a basic protein) or zinc or both, the resulting preparation having a slower onset but longer duration of action. A further modification in the rate of absorption depends on whether the insulin preparation is amorphous or

INSULIN FORMULATIONS

Duration of action	Examples	Peak effect (h)	Duration of action (h)
Short	Insulin injection (soluble insulin)	2–4	6–12
Intermediate	Isophane insulin	5–12	12–24
	Insulin zinc suspension (amorphous)	3–6	12–16
Long	Insulin zinc suspension (crystalline)	5–14	24–30
Mixed	Variable portions of soluble and isophane insulins	2–10 3–8	18–20 16–24

Table 21.1 Insulin formuations.

crystalline, the latter dissolving more slowly. Broadly speaking, insulin preparations can be divided into four categories—short, intermediate, long and mixed—depending on their onset and duration of action following subcutaneous administration (Table 21.1).

Dose

Insulin is available in the uniform strength of 100 units/ml. The dose, frequency of administration and combination of insulin formulations depend on numerous factors that vary greatly between individuals. The majority of patients need a long-acting insulin given either once or twice daily to provide basal blood sugar homeostasis, as well as more frequent injections of a short-acting insulin to mimic the physiological increase of insulin secretion associated with meals. A typical regimen would include administration of a short-acting insulin with main meals and a longer acting insulin either once or twice daily. Insulin is given via convenient, commercially available pen injector devices. Patients monitor glycaemic control by measuring capillary blood glucose levels using glucose oxidase impregnated sticks. In this way patients can adjust their own dose of insulin to maintain blood sugar levels as near normal as possible during the day. Long-term glycaemic control is assessed by measuring the concen-tration of a glycosylated form of haemoglobin (HbA_{1c}).

Oral hypoglycaemic drugs

Sulphonylureas

Mechanism

Sulphonylureas act primarily by stimulating pancreatic beta cells to produce more insulin. Functioning pancreatic tissue is therefore necessary for their action. In addition, they inhibit both gluconeogenesis and insulin degradation in the liver and possibly increase insulin receptor density.

Adverse effects

All sulphonylureas can cause symptomatic hypoglycaemia, which is the most frequent adverse reaction. This is most troublesome with drugs that have a long elimination half-life and are excreted via the kidney. Chlorpropamide, which should no longer be used because of this problem, was particularly troublesome in this respect but all sulphonylureas have the potential to cause hypoglycaemia. Sulphonylureas are also associated with allergic reactions (mainly rashes) gastrointestinal symptoms, bone marrow suppression and cholestatic jaundice, which can be either allergic or dose related.

Drug interactions

The interactions described for insulin apply also to sulphonylureas. It is important to warn patients that alcohol may potentiate the hypoglycaemic effect. In addition, sulphonamides (including cotrimoxazole) can enhance the hypoglycaemic effect of sulphonylureas.

Clinical use and dose (Table 21.2)

The majority of patients should be started on a drug with a short half-life (e.g. gliquidone, glipizide, gliclazide or glibenclamide). This helps minimize the risk of hypoglycaemia, although all of these agents may still cause this problem, particularly in elderly patients and in subjects with renal, cardiac and hepatic dysfunction. Sulphonylureas can be combined with other oral hypoglycaemic agents (for example, metformin or acarbose), and can also, occasionally, be combined with insulin in patients with type 2 diabetes to optimize blood glucose control.

Biguanides (metformin)

Mechanisms

The mechanisms are uncertain, but the following effects are likely to contribute:

1 Decreased glucose absorption from the gut.
2 Increased glucose entry to cells.
3 Anorectic effects.

Pharmacokinetics

Metformin is excreted unchanged by the kidney.

Adverse effects

Lactic acidosis is the most serious, although uncommon, problem. It carries a high mortality and is more common in patients with renal, hepatic or cardiac dysfunction. The more frequent adverse effects affect the gastrointestinal tract: nausea, vomiting and diarrhoea.

Dose

Metformin: 0.5–1 g 8-hourly.

Glucosidase inhibitors (acarbose)

Inhibition of α-glucosidase activity in the gastrointestinal tract reduces breakdown of more complex sugars to glucose. This limits glucose absorption following carbohydrate ingestion and can be used in treatment of patients with type 2 diabetes. Acarbose can be given as adjuvant therapy with either sulphonylurea agents or metformin. Unfortunately, failure to digest carbohydrate adequately results in bacterial fermentation within the gut resulting in excessive flatus production, which many patients find uncomfortable. For this reason, the use of this drug is relatively limited.

SULPHONYLUREAS				
	Half-life (h)	Clearance route	Dose (mg)	Frequency of daily dose
Glibenclamide	6	M	5	1–3
Gliclazide	12	M	40–320	1
Glipizide	2–4	M	2.5–7.5	2–3
Gliquidone	1.5	M	15–45	2–3
Glymidine	5–8	M (A)	500	1–3

M, metabolized by liver; A, active metabolites.

Table 21.2 Sulphonylureas currently in clinical use.

Repaglinide

Repaglinide is a drug that is chemically different from sulphonylureas but which increases pancreatic insulin release. It has a very short duration of action, and is taken along with meals to improve insulin release and maintain euglycaemia. Its short duration of action make it less likely to cause hypoglycaemia. It can be combined with metformin. Its place in the overall management in patients with type 2 diabetes has still to be defined.

Thiozolidinediones

This new class of drugs acts to increase insulin sensitivity (i.e. increase insulin-stimulated glucose uptake by key target tissues such as skeletal muscle). Although the mechanism of action is not fully understood, these drugs activate nuclear receptors (PPARγ). In research studies, they have been shown to improve insulin sensitivity. The first drug of this class to be released (Troglitazone) causes severe hepatic dysfunction in a small number of patients and has now been withdrawn from use in the UK. However, other agents of this class are likely to become available for clinical use, although their role in the management of patients with type 2 diabetes mellitus is still undefined.

Clinical use, benefits and risks of insulin and oral hypoglycaemic drugs

Variable insulin formulations, the technology of insulin delivery (infusion pumps and pen injector devices) and technology for home monitoring of blood glucose allow strict control of glucose homeostasis in insulin-taking patients. There is evidence that strict control of blood glucose will retard the progression of the microvascular complications in patients with both type 1 and type 2 diabetes mellitus. This does, of course, place patients at greater risk of insulin-induced hypoglycaemia. In patients with type 2 diabetes mellitus, dietary restriction of refined carbohydrate allied to overall weight reduction are often used as initial therapeutics approaches. Patients whose control is not satisfactory with this measure can be treated with metformin (particularly effective in overweight patients) or sulphonylureas. The two drugs can be safely combined. Insulin can, on occasion, also be combined with oral hypoglycaemic agents to improve glycaemic control further. With time, however, as pancreatic insulin production declines, many patients require insulin on its own to maintain reasonable glycaemic and metabolic homeostasis.

Additionally, there is very good evidence that effective antihypertensive therapy will reduce the progression of diabetic nephropathy, and that ACE inhibitors are particularly effective in this regard.

Increasing understanding of the links between NIDDM, essential hypertension, obesity and atherosclerosis and identification of hyperinsulinaemia as a risk factor for atherosclerosis may account for the failure of hypoglycaemic therapy to reduce the high cardiovascular mortality in patients with type 2 diabetes mellitus. However, recent data convincingly shows that blood pressure lowering treatment will reduce the morbidity and mortality from macrovascular disease in patients with type 2 diabetes and this should be regarded as a primary therapeutic goal in this disorder. Furthermore, the absolute importance of weight reduction as a means of improving insulin sensitivity and reducing hyperinsulinaemia in these patients should be emphasized.

Diabetic emergencies

Hypoglycaemic coma

Causes
Coma is usually precipitated by missing a meal, unaccustomed exercise or taking too much insulin or sulphonylurea.

Clinical features
Coma can present with a wide range of neurological signs. Every medical emergency arriving with mental impairment, coma or other

neurological signs must have capillary glucose checked on arrival.

Treatment

A 50 ml dose of 50% dextrose is given intravenously and repeated as necessary. Alternatively, I mg glucagon is given intravenously or intramuscularly which is useful if the patient is difficult to restrain. Glucagon may be given to patients to retain at home for administration by relatives as emergency treatment for hypoglycaemia.

Ketoacidosis

Causes

Infections are the most common identifiable cause. Myocardial infarction, trauma and inadequate insulin dosage are other causes.

Clinical features

Typically these patients are dehydrated, hyperventilating and may have impaired consciousness. Blood glucose is usually markedly elevated and arterial hydrogen ion concentration is low. Body potassium content is decreased although the plasma potassium concentration is high, reflecting the need for insulin to transport potassium across cell membranes.

Treatment

This is based on four measures:
1 Fluid to replace dehydration.
2 Insulin to control hyperglycaemia.
3 Potassium to counter hypokalaemia.
4 Bicarbonate to counter acidosis.

Typical deficiencies would be: water, 6 l; sodium, 600 mmol (mEq); potassium, 400 mmol (mEq).

Fluid. 1000 ml isotonic saline in 30 min.
1000 ml isotonic saline in I h.
1000 ml isotonic saline in 2 h.
1000 ml isotonic saline in 4 h.
500 ml isotonic saline 4-hourly.

Note. Use a central venous pressure line in the elderly or those with cardiac disease. If serum sodium rises above 155 mmol/l (mEq/l), use half normal saline.

Insulin. Soluble insulin, 6 units/h, is given by infusion pump. A double rate is given if the glucose level is not falling at 2 h.
When blood glucose is <15 mmol/l (270 mg/100 ml), change to 5% glucose infusion at the rate of 500 ml 4-hourly (add 13 mmol/l potassium chloride) and give 3 units/h insulin; continue insulin parenterally with intravenous dextrose until the patient is eating.

Potassium. Giving insulin and correcting acidosis lowers plasma potassium. Hypokalaemia is a major cause of morbidity in treating ketoacidosis. Give 20 mmol/h from the beginning, adjusting as shown in Table 21.3 for plasma potassium. Continuous monitoring of the electrocardiogram should be undertaken; changes in T-waves give an early indication of important changes in plasma potassium.

Bicarbonate. The above treatment is normally sufficient to restore normal acid–base

POTASSIUM IN DIABETIC ACIDOSIS

mmol (mEq)/h	Plasma K+ mmol (mEq)/l
39	< 3
26	3–4
20	4–5
13	5–6
0	> 6

Table 21.3 Potassium regimen in patients with diabetic acidosis.

balance, correct dehydration and normalize blood sugar concentrations. Severely acidotic patients can be given bicarbonate, although this has been associated with serious fluid disequilibrium and development of cerebral oedema. For this reason the use of bicarbonate is not routinely recommended.

Comment. Successful treatment of ketoacidosis depends on frequent monitoring, and rapid response to, biochemical and haemodynamic indices.

Remember that there is often an underlying cause. If you suspect infection, treat with antibiotics after relevant culture specimens have been obtained.

Hyperosmolar, non-ketotic hyperglycaemic coma

Cause
The cause is obscure. It usually occurs in the elderly or non-insulin dependent diabetic person.

Features
Typical laboratory findings are very high blood glucose raised urea, raised sodium and a high plasma osmolality.

Treatment
Isotonic saline is given or half normal if plasma sodium is >150 mmol (mEq)/l. Adjust the rate of infusion with a central venous pressure line. Give insulin as for ketoacidosis and possibly heparin, as these patients are prone to thrombosis.

21.2 Thyroid disease

Hyperthyroidism

Pathophysiology
The majority of patients with hyperthyroidism have Graves' disease, which is an autoimmune disorder characterized by antibodies directed against and stimulatory for the thyroid stimu-

lating hormone (TSH) receptor. The peak incidence is in middle-aged females. The disorder can be chronic, but in a substantial proportion of patients a single episode of hyperthyroidism may enter remission either spontaneously or following treatment with antithyroid drugs. Remission is more likely in patients who have mild disease with minimal enlargement of the thyroid gland.

Toxic multinodular goitre and solitary toxic thyroid adenoma can also cause hyperthyroidism. Patients with these disorders will not enter remission following a course of treatment with antithyroid drugs and are best managed by destructive therapy (either surgery or radioactive iodine).

General principles of treatment
1 Symptomatic therapy: some of the peripheral manifestations of thyroid hormone excess, such as tachycardia and tremor, will respond to beta-adrenoreceptor blockade. Non-selective beta-blockers (such as propranolol) are of value, as the tremor of thyrotoxicosis responds to $beta_2$-but not $beta_1$-antagonists.
2 Radioactive iodine (^{131}I) causes a radiation thyroiditis and so reduces hormone reduction by the gland.
3 Thyroid hormone synthesis can be interrupted by drugs such as carbimazole.

Drugs that block iodine uptake by the thyroid (potassium perchlorate) or block thyroid hormone release (potassium iodide) can cause hypothyroidism but are not routinely used in the treatment of thyrotoxicosis.

Thiourylene antithyroid drugs
These drugs (carbimazole, methimazole, propylthiouracil) all share a similar chemical structure. Methimazole is a product of carbimazole metabolism and is the active compound. Methimazole is widely used in the USA and Europe while carbimazole is available in the UK.

These drugs act to inhibit thyroid hormone synthesis by:
1 Inhibition of iodide oxidation.

2 Inhibition of iodination of tyrosine.

3 Inhibition of coupling of iodotyrosines.

Propylthiouracil also inhibits the conversion of T_4 to T_3; as T_3 the active hormone, this may have some additional therapeutic benefit. It is unlikely that antithyroid drugs have any effect on the underlying course of Graves' disease.

As antithyroid drugs do not alter the secretion of preformed thyroid hormone, the effects on circulating thyroid hormone levels and on the symptoms of thyrotoxicosis are not apparent for some time (2–4 weeks).

Pharmacokinetics

Carbimazole is hydrolysed in plasma to methimazole. Methimazole is accumulated in thyroid tissue, and as the intrathyroidal duration of action is at least 12 h the drugs need only be given twice daily. Carbimazole/methimazole and propylthiouracil cross the placenta and can therefore result in fetal hypothyroidism and goitre development. Pregnant patients given antithyroid drugs need to be given the lowest dose possible for this reason. Use of carbimazole in pregnancy has been associated with a very rare occurence of aplasia cutis, a congenital abnormality of scalp skin development. The drugs are secreted in breast milk (propylthiouracil to a lesser extent than carbimazole/methimazole), and this can result in neonatal hypothyroidism.

Adverse effects

1 All the drugs will cause hypothyroidism and goitre enlargement when given chronically. This can be prevented by reducing the dose of the drug or by giving the patient thyroid hormone (see below).

2 The most common side effect is urticarial rash. A substantial proportion of patients who develop a rash when on carbimazole will also do so on propylthiouracil.

3 The most serious side effect is granulocytopenia, which may progress to agranulocytosis. Although potentially serious, these problems generally resolve on stopping therapy. Patients should be given a written warning at the start of treatment about this possible side effect

(which is rare) and should be instructed to report any sore throat or fever immediately.

4 Arthralgia, hepatitis and serum sickness type reactions are all rarely seen with these drugs.

Clinical use and dose

Carbimazole: 30–60 mg daily is normally used. Most patients will respond to 20 mg twice daily. To prevent hypothyroidism, the dose can be reduced thereafter to around 5–10 mg per day. A more efficient procedure is to continue with the initial dose and to add thyroid hormone (thyroxine, 0.1–0.15 mg per day) once the patient has become euthyroid.

Methimazole: this drug is not available in the UK. A dose of 10–15 mg twice daily will control the majority of patients with thyrotoxicosis.

Propylthiouracil: an initial dose of 100 mg three times per day will control the majority of patients.

Patients with Graves' disease who may enter remission are often given antithyroid drugs for up to 1 year. If remission seems likely at that point, drugs may be withdrawn and the patients followed to detect subsequent relapse. This approach is not appropriate for patients who do not have disease which will enter remission (e.g. multinodular goitre), for patients in whom relapse of thyrotoxicosis would be harmful (e.g. patients with cardiac disease) or in patients in whom remission is very unlikely (patients with very large goitres or where the immune markers of Graves' disease are very high). Antithyroid drugs may also be used to prepare patients before destructive therapy in the form of either thyroid surgery or radioactive iodine.

Radioactive iodine

Radioactive iodine is well absorbed orally and causes a radiation thyroiditis. There is little radiation dose to other tissues. The advantages of radioactive iodine are its simplicity (normally a single dose), low cost and safety.

The major disadvantage is the occurrence of hypothyroidism. Early hypothyroidism (within a few months) is a dose related phenomenon. Where large doses are given, up to 90% of patients may become hypothyroid after the first dose. With lower doses, between 10 and 20% of patients will be hypothyroid. Thereafter, late hypothyroidism will affect between 2 and 4% of patients per year. This is an inexorable phenomenon and the majority of patients given radioactive iodine will eventually become hypothyroid. For this reason some centres prefer to give a large ablative dose at the outset. There is no evidence of any carcinogenic risk following radioactive iodine treatment. There is no evidence of any harm to germinal tissue, although patients are advised to avoid conception within 6 months of radioactive iodine therapy (male patients are advised not to father children for a similar period of time).

Potassium iodide
Iodide has multiple actions on the thyroid. The most important is an immediate reduction in thyroid hormone release and for this reason potassium iodide is used in thyroid crisis. The drug will also inhibit thyroid hormone formation and iodide trapping.

Potassium perchlorate
This drug prevents thyroid iodide uptake. It has been associated with the development of aplastic anaemia and is not used in routine clinical practice.

Beta-adrenoreceptor blockade
This has been discussed above. Propranolol reduces peripheral conversion of T_4 to T_3, and also provides some symptomatic relief. It should be emphasized that beta-blockers have no effect on the underlying process of Graves' disease or on thyroid hormone secretion.

Thyroid crisis
This condition has a high mortality and is characterized by fever, tachycardia, dehydration

and confusion. Potassium iodide along with carbimazole are used: patients also require general supportive measures, including rehydration, intravenous beta-blocker therapy and steroids.

Hypothyroidism
This can result as a consequence of previous treatment of thyrotoxicosis, congenital dysfunction or as a consequence of autoimmune thyroiditis. Lithium (used in the treatment of bipolar affective disorders) inhibits thyroid hormone release and can result in hypothyroidism requiring treatment.

Thyroid replacement therapy
Treatment is directed at replacing thyroid hormone levels in the circulation: pituitary secretion of TSH can be used as a guide to the adequacy of therapy. Two preparations are available: thyroxine (T_4) and triiodothyronine (T_3), although the latter is rarely used.

Mechanism
T_3 binds to nuclear receptors and regulates gene transcription. This leads to multiple metabolic actions. T_4 is converted to T_3 in cells by a deiodinase enzyme. In some tissue (e.g. the pituitary) there is an obligatory requirement for a high percentage of T_3 to be derived from intracellular T_4 conversion. For this reason T_4 is a more effective hormone in suppression of TSH than T_3 and is therefore the preferred thyroid hormone for replacement.

Pharmacokinetics
Both T_4 and T_3 are adequately absorbed following oral administration. T_4 has a half-life of about a week and T_3 about 2 days. Both undergo conjugation in the liver and enterohepatic circulation.

Adverse effects
These are related to the physiological and pharmacological actions of thyroid hormone. Elderly patients, or those known to have ischaemic heart disease, are given low initial

doses with slow increments since angina or myocardial infarction can be precipitated. In patients at risk of these problems it may be sensible to prescribe beta-blocker therapy when starting thyroid hormone replacement. Thyroid hormone excess produces the usual clinical features of thyrotoxicosis.

The correct dose of thyroxine is assessed by measurement of serum TSH concentrations.

Dose

Thyroxine: starting dose is 0.05 mg/day (0.025 mg/day if elderly or with heart disease), with dose increments every 2–3 weeks depending on thyroid function. The average dose in patients is 0.125 mg/day. Thyroxine is also used postoperatively in thyroid carcinoma:

1 To replace endogenous thyroxine.
2 To suppress TSH, as many tumours are TSH dependent.

The dose of thyroxine used under these circumstances is higher than that given as replacement therapy, and is normally in the region of 0.2 mg/day.

21.3 Bone metabolism

Hormone replacement therapy (HRT)

Clinical use

Oestrogen prevents menopause-associated bone loss (potential loss of ~25%) when started at the menopause but also increases spine bone mineral density (BMD) by between 5 and 10% when started several years after the menopause. Use of hormone replacement therapy (HRT) is associated (consistent across several retrospective case-control studies) with 50% reduction in hip, vertebral and forearm fractures.

The commonest use of HRT is for the relief of post-menopausal symptoms including vasomotor symptoms (e.g. flushing). Longer term use to prevent or treat osteoporosis requires consideration of the wider risks (slight increase in risk of breast carcinoma, see below) vs. benefits (probable reduction in incidence of deaths from ischaemic heart disease, although the current data are conflicting regarding this issue).

Within a few years of stopping HRT the skeletal benefit from HRT (BMD and fracture risk reduction) is lost.

Mechanism

Oestrogen suppresses osteoclast-mediated bone resorption.

Pharmacokinetics

Half-life 10–18 h. Orally administered oestrogens undergo extensive first-pass metabolism by the liver.

Side effects

Generally well tolerated but oestrogen dose-dependent side effects include breast tenderness, fluid retention and weight gain. There is a small but significant increase in risk of deep vein thrombosis (DVT) and pulmonary thromboembolism (PTE) (about 5–10 cases per 100 000 woman years' use). There is a small increase in breast carcinoma incidence with long-term use (12 extra cases of breast cancer are likely to accrue when treating 1000 post-menopausal women with HRT for 15 years).

Oestrogen should be avoided when there is a past history of oestrogen-dependent cancer such as cancer of breast or endometrium, of DVT or PTE, or when there is undiagnosed vaginal bleeding. There are a number of relative contraindications including history of migraine.

Drug interactions

Clinical use and dosage
The usual dose for prevention and treatment of bone loss is 0.625 mg/day of conjugated equine oestrogen, although there is a dose response between 0.3 and 1.25 mg/day, and as little as 0.3 mg/day may prevent bone loss.

Oestrogen for systemic benefit may be administered orally (once daily), subcutaneously (implants, given 6-monthly) or trans-dermally(once or twice per week). Oestrogen may be administered topically, e.g. per vaginam for local symptom relief.

Oestrogen without progesterone may be safely given to women who have undergone hysterectomy, but if the uterus is present unopposed oestrogen is associated with risk of endometrial hyperplasia or carcinoma; this risk is avoided by giving progesterone also. When oestrogen and progesterone are given cyclically, this results in monthly period-like withdrawal bleeding; this can be avoided by giving daily concurrent oestrogen and progesterone ('non-bleed HRT'). Alternatively, oestrogen analogues with progestogenic properties (e.g. tibolone) achieve the benefits of oestrogen without the need for bleeding.

Selective oestrogen–receptor modulators (SERMs)

Raloxifene
Raloxifene is a non-steroidal synthetic drug that exhibits oestrogen-like effects in some tissues with oestrogen receptors and lacks effects in others.

Use
It is effective in reducing the incidence of vertebral fractures in osteoporotic women, and although it does this partly through changes in BMD, the gains in BMD are less than those seen with oestrogen. However, it does not cause endometrial proliferation (no vaginal bleeding), nor does it increase the risk of breast cancer (this risk may even be reduced with raloxifene). Like oestrogen raloxifene is associated with a favourable influence on lipid profile.

Mechanism
Tissue-specific differential expression of oestrogen-regulated genes.

Pharmacokinetics
Sixty per cent of the oral dose is absorbed. Extensive first-pass metabolism and 2% bioavailability.

Side effects
Incidence of post-menopausal vasomotor symptoms, including flushing, is increased with raloxifene. It shares with oestrogen the increase in risk of DVT and PTE and is contraindicated where there is a past history of either.

Drug interactions
Colestyramine interferes with absorption.

Clinical use and dosage
60 mg/day orally.

Calcium

Use
Calcium supplements are used when calcium intake is deficient. Supplementation is more likely to be required during pregnancy and lactation when demand is higher, and in older age, when intake and absorption are lower.

Drug interactions
Calcium should not be ingested concurrently with bisphosphonates as the absorption of the latter will be reduced. If calcium is taken concurrently with thiazide diuretics there is a risk of hypercalcaemia.

Clinical use and dosage
Calcium may be given as supplement in association with antiresorptive therapy in the treatment of osteoporosis. Typically 1 g calcium is given. To achieve 1 g of elemental calcium (25 mmol Ca^{2+}) 2.5 g/day calcium carbonate should be given (which is equivalent to 7.5 g/day of calcium lactate or 6.7 g calcium gluconate).

Vitamin D
Vitamin D is an endogenous vitamin/hormone that is derived primarily from the action of ultraviolet light on dehydrocholesterol in the skin; synthesis requires hydroxylation steps in the liver (25-hydroxylase) and kidneys (1α-hydroxylase). The active form of vitamin D is 1,25-dihydroxycolecalciferol or calcitriol

(1,25DHCC). Some vitamin D is obtained from the diet.

Mechanism

Prime action is to facilitate intestinal absorption of calcium. 1,25DHCC promotes calcium mobilization from bone and may also increase renal calcium and phosphate reabsorption.

Pharmacokinetics

Vitamin D is fat soluble and bile is necessary for absorption. Vitamin D undergoes enterohepatic circulation.

Side effects

Hypercalcaemia is a feature of vitamin D toxicity. This is most likely with potent vitamin D analogues such as 1,25DHCC or with 1α-hydroxycholecalciferol (alphacalcidol): toxicity can last several days with these preparations but can last substantially longer with ergocalciferol. Use of 1,25DHCC and alphacalcidol requires monitoring of serum calcium.

Drug interactions

Anticonvulsants and other drugs can induce the enzymes that metabolize vitamin D and may result in vitamin D deficiency syndromes such as osteomalacia.

Clinical use and dosage

See Table 21.4 (below).

Bisphosphonates

Bisphosphonates are a family of carbon-substituted pyrophosphates that bind avidly to bone. When released from bone they inhibit osteoclast-mediated bone resorption.

Indications (Table 21.5)

a Osteoporosis (post-menopausal)

Significant increases in lumbar spine BMD (6–8% gains) (etidronate, alendronate and risedronate) and in femoral BMD (4–6%) (alendronate and risedronate) and a significant reduction in risk of vertebral (etidronate, alendronate and risedronate) and other other fractures including hip fractures (alendronate

VITAMIN D ANALOGUES

	Ergocalciferol, calciferol	Alphacalcidol	Calcitriol
Vitamin D deficiency	400–5000 IU/day		
Prevention of hip fractures in elderly*	800 IU/day (+calcium)		
Vitamin D deficiency malabsorption hepatic cirrhosis	≤ 40000 IU/day	0.5–2 µg/day	0.25–1 µg/day
Hypoparathyroidism	25 000–10 000 IU/day	0.5–2 µg/day	0.25–1 µg/day
Renal osteodystrophy			0.25–1 µg/day
Osteoporosis† post-menopausal steroid-induced			0.5–1 µg/day

* 800 IU/day vitamin D3 (with 1.2 g calcium carbonate) has been shown to reduce the incidence of hip fractures (by about 27%) in elderly female residents in sheltered housing or nursing homes (likely to be a consequence of treating vitamin D deficiency and hypocalcaemia-associated secondary hyperparathyroidism).
† Limited evidence of efficacy.

Table 21.4 Vitamin D analogues.

and risedronate) are seen with oral bisphos-phonates used in association with calcium supplementation (generally 500–1000 mg/day) when treating osteoporotic women with pre-valent vertebral fractures.

Osteoporosis (corticosteroid): Significant in-creases in lumbar spinal BMD with trends to-wards a reduction in the incidence of vertebral fractures are seen with etidronate, alendronate and risedronate in patients initiating or already receiving corticosteroid treatment at doses with a potential to adversely affect BMD (>7.5 mg/day prednisolone for more than 3 months).

b *Paget's disease*
In Paget's disease bisphosphonates have been shown to suppress disease activity (bone alka-line phosphatase normalized in up to 70%), treat bone pain (~70%).

c *Hypercalcaemia:*
Intravenous (etidronate, pamidronate) bispho-sphonates are used in association with rehy-dration, furosemide–saline diuresis, and calcitonin (optional) to reduce calcium levels when hyercalcaemia is severe and sympto-matic. This effect of bisphosphonates is appar-ent 48–72 h after administration. It is most effective in hypercalcaemia of malignancy, less so in hyperparathyroidism.

d *Metastatic bone disease*
There are reports that skeletal complications (including fracture) in advanced multiple mye-loma and in metastatic breast carcinoma are reduced with bisphosphonates. Survival is not prolonged.

Pharmacokinetics
Between 20 and 50% of absorbed (see below) bisphosphonate binds to bone within 24 h; it remains bound to bone for many months, possibly years. Unbound (to bone) drug is excreted unchanged by the kidneys (caution in renal impairment).

Side effects
Generally well tolerated. Aminobisphosphon-ates are associated with risk of oesophageal irritation and ulceration (direct chemical effect). Acute phase reactions (commonly fever, occasionally lymphopenia) occur in up to 30% with intravenous use (but are harmless).

BISPHOSPHONATES

Drug	Relative antiresorptive potency	Uses
First generation (with short alkyl or halide side chain)		
Etidronate	1	a,b,c
Clodronate	10	b,c,d
Second generation (generally with amino-terminal group)		
Tiludronate	10	b
Pamidronate	100	a,b,c,d
Alendronate	100–1000	a,b
Third generation (cyclic side chain)		
Risedronate	1000–10 000	a,b
Ibandronate	1000–10 000	a
Zoledronate	10 000+	

Underlining denotes current licensed indications for use in the UK.

Table 21.5   Indications for bisphosphonates.

Drug interactions
Calcium and other chelating agents will reduce the absorption of bisphosphonates from the gastrointestinal tract.

Clinical use and dosage
Orally administered bisphosphonates are absorbed from the upper small intestine, but absorption is poor, typically ranging from 0.7% to 6%. Absorption is reduced by calcium and by food in general. Consequently oral bisphosphonates are usually given either first thing in the morning after overnight fast (with nothing to eat for the next 30 min) or 2 h after the last meal and 2 h before the next meal. They should only be taken with plain water.

Calcitonin
Peptide hormone synthesized by the parafollicular cells within the thyroid gland. Synthetic forms (salmon and human calcitonin) are available for therapeutic use.

Use

Osteoporosis
Calcitonin is associated (at 200 IU/day intranasally) with a slight reduction in incidence of osteoporotic vertebral fractures with minimal influence on BMD. It is less efficacious than HRT and bisphosphonates. It appears to have an analgesic action (possibly mediated via endogenous endorphins) in osteoporotic vertebral collapse.

Paget's disease
Calcitonin is effective in relieving bone pain in Paget's disease, and can suppress Pagetic disease activity (but unlike bipshosphonates doesn't induce remission).

Hypercalcemia
Calcitonin can be used along with rehydration, furosemide–saline diuresis, and parenteral bisphosphonates to reduce serum calcium levels in severe and symptomatic hypercalcemia.

Mechanism
Calcitonin reduces bone resorption by reducing both the number and activity of osteoclasts.

Pharmacokinetics
Administration either by subcutaneous or intramuscular injection or by intranasal spray. Half-life 40 min. Metabolized by kidneys.

Side effects
Nausea, vomiting and flushing occur in about 10% of cases. Subcutaneous injection may be associated with local discomfort at the injection site. Nasal irritation and ulceration may occur. Antibodies may develop when calcitonin is used for prolonged periods; these may attenuate its actions. Rarely allergic reactions occur.

Clinical use and dosage
Calcitonin is very expensive. Intranasal calcitonin (for osteoporosis) is administered at 200 IU/day. Subcutaneous dose: 50–100 IU/day.

Anterior and posterior pituitary

Hormones
Hypopituitarism results in failure to produce thyroid, adrenal, ovarian and testicular steroids; therapy with these preparations is considered elsewhere. Growth hormone deficiency requires growth hormone replacement treatment in childhood—genetically engineered growth hormone is available and is administered in a dose of 0.5–0.7 IU/kg/week. Adult hypopituitary patients are also growth hormone deficient and there is some evidence that growth hormone replacement in this circumstance can exert beneficial effects on the pathophysiological abnormalities present in this circumstance. These include dyslipidaemia, osteoporosis and neuropsychiatric morbidity. However, growth hormone therapy has not been shown to alter mortality. This treatment is given by daily subcutaneous injection.

Adrenal steroid replacement therapy

Patients with anterior pituitary failure have a deficiency in the production of adrenocortico-trophic hormone (ACTH) and, consequently, are unable to produce adequate amounts of the glucocorticoid hormone cortisol. Production of the mineralocorticoid hormone, aldosterone, is generally not significantly abnormal in this circumstance as the zona glomerulosa of the adrenal cortex is regulated by the activity of the renin–angiotensin system. Patients with primary adrenal failure are, of course, deficient in both cortisol and aldosterone.

Patients with pituitary failure are generally given hydrocortisone as their replacement glucocorticoid. This is chemically identical to the physiological hormone. It is well absorbed orally. The replacement dose is between 20 and 30 mg hydrocortisone per day, which will mimic normal physiological adrenal steroid output. The dose is generally divided into 15–20 mg taken in the morning and 5–10 mg taken later in the day, in an attempt to reproduce the normal diurnal pattern of cortisol production. Patients taking glucocorticoid replacement need to increase the replacement dose during intercurrent illness or major physiological stress (patients are generally advised to double the dose for several days and to seek medical advice). All patients taking steroid replacement therapy should carry a form of identification that gives details of their medical condition and current therapy. Other synthetic glucocorticoids, such as prednisolone (5–7.5 mg/day) and dexamethasone (500–750 μg/day) can be used as an alternative to hydrocortisone as replacement therapy.

Patients with primary adrenal failure also need to take a mineralocorticoid hormone. Fluodrocortisone is a synthetic steroid with high affinity for the mineralocorticoid receptor. This can be given in a dose of between 100 and 300 μg/day: the dose can be titrated against blood pressure (patients who are deficient in mineralocorticoids show a substantial fall in blood pressure on standing) and plasma electrolytes. Mineralocortoid excess is associated with hypocalaemia and alkalosis.

Diabetes insipidus

This can arise as a consequence of hypothalamic or pituitary dysfunction. Patients with intact thirst sensation present with polyuria and polydipsia; those with absent thirst (sometimes seen following head injury and hypothalamic syndromes) can have marked polyuria without polydipsia, resulting in severe hypernatraemia. Treatment is with synthetic antidiuretic hormone arginine vasopressin (DDAVP), given either intramuscularly or by nasal spray. An oral formulation of DDAVP is available, although its absorption is less good than that of the nasal preparation. However, it may be used in patients who are unable to utilize the nasal preparation.

Pharmacokinetics

DDAVP is broken down by vasopressinase, and the activity of this increases during pregnancy leading to an increase in dosage requirement.

Dosage

DDAVP: 10–20 μg/day by nasal spray; 1–4 μg by intramuscular injection.

Dopamine agonists for hyperprolactinaemia and acromegaly

Medical therapy for the treatment of prolactin excess and acromegaly using dopamine agonists (such as bromocriptine or the longer acting agent, cabergoline) is considered in detail in Chapter 15.

Somatostatin analogues

The hypothalmic hormone, somatostatin, inhibits release of other hormones from a variety of endocrine tumours. Synthetic analogues of somatostatin are of value in treatment of several neuro-endocrine tumours, including those derived from pancreatic endocrine tissue (for example, glucagonomas and VIP-omas). In addition, these agents have been used in the treatment of carcinoid syndrome: in these circumstances there is no evidence that therapy reduces tumour growth, but there is a valuable effect on limiting release of serotonin. Finally, use of somatostatin analogues is of value in the medical management of patients with acromegaly. In these circumstances, the drugs can be given as initial therapy or as adjuvant treatment after surgery and radiotherapy. The drugs can cause marked suppression of growth hormone secretion; their use is associated with shrinkage of the tumour.

Octreotide is a short-acting formulation that is given by subcutaneous injection (50–200 µg three times daily). A long-acting preparation is now available which can be given intramuscularly once per month in a dose of 20 mg/daily. An alternative agent (lanreotide) has similar actions.

Side effects
Side effects of somatostatin analogues include gastrointestinal upset and fat malabsorption. The development of gallstones has been recorded with these agents.

CHAPTER 22

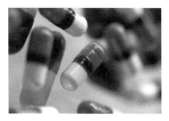

Travel Medicine and Tropical Disease

Over 45 million Britons travel abroad each year. Many travelling to Europe, the USA and Australia require no special prophylaxis against infections different to those in Britain as the risks and public health are similar. However, travel to many other countries, especially in the Tropics and Subtropics, can expose the traveller to new health risks. Making a sound risk assessment for each traveller is the first stage of any pre-travel consultation.

It must be remembered that most illness encountered by travellers is not preventable by prophylaxis and much morbidity and mortality encountered abroad is not infection related (e.g. sunburn, alcohol excess, road-traffic accidents, human immunodeficiency virus (HIV) infection and many types of diarrhoea). To prevent infections it is always important to emphasize other health precautions, including care with food and water hygiene, safer sex and the avoidance of mosquito bites.

There are a number of sources of continually updated information on disease prevalence within different countries combined with other information necessary to make these risk assessments. The TRAVAX (A–Z of Healthy Travel) database is provided within the NHS by the Scottish Centre for Infection and Environmental Health (http://www.axl.co.uk/scieh) and it is available through the NHS Net. A public site is also available (http://www.fitfortravel.scot.nhs.uk).

22.1 Assessing the need for prophylaxis

- The significance to the individual traveller relates to the potential seriousness of the disease itself but it must not be forgotten that infected asymptomatic carriers can often, after return home, transmit serious illness to other family members and close contacts (e.g. hepatitis A, HIV infection).
- The likelihood of contracting any infection depends upon multiple factors including the prevalence of the infection in the countries being visited, the length of time abroad and activities to be undertaken (e.g. rural or safari trips where malaria and rabies need to be given extra consideration and sporting activities such as rugby football where injury, with bleeding and the possibility of blood-borne infection, is common).
- The value of any immuno- or chemoprophylaxis depends upon the level of protection it provides, ease of administration (e.g. number of doses) and cost in relation to the protection provided.
- Sometimes peer pressures and less logical considerations enter into the decision making process and these cannot be ignored. For example, there is a lot of understandable and sometimes exaggerated fear over the risk of contacting rabies and while the risk of yellow fever in East Africa is negligible for

the package tourist the vaccine is usually given in line with national directives. The media can also have a positive role to play in increasing the traveller's awareness of real risks such as the recent increase in diphtheria in countries of the former Soviet Union or the risk of food- and water-borne diseases following natural disasters such as earthquakes.

These points are shown schematically below in Table 22.1. They can help the advisor and traveller make decisions only after balancing these various factors. A high score makes it likely that a particular form of prophylaxis will be worthwhile and a low score makes it questionable.

The decision whether to give a particular traveller prophylaxis should be the result of an informed decision and this may also involve the patient and when appropriate parents or other family and party members or group leaders.

22.2 Principles of immunization

Passive immunization

Passive immunization uses existing antibodies in human immunoglobulin, prepared from pooled human blood donations, to provide protection.

Human normal pooled immunoglobulin (HNIG) is almost entirely IgG, and can provide pre-exposure protection against diseases prevalent in the blood donating population such as hepatitis A.

Human specific immunoglobulin is obtained from convalescent patient sera or taken from those recently actively immunized. This is used as post exposure treatment for rabies, tetanus and hepatitis B to prevent or modify any subsequent illness. It should always be given as soon as possible following exposure.

Occasionally HNIG, against hepatitis A, and specific hepatitis B immunoglobulin are given to those going to be a high risk when there is no time to give effective active vaccination.

However the indications for this are now few with more rapidly effective, and often single dose, active vaccines.

Passive immunity following the administration of NHIG wanes within a few months related to the half-life of the product. Thus it should be given close to the date of travel.

Live vaccinations should ideally be given 3 weeks before or 3 months after normal human immunoglobulin, which may contain antibodies to the relevant live vaccine, preventing an optimal vaccine response. Yellow fever vaccine is an exception to this rule, because HNIG does not contain significant specific antibodies to yellow fever.

Active immunization

Active immunization is achieved when the immune system is challenged by immunogens to produce humoral or cellular responses. Should infection subsequently rechallenge the immune 'memory', it will provoke a rapid and specific response to that antigen.

- Active immunization may be induced by inactivated organisms, inactivated toxins (toxoids), immunogenic components of organisms or live attenuated organisms (Table 22.2).
- Active vaccines can be absorbed onto an adjuvant such as aluminium salts to increase their immunogenicity.
- Oral vaccines can provide gut immunity through stimulating IgA in enteral secretions.
- The length of protection of active vaccination varies but is usually longer with live vaccines.

Most active vaccines induce humoral (antibody related immunity), however, intradermal attenuated mycobacterium, bacillus Calmette–Guérin (BCG), provides protection against *Mycobacterium tuberculosis* infection by inducing cell-mediated immunity.

Following administration of a live or inactivated vaccine, there is a primary delay before appreciable levels of antibody are manufactured by the immune system. Therefore, for maximum protection primary active immunization courses require to be in advance of possible exposure, and in some instances

RISK ASSESSMENTS ABOUT PROPHYLAXIS FOR TRAVELLERS

Grade	Qualifier	Description
1	Significance to the individual traveller	
How serious could the specific infection be for the individual if infected?		
0	Minor	Rarely a severe illness
1	Moderate	Serious illness, complete recovery usual, death rare
2	Major	Severe illness, complications and death possible
3	Critical	Severe illness, serious or long-term complications common
4	Grave	Severe illness, complications and death are usual
2	Significance to the community	
How serious are the public health implications if the traveller was to be infected?		
0	Minor	Minimal or no risk to public health
1	Moderate	Potential for spread to close contacts but usually confinable
2	Major	Potential for spread within the population
3	Critical	High probability of spread within a population
4	Grave	Certainty of spread within the exposed population
3	Likelihood of exposure	
How likely is the traveller to become infected—considering destination and intended lifestyle?		
0	Very unlikely	Disease not normally present at destination
1	Unlikely	Disease present, intended lifestyle makes infection unlikely
2	Possible	Disease widespread but traveller likely to be able to avoid infection
3	Probable	Disease widespread; traveller's lifestyle makes avoiding infection difficult
4	Almost certain	Disease widespread and highly contagious
4	Evaluation of active intervention	
How effective and practical is the available prophylaxis (vaccine or tablets) also considering side effects, cost and time available for completing optimal schedule?		
0	Passable	Marginal benefits, acceptable side effects, may be difficult to deliver
1	Satisfactory	Significant benefits, possible side effects, may be difficult to deliver
2	Useful	Useful and feasible intervention with some measurable benefits and few adverse side effects
3	Effective	Useful and feasible intervention with significant measurable benefits and few or no adverse side effects
4	Ideal	Highly effective and feasible intervention with side effects very unlikely
5	Context	
Could the 'best' decision about prophylaxis be influenced by current public concerns, peer or media pressure?		
0	Indifferent	Little public interest or likely media response
1	Unsettled	Some public or media unease. Potential for repercussions if intervention fails
2	Sensitive	A publicly sensitive issue, press interest. Risk of serious repercussions if intervention fails
3	Adverse	Considerable public concern, political and emotional pressure, unhelpful and antagonistic media reports
4	Hostile	A lot of public and media interest, political involvement. Inappropriate demands may lead to inappropriate responses

Table 22.1 Scheme for helping to make risk assessments on the need for prophylaxis for a traveller.

VACCINES

	Viral	Bacterial
Live attenuated vaccines	Oral polio Measles Mumps Rubella Yellow fever	BCG Oral typhoid
Inactivated organisms	Inactivated polio Hepatitis A Rabies Japanese B encephalitis (not licensed in UK) Tick-borne encephalitis (not licensed in UK)	Pertussis Typhoid Cholera
Immunogenic components of organisms	Influenza Hepatitis B	*Haemophilus* *influenzae* type B Pneumococcal (polysaccharide) Meningococcal A + C Typhim Vi (polysaccharide)
Inactivated toxoids		Tetanus Diphtheria

Table 22.2 Current vaccines available in Britain.

quite long periods (e.g. toxoids of diphtheria and tetanus) and with rabies (see Table 22.3).

If a definite exposure occurs before these intervals have passed extra immediate doses of vaccine may have to be considered (e.g. following a potentially rabid bite) or a dose of specific immunoglobulin (e.g. after a tetanus prone wound or exposure to hepatitis B).

In time, most vaccine-induced antibody responses decline and may require to be boosted. These intervals can vary greatly (e.g. a few years with typhoid and more than 10 years with hepatitis A). Increasingly it is being recognized that real protection can be achieved for much longer than the detectable presence of antibodies because a very rapid amnestic response can still occur after exposure to infection.

Boosters normally give maximum protection after a few days although this may be longer with intradermal vaccinations. If the booster dose interval has been substantially delayed the interval may be longer.

Live vaccines

Live vaccines are usually best stored at cool temperatures (0–5°C) and are heat and light labile once reconstituted. Thus provision of a 'cold chain' of refrigeration is important but may be difficult, especially in poorer and tropical developing countries.

When more than one live vaccine is required, they are best given simultaneously or at least 3 weeks apart to prevent the

PROTECTION AFTER VACCINATION

Vaccine	Interval required after primary course for maximum protection
Poliomyelitis (oral)	1–2 weeks after 3 doses
Poliomyelitis (parenteral)	1–2 weeks after 3 doses
Tetanus	1–2 weeks after 3 doses
Diphtheria	1–2 weeks after 3 doses
BCG	6 weeks after 1 dose
Typhoid Vi	2 weeks after 1 dose
Hepatitis A	2 weeks after 1 dose
Immunoglobulin	Immediate
Hepatitis B	1 month after 3 doses
Japanese B encephalitis	1–2 weeks after 3 doses
Rabies intramuscular	1–2 weeks after 3 doses
Rabies intradermal	4 weeks after 3 doses
Tick-borne encephalitis	2 weeks after 2 doses
MMR	2 weeks after 1 dose
Yellow fever	10 days after 1 dose

Table 22.3 Approximate time interval required for maximum protection after primary course of vaccination.

interferon response from the first vaccine reducing the effectiveness of subsequent vaccines.

Vaccine contraindications

Live vaccines should usually be avoided in pregnancy, as a result of a theoretical risk of fetal damage, and also in patients who are significantly immunosuppressed from either illness or medication. Manufacturers often also advise that inactivated vaccines are best avoided in pregnancy although there is little evidence of them causing any harm to the fetus. They can be administered if the risk of infection is substantial. Febrile reactions can sometimes precipitate a miscarriage.

During an acute febrile illness, vaccination should be postponed, as it will be difficult to recognize a vaccine 'reaction'. Mild afebrile or non-systemic illnesses are not normally contraindications.

If there has been a severe local, or systemic reaction such as anaphylaxis, to a previous dose of vaccine then further doses of that vaccine must be avoided.

Some vaccines contain traces of egg proteins or antibiotics and should be avoided in those who have serious allergy to these components.

As vaccines may induce severe allergic reactions, all vaccination centres should have facilities for dealing with anaphylaxis. Vaccinated patients should ideally be observed in the vaccination centre for 30 min. Vasovagal reactions are much more common and these can be quite alarming, sometimes with anoxic convulsions. A previous history of faints should alert the advisor to this possibility.

22.3 Vaccines used for preventing infection in travellers

Poliomyelitis

Poliomyelitis is an enterovirus spread by the faecal–oral route and is associated with poor sanitation. It is a hardy virus, resistant to lower concentrations of chlorine and can survive for long periods outside the host. The virus has a predilection for central nervous system (CNS) tissue. There are three strains of poliovirus.

Disease risk areas. Poliomyelitis used to be of worldwide distribution but intensive immunization campaigns supported by the World Health Organization (WHO) have resulted in the disease being eliminated from the Americas, and the Far East is close to being declared infection free. Main foci are now the Indian subcontinent and parts of Africa.

Vaccines

Oral polio vaccine (OPV) is included in the British vaccination schedule. Booster doses should be given to travellers to risk areas who have not had OPV for more than 10 years. OPV is a live vaccine and contains all three viral types. Attenuated strains of OPV may rarely revert to pathological 'wild' virus after transit through the bowel and cause a polio-like illness. Therefore, scrupulous attention to hygiene following toileting or nappy changes should be practiced when children have received the vaccine and close contacts should receive a booster dose of OPV at the same time. OPV drops are often given on sugar lumps to disguise its oily taste.

Inactivated polio vaccine (IPV) is a whole cell virus vaccine inactivated by formaldehyde. It is given by intramuscular or subcutaneous injection; booster doses are required at 10-yearly intervals. If oral polio is contraindicated (immunosuppression or pregnancy) IPV may be given instead. Some countries now give IPV (often in combination with other childhood vaccines) instead of OPV to try and eliminate the rare cases of vaccine-associated disease.

Tetanus

Clostridium tetani is a Gram-positive anaerobe that lives in soil and arises from bird and animal faecal contamination. Contaminated wounds, which may often be minor such as from thorns, lead to muscular spasms secondary to CNS changes induced by tetanus toxin. It is the toxin, not the organism itself, which leads to disease.

Disease risk areas. Worldwide. Herd immunity is not helpful since the disease is not spread from person to person and every individual must be vaccinated. In countries where childhood vaccination schedules have been introduced recently it has become a disease of unimmunized adults. While 10-yearly boosters are not currently advised in Britain, after the full five doses have been received in childhood and adolescence, extra boosters for travellers going to countries with poor hygiene can be given.

Vaccine

Tetanus toxoid vaccine is tetanus toxin inactivated by formaldehyde and adsorbed on aluminium phosphate or aluminium hydroxide. Medical attention should be sought for a wound possibly contaminated by tetanus when tetanus toxoid boosters or tetanus specific immunoglobulin may be required. Local reactions may occur, but systemic febrile reactions are rare. Their incidence increases, however, if fully immune individuals have been given unnecessary extra doses of vaccines (e.g. for repeated wounds requiring attention in accident and emergency departments). Vigorous local inflammatory reactions at the site of injection suggest that the individual may be becoming hypersensitive.

Typhoid

Salmonella typhi is a Gram-negative bacillus that causes a septicaemic illness. Untreated illnesses can lead to serious complications and death in around 10% of instances. Spread is through the faecal–oral route from contaminated food or water and occasionally from person-to-person. Typhoid vaccines do not protect against other enteric fevers, including *S. paratyphi*.

Disease risk areas. Typhoid is endemic in developing countries with poor sanitation.

Vaccine

Two options are available:

1 Typhoid Vi polysaccharide capsular vaccine (typhim Vi) contains the Vi antigen of the *S.*

typhi capsule and is preserved with phenol. One dose is given intramuscularly or subcutaneously with 3-yearly boosters.

It should only be used in pregnancy when the risk of infection is high and there is often a suboptimal response in children younger than 18 months. Local and febrile reactions lasting 24 h are much less marked with typhoid Vi capsular vaccine than with a previously available injectable heat killed vaccine.

This vaccine is now available combined with one for hepatitis A.

2 Oral live attenuated strain of *S. typhi* in an enteric capsule offers an added theoretical advantage of inducing gut immunity. Three doses are given on alternate days on an empty stomach with a cool drink and should not be given concurrently with OPV or when the recipient is on antibiotics or mefloquine. Boosters are required yearly, although there is evidence that if more doses are used for the primary course boosters are needed less frequently. Rarely, oral typhoid vaccine causes a mild gastrointestinal upset.

Cholera

Cholera is characterized by profuse watery non-bloody diarrhoea and is caused by the enterotoxin of *Vibrio cholerae*. A high infective dose of organisms is required and it is rare in travellers taking sensible precautions with their water hygiene. Disease is spread through contaminated water and less commonly, food. A new pathogenic serotype has emerged in recent years (O 139).

Disease risk areas. India, South-east Asia, Africa and Central and South America.

Vaccine

The cholera vaccine, consisting of heat-killed organisms preserved with phenol, is now no longer available in Britain. It gave only 50% protection for 6 months and was ineffective in preventing serotype O 139. It is no longer recommended for travellers by the WHO.

Some countries now have available a more effective oral vaccine which may eventually be combined with a vaccine against enterotoxigenic *Escherichia coli*, the most common cause of travellers' diarrhoea.

Hepatitis A

Hepatitis A is a hepatotropic virus spread by the faecal–oral route and also person-to-person when hygiene is poor. Asymptomatic infections are common, especially in children. In countries with poor hygiene 90% of children have been naturally infected by the age of 10 years.

Hepatitis IgG antibodies from natural infection confer life-long immunity. Therefore it is worthwhile checking the immune status of older people (above 60 years), those with a previous history of unexplained jaundice and those who have lived in endemic areas before immunization.

Disease risk areas. Worldwide but greater risk in developing countries with poor sanitation.

Vaccine

Hepatitis A vaccine is a whole cell virus vaccine inactivated with formaldehyde and is given intramuscularly.

A single monodose vaccine is available for primary immunization, with a booster in 6 months to 1 year conferring protection for at least 10 years. Following immunization, transient local reactions rarely occur and less commonly fever, fatigue or loss of appetite.

If vaccine is contraindicated passive immunity can be conferred using human normal immunoglobulin. This will protect for 2–6 months depending on the dose.

Hepatitis A vaccine is available combined with one for hepatitis B.

Diphtheria

Diphtheria is caused by toxin-producing *Corynebacterium diphtheriae* and is spread by respiratory droplets.

It causes upper respiratory tract symptoms characterized by the development of a thick grey membrane over the tonsils and pharynx and marked lymphadenopathy, which may lead to respiratory obstruction. Toxin-mediated damage affects the myocardium and nervous system.

Disease risk areas. Worldwide but becoming rarer as vaccination of children becomes more widespread. As was seen recently in the countries of the former Soviet Union, if vaccination coverage declines large outbreaks can follow.

Vaccine
Diphtheria vaccine is prepared from formaldehyde-inactivated diphtheria toxin adsorbed onto aluminium phosphate or aluminium hydroxide. The primary course is three doses and low-dose vaccine is used for primary and booster doses in adults. Boosters are required 10-yearly.

Vaccination is recommended for travellers likely to be in close contact with the local population in risk areas.

Swelling and redness may occur at the injection site, with fever and headache occurring less frequently.

Yellow fever
Yellow fever is a mosquito-borne arbovirus infection. The responsible mosquito is *Aedes aegypti*. It causes high fever, widespread haemorrhage, jaundice and death around 50% of cases. Precautions against mosquito bites should be taken.

Disease risk areas. Sub-Saharan Africa and South America. The disease is not present in Asia.

Vaccine
Yellow fever vaccine is a very effective live attenuated vaccine containing the 17D strain of yellow fever, grown within live chick embryos.

A single subcutaneous dose is given. A vaccination certificate is issued for immigration purposes, which is valid 10 days after vaccination or immediately after boosters. Booster doses are required 10-yearly.

Yellow fever vaccination is recommended and is sometimes mandatory for entering countries with yellow fever. A certificate may also be required if travelling from a yellow fever area to uninfected country which has *Aedes* mosquitoes.

Vaccination is only administered in WHO-designated centres. Mild local or systemic reactions may appear 5–10 days post-vaccination. Severe reactions are rare.

Yellow fever vaccine contains live attenuated virus and is contraindicated in pregnancy (although no fetal damage has been recorded), immunocompromised people, children under 6 months of age (encephalitis may occur in young infants) and in patients with serious egg allergy.

Japanese B encephalitis
Japanese B encephalitis is a mosquito-borne flavivirus. Infection is often asymptomatic in endemic areas, but symptomatic cases develop encephalitis with a high mortality and incidence of residual neurological deficit. Precaution against mosquito bites should be taken.

Disease risk areas. South-east Asia including China, Thailand, India and low-lying areas of Nepal. Epidemics occur following the rainy season when mosquitoes are most active.

Vaccine
Japanese B encephalitis vaccine is a formaldehyde-inactivated whole cell virus. Two or three doses are given subcutaneously over a period of 4 weeks for maximum protection. Boosters are required 2- to 3-yearly.

Vaccination is recommended especially for those going to rural areas, staying for long periods (e.g. more than 1 month) or for repeated visits. It is especially recommended for infants and children in whom the illness can be more severe. Vaccine is available on a named patient basis as it is not licensed in Britain.

An urticarial rash sometimes occurs usually 1–2 days after the inoculation. It may be severe enough to warrant a short course of steroids and antihistamines.

Tick-borne encephalitis

Tick-borne encephalitis is caused by a flavivirus transmitted to humans by a bite from an infected tick. Ticks are most active in the spring and autumn. A meningoencephalitis with paresis may be seen in the acute illness and recovery may be slow. Death is rare.

Passive vaccination with specific hyperimmune globulin is protective if given within 4 days of the tick bite.

Disease risk areas. Tick-borne encephalitis is endemic in forested areas of Scandinavia, Austria and Germany, Eastern Europe and countries of the former Soviet Union.

Vaccine

Tick-borne encephalitis vaccine virus is grown in chick embryo cells and is inactivated with formalin.

Two doses of vaccine are given intramuscularly with an interval time of 2–4 weeks. Initially a booster is required after 1 year, but subsequently only 3-yearly. The vaccine is given in Bavaria as part of the routine childhood vaccination schedule.

Vaccine is recommended for those likely to be exposed to tick bites in forested infected areas, for example campers and rural workers. Efforts should be made to avoid bites, but if bitten to carefully and promptly remove ticks.

Local reactions may occur post-vaccination. Vaccination should be avoided if there is serious egg allergy.

Hepatitis B

Hepatitis B has a mortality of 0.1% in the acute phase. Five per cent of those infected become long-term carriers (greater than 6 months) and carriers may be at risk of future chronic liver disease and hepatocellular carcinoma.

Spread is perinatally (mother to child), by blood to blood contact or by sexual intercourse.

Disease risk areas. Worldwide but there is a higher incidence of carriers in West Central Africa, South-east Asia and South America.

Vaccine

Hepatitis B vaccine is a recombinant vaccine containing hepatitis B surface antigen (anti-HbS) produced from yeast cells. The prepared vaccine is adsorbed onto aluminium hydroxide as an adjuvant. The vaccine is advised for those at occupational risk and also for long-stay expatriates. A history of recent exposure in the unimmunized is an indication for specific immune globulin while a course of active vaccine is commenced.

Three doses of intramuscular vaccine are given over a period of 6 months (0.1 and 6 months). An accelerated course can be given with four doses of vaccine over 6 months (0, 1, 2 and 6 months). Anti-HbS levels are usually checked for those at occupational risk to ensure an adequate level of protection has been achieved ($>100\,IU/l$).

Of those vaccinated 5–10% fail to develop an adequate response even after three or more doses.

Further boosters are usually given at 3- to 5-yearly intervals or depending upon the level of anti-HbS.

Possible adverse reactions include fever, arthralgia, myalgia and mildly deranged liver function tests.

Meningococcal meningitis

Meningococcal meningitis can be rapidly fatal, and is caused by an invasive Gram-negative bacillus (*Neisseria meningitidis*), leading to septicaemia and meningitis. In the UK the most common antigenic groups are B and C, but group A is commonly associated with large epidemics in sub-Saharan Africa. Transmission is by respiratory droplet spread and epidemics occur in the dry season.

Disease risk areas. Epidemics occur in sub-Saharan Africa and have occurred unpredictably in northern India, Nepal and parts of Brazil.

Vaccine

Meningococcal A and C polysaccharide vaccine is advised for travellers visiting areas with epidemic meningococcal disease who are going to be in close contact with the local population, especially if they are likely to be away from medical services, e.g. trekking in Nepal. It is not normally used for package tourists staying in hotels with other expatriates.

One dose of vaccine is required subcutaneously or intramuscularly, which is effective in 7 days. Boosters are required 3- to 5-yearly. Vaccine response is poorer in children under 2 years of age.

Rabies

Rabies is a neurotropic rhabdovirus with an animal reservoir in canines and bats. Infection is usually by inoculation of infected saliva from a bite of a rabid animal. Once symptomatic, rabies is invariably fatal. It occurs in all continents except Australasia and Antarctica.

Vaccine

The rabies vaccine licensed in Britain is a whole cell virus cultured on human diploid cells and inactivated by propiolactone. Pre-exposure vaccine is offered to those involved in animal husbandry in infected areas, or to travellers who may be more than 24 hours away from a source of post-exposure vaccine. The vaccine gives protection if given immediately after exposure but should ideally be used in conjunction with specific immune globulin.

Three injections over a period of 1 month (0, 7 and 28 days) provide protection, but the traveller should still seek urgent medical advice if put at risk for extra doses to ensure maximum antibody levels. Specific immune globulin is not needed in these circumstances. Boosters are required 3-yearly.

Local reactions rarely occur, with systemic reactions such as fever, headache and rashes being occasionally reported.

Plague

Yersinia pestis causes bacteraemic or pneumonic plague. The disease is associated with flea-infested rats and, therefore, travellers are rarely at risk. It occurs in India, Vietnam, Madagascar, rural South America and Central Africa.

Vaccine

Two doses of killed plague vaccine are given subcutaneously over 1 month. Boosters are required 6-monthly. Vaccine is no longer available in the UK and has to be imported from USA. It is usually more practical to give tetracycline to travellers unavoidably exposed to plague, with advice to start treatment promptly if they become ill.

22.4 Preventing malaria

Malaria is a rapidly fatal tropical disease causing more than 1 million deaths per year. There are 2000 cases of imported malaria each year in Britain with approximately 10 deaths.

Malaria is caused by the *Plasmodium* genus of protozoans. The parasite is introduced into humans via the bite of the female anophiline mosquito. After a development phase in the liver, the parasite invades erythrocytes leading to intravascular haemolysis and multisystem organ failure.

There are four species of human malaria.
1 *P. falciparum* is the life-threatening form of malaria and is also called malignant malaria. Fevers may be erratic or almost constant.
2 *P. malariae* causes quartan malaria as it produces fever every 3rd day.
3 *P. vivax* and *P. ovale* are known as tertian malaria giving fever on alternate days after the disease has become established. These species of malaria have a hypnozoite stage, where the parasite has the ability to lie dormant in the liver for months before reactivating.

P. malariae, *P. vivax* and *P. ovale* are rarely life threatening and are referred to as benign malaria.

The cardinal symptom of malaria is fever often with rigors, followed by profuse sweating, headache and myalgia. Falciparum malaria may result in jaundice and encephalitis leading to confusion, coma and death. Later complications in those who survive include renal and respiratory failure.

Disease risk areas. Malaria is endemic in the Tropics and Subtropics below altitudes of 1500 m (see Fig. 22.1). The most serious risk areas for malignant malaria are sub-Saharan Africa and Amazonia in South America.

Chemoprophylaxis against malaria

Malaria prevention through chemoprophylaxis is not absolute. Avoidance of mosquito bites is fundamental in preventing malaria. Therefore, long sleeves and trousers should be worn, especially after sunset when the female mosquito is most active. The importance of insect repellents and mosquito nets impregnated with an insecticide should be emphasized.

The choice of antimalarial is decided by the likelihood of exposure, the prevalent species and local resistance patterns of the parasite. Resistance to chloroquine is now widespread and it is rarely used alone.

Prophylaxis should be commenced 1 week before travel (3 weeks for mefloquine) to ensure adequate blood levels and to detect those likely to get side effects, during the whole time of exposure and for 4 weeks after visiting a malaria area to cover the 'incubation' phase of malignant malaria.

Despite adequate precautions, malaria infection remains possible; thus any febrile illness should be promptly investigated and treated, sometimes empirically, within 1 year of return from a malarious area.

Chloroquine

Chloroquine is a 4-aminoquinolone that binds to and alters plasmodium DNA, causes lysis of the plasmodial membrane and inhibits the erythrocytic phase of plasmodia development.

It is well absorbed with bioavailability approaching 90%. The volume of distribution is large, and chloroquine is slowly excreted in the urine, which allows for once weekly dosing. Tissue penetration, especially of erythrocytes, is good.

Each chloroquine tablet comprises 250 mg chloroquine phosphate (Avloclor), equivalent to 155 mg of chloroquine base, or 200 mg of chloroquine sulphate (Nivaquine), equivalent to 150 mg of chloroquine base.

The adult prophylaxis dose is 2 tablets/week (for childhood doses, see Table 22.4).

Adverse effects

Gastrointestinal upset (nausea, vomiting), skin reactions with generalized pruritis, worsening of psoriasis, headache and transient blurring of vision may occur, but serious reactions are rare.

Cautions

Chloroquine should be used with caution in hepatic and renal impairment and avoided in epilepsy. In antimalarial doses, it poses no observed risk to a fetus. Concurrent administration with halofantrine and hepatotoxic drugs should be avoided.

Overdosage

In overdose chloroquine is highly toxic causing life threatening arrhythmias and seizures. Advice from poison centres is recommended.

Proguanil

Proguanil is a synthetic biguanide that inhibits dihydrofolate reductase, preventing malarial development in tissues. It is well absorbed, has a half-life of 20 h and 200 mg (adult dose) is taken daily.

Adverse effects

Taking proguanil after food eases associated nausea and vomiting. Aphthous mouth ulceration may occur.

Cautions

Proguanil appears to be safe in pregnancy, but folic acid supplements should be given. Caution with severe renal failure and when taking warfarin as the prothrombin time can be increased.

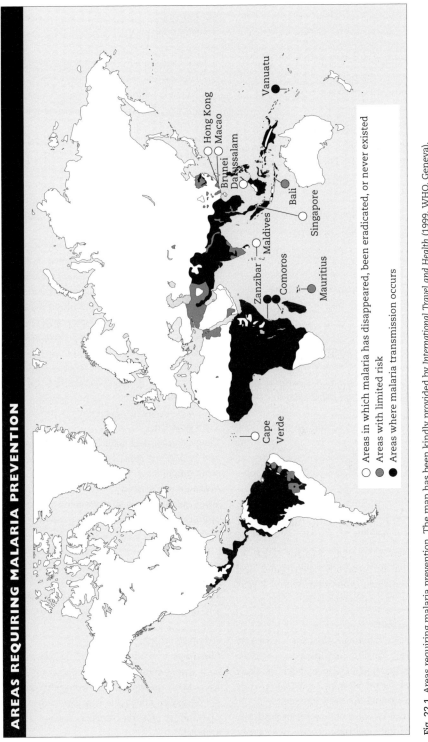

Fig. 22.1 Areas requiring malaria prevention. The map has been kindly provided by *International Travel and Health* (1999, WHO, Geneva).

ANTIMALARIALS IN CHILDREN

Weight (kg)	Age (years)	Proportion of adult dose
<5	<1	0.25 chloroquine/proguanil
5–20	1–5	0.5 chloroquine proguanil
20–39	6–11	0.75 chloroquine/proguanil
20–39	6–11	0.5 maloprim/mefloquine
>40	>12	Adult dose:
		chloroquine base 300 mg/week
		proquanil 200 mg/day
		Maloprim 1 tablet/week
		mefloquine 250 mg/week
		doxycycline 100 mg/day

Mefloquine not recommended for children less than 15 kg.

Table 22.4 Childhood doses of antimalarials.

Overdosage

Proguanil is the safest of all antimalarials. In overdose renal discomfort, haematuria, vomiting and epigastric pain may occur.

Mefloquine

Mefloquine is used in areas where chloroquine and proguanil fail to offer sufficient protection against falciparum malaria. It is a 4-quinoline methanol drug that was developed by the US army.

Mefloquine is active against all human species of malaria, and acts by destroying the asexual blood forms. Unfortunately, falciparum resistance has already been reported in some areas of South-east Asia and Africa.

Mefloquine is well absorbed, with 98% plasma bound. It is slowly eliminated by urine, has a half-life of 21 days and can be taken once weekly. It is advisable to commence mefloquine 3 weeks before travel in those who have not used it before, to allow drug elimination if adverse effects occur.

Adverse effects

Nausea and vomiting, dizziness, erythema multiforme, cardiac conduction defects. Neuropsychiatric disturbances such as sleep disturbance, vivid dreams, unusual anxiety and depression, have been reported.

Mefloquine is contraindicated in renal and severe hepatic impairment, those with a past history or serious psychiatric illness, epilepsy, cardiac conduction defects, lactation and pregnancy. While there is increasing evidence that the drug is safe in pregnancy, caution is advised in the first trimester and pregnancy is best avoided during the 3 months following treatment.

Concurrent halofantrine therapy should be avoided and subsequent quinine doses if used for treatment may need to be reduced.

Doxycycline

Doxycycline is used for areas with chloroquine and mefloquine resistant falciparum malaria or when mefloquine as a first choice, is contraindicated. It is also a useful choice in epilepsy when chloroquine and mefloquine are contraindicated. It acts by inhibiting protein synthesis.

Doxycycline is almost completely absorbed and has a peak serum level at 2 h. Absorption is unaffected by food or milk. The half-life is 18–22 h, it is concentrated in the urine and bile and is excreted in a biologically active form.

Adverse effects

Nausea and vomiting, photosensitivity rashes, and interactions with anticoagulant drugs have been reported. Oesophagitis can be prevented by taking the capsules with a glass of water to ensure compete passage to the stomach.

Doxycycline is contraindicated in pregnancy, lactation and in children under 12 years of age.

Maloprim

Maloprim contains pyrimethamine 12.5 mg and dapsone 100 mg. It is occasionally used in conjunction with chloroquine for falciparum malaria, when mefloquine is contraindicated.

The adult dose is one tablet/week and must not be exceeded. No paediatric formulation is available.

Adverse effects
Methaemoglobulinaemia resulting in cyanosis, haemolysis if glucose 6-phosphate dehydrogenase deficient, insomnia and bone marrow depression, especially if the dose is exceeded.

Fansidar

Fansidar contains sulfadoxine 500 mg and pyrimethamine 25 mg and has been used for prophylaxis of falciparum malaria, but as a consequence of its side effects and the risk of Stevens–Johnson syndrome it is no longer recommended by most authorities.

Malarial prophylaxis recommendations alter as a result of changing patterns of resistance; therefore, up to date advice should be sought from specialist centres or continually updated on-line databases such as TRAVAX (described above). Current guidelines for the prevention of malaria in travellers from the UK are in the *Communicable Diseases Review of the Public Health Laboratory Service (1997)* **7**(10): R137–R152 (also available on-line through TRAVAX).

22.5 Further reading

Bell, D.R. (1995) *Lecture Notes on Tropical Medicine*, 4th edn. Blackwell Science Ltd, Oxford.

Kassianos, G. C. (1998) *Immunization: Precaution and Contraindication*, 3rd edn. Blackwell Science Ltd, Oxford.

Walker, E., Williams, G. & Raeside, F. (1997) *ABC of Healthy Travel*, 5th edn. BMJ Publishing Group, London.

World Health Organization (1999; updated annually) *International Travel and Health*. WHO, Geneva.

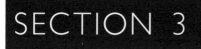

SECTION 3

Drug Use, Misuse and Regulation

CHAPTER 23

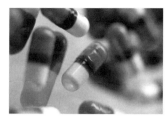

Poisoning and Drug Overdose

Acute poisoning is a common and important emergency that accounts for about 10% of acute medical admissions. Causes of poisoning may be classified in order of frequency into three groups:

1 Intentional.

2 Accidental (common in children).

3 Homicidal (rare).

Intentional poisoning includes both genuine suicidal attempts, which are associated with depression or other psychiatric disease, and so-called parasuicide, where the patient is attempting to modify the social circumstances.

Accidental poisoning includes iatrogenic incidents and cases where parents administer an excessive dose in treating a childhood illness. There are also infrequent cases where young children have been deliberately overdosed by their parents as a manifestation of child abuse.

23.1 General management of the poisoned patient

Overdose with more than one drug or with a drug plus alcohol is common and in clinical presentation can be variable depending upon the relative doses. The management of poisoning should always follow a general plan:

1 Assessment and diagnosis.

2 Supportive care.

3 Treatment:

(a) measures to reduce absorption or increase excretion of the poison.

(b) antidotes to specific poisons.

4 Psychiatric assessment.

Assessment and diagnosis

Apart from some incidents in children where a lack of risk can be established with absolute certainty, almost all poisoned or overdosed patients need to be admitted at least for a period of observation. Assess and treat according to clinical findings rather than according to the alleged poison. If respiratory and cardiovascular functions are impaired, resuscitation and life-support measures should be instituted immediately, especially in semi-comatose and comatose patients. Specific treatments can then be given later.

The signs and symptoms may vary depending on the type of poison, its formulation (e.g. sustained release drugs), time elapsed since ingestion, the amount taken and the route of exposure (e.g. oral, intravenous or inhaled). The level of consciousness should be assessed and classified according to the simple grading scale listed in Table 23.1. There are relatively few physical signs associated with specific poisons but important examples are listed in Table 23.2. Once the necessary resuscitation has been performed, it is important to document the history, including past and present illnesses as well as drug impaired consciousness. It is also important to seek information

EDINBURGH COMA SCALE

Grade I	Drowsy; responds to verbal commands
Grade II	Unresponsive to verbal commands
Grade III	Unconscious, responsive to maximal painful stimuli
Grade IV	No response to stimuli

Alternatively, on an Intensive Care ward, the more detailed Glasgow coma scale may be used

Table 23.1 The Edinburgh coma scale.

CLUES TO SUBSTANCE INGESTION

Coma	Barbiturates; benzodiazepines; ethanol; ethylene glycol; methanol; opiates; trichloroethanol; tricyclic antidepressants
Convulsions	Amfetamine (amphetamine); Ecstasy; phenothiazines; theophylline; tricyclic antidepressants
Constricted pupils	Organophosphates; opiates and trichloroethanol
Dilated pupils	Cocaine; phenothiazines; quinine; sympathomimetics and tricyclic antidepressants
Cardiac arrythmias	Antiarrhythmics; anticholinergics; phenothiazines; quinine; sympathomimetics; and tricyclic antidepressants
Pulmonary oedema	Aspirin; ethylene glycol; irritant gases; opiates; organophosphates; tricyclic antidepressants; and paraquat
Metabolic acidosis	Aspirin; ethanol; ethylene glycol; methanol and tricyclic antidepressants
Hyperthermia	Anticholinergics; Ecstasy and monoamine oxidase inhibitors
Hepatic failure	Paracetamol
Renal failure not related to hypotension or rhabdomyolysis	Ethylene glycol; methanol; paracetamol and aspirin

Table 23.2 Clues to the substances ingested.

from relatives or friends, or whoever brought the patient to hospital including ambulance personnel or police. Unfortunately, information thus collected is often unreliable or incomplete. In such cases toxicological analysis of biological samples from the patient or samples of the suspect poison may be needed to establish the presence or absence of toxic substances.

Once the vital functions are checked and supported it is possible to complete the physical examination including assessment of the pupils, neck, heart, lungs, abdomen and central nervous system. Particular efforts should be

ACUTE POISONING: CLINICAL AND BIOCHEMICAL CONSEQUENCES

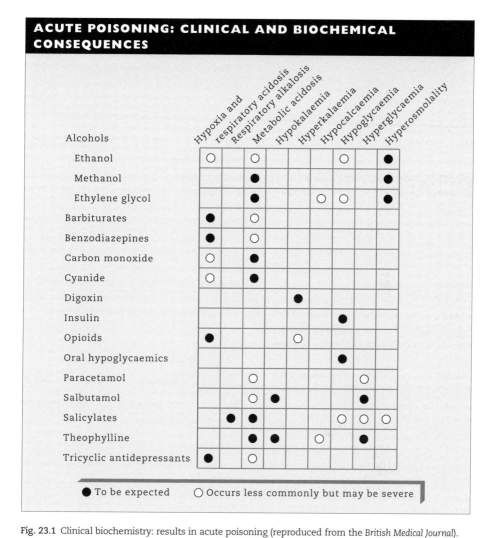

	Hypoxia and respiratory acidosis	Respiratory alkalosis	Metabolic acidosis	Hypokalaemia	Hyperkalaemia	Hypocalcaemia	Hypoglycaemia	Hyperglycaemia	Hyperosmolality
Alcohols									
Ethanol	○		○				○		●
Methanol			●						●
Ethylene glycol			●			○	○		●
Barbiturates	●		○						
Benzodiazepines	●		○						
Carbon monoxide	○		●						
Cyanide	○		●						
Digoxin					●				
Insulin							●		
Opioids	●			○					
Oral hypoglycaemics							●		
Paracetamol			○					○	
Salbutamol			○	●				●	
Salicylates		●	●				○	○	○
Theophylline		●	●	○				●	
Tricyclic antidepressants	●		○						

● To be expected   ○ Occurs less commonly but may be severe

Fig. 23.1 Clinical biochemistry: results in acute poisoning (reproduced from the *British Medical Journal*).

made to look for jaundice, injection marks, scars and skin blisters or necrosis. Laboratory investigations can be helpful both for diagnosis and treatment (as shown in Fig. 23.1). In addition, any vomitus should be saved, together with samples of blood and urine, for possible toxicological analysis.

Supportive therapy

Food, vomitus, secretions or dentures should be removed from the mouth and the tongue prevented from falling backwards where it can obstruct the airway. This is achieved by placing the patient in the coma (left lateral) position. If a gag reflex is absent the airway should be protected by using either a Guedal or Brooke's airway or inserting a cuffed endotracheal tube. The respiratory cardiovascular central nervous system (CNS) and body temperature can then be checked in more detail so that appropriate action can be taken. For the majority of cases general nursing care is all that is required. Providing that adequate attention is given to pressure areas, the eyes, mouth and the care of any injuries, the patient can be expected to fully recover.

The care of more serious cases should follow the following guidelines.

Respiratory system

Aspiration of the gastric contents could have occurred before treatment started and sometimes may occur even in the presence of an airway or an endotracheal tube. It is therefore important to check the lungs frequently and to X-ray the chest if appropriate. Respiratory function should be monitored and assisted ventilation is indicated if the tidal volume falls below 300 ml or if arterial blood gases demonstrate hypercapnoea (Pco_2 exceeds Po_2).

Cardiovascular system

The blood pressure and electrocardiogram should be monitored and cardiac output supported as necessary to maintain tissue perfusion. Hypotension is a common accompaniment of severe overdose and cardiac arrhythmias complicate some cases. Intravenous access should be established as soon as possible in order to permit administration of fluids for the treatment of hypotension and to facilitate intravenous administration of drugs. Inotropic agents such as dopamine, dobutamine or isoprenaline may be used to counteract the cardiac depressant effects of the poisons. These drugs also protect renal perfusion and can help to avoid or reduce impairment of renal function. It should be remembered that as all antiarrhythmic drugs can produce toxic arrhythmia they should be used cautiously and only if other treatments have failed.

Urinary system

Renal function should be monitored and it is reasonable to catheterize the bladder in severely poisoned and unconscious patients. Fluid intake and output should be carefully recorded. If the patient is in renal failure haemodialysis should be used to support renal function, recognizing that only occasionally will it actually help in removing the poison.

The CNS

Convulsions can usually be controlled either by intravenous diazepam or clomethiazole. If convulsions are occurring during assisted ventilation then infusion of thiopenthone may be used.

Temperature

It is essential to ensure that the core temperature is recorded with a low reading thermometer because hypothermia contributes to shock, acidaemia and hypoxia. In order to conserve heat the patient should be wrapped in a foil or plastic blanket and nursed in a warm atmosphere. The use of humidified air is essential if the patient is on mechanical ventilation. In cases of hyperthermia (i.e. rectal temperature above 39°C) and muscle spasms, elective paralysis with pancuronium should be used and mechanical ventilation instituted.

23.2 Specific treatment for poisoning

Measures to prevent the absorption of a drug or poison

Measures that may reduce the absorption of a drug or poison include emesis, gastric lavage, oral adsorbents or cathartics. Both emesis and gastric lavage can be hazardous and their efficacy is limited. They should be used only when clearly indicated, that is:

1 A clinically significant dose of the poison is thought to have been ingested.

2 Ingestion occurred less than 2 h before treatment. Exceptions include aspirin and drugs with an anticholinergic effect, since in both cases the drug may persist in the stomach for several hours.

3 The time of ingestion is not known but the patient is unconscious with signs of serious poisoning. In the latter case only the lavage is indicated and the airway must be protected by an endotracheal tube.

Lavage and emesis are contraindicated if the suspected poison is corrosive or if there is a past history of oesophageal varices.

Emesis

Emesis has long been a favoured method of gastric emptying, particularly in children, on the grounds that it is easy to administer and reliably causes vomiting. However, the use of Ipecac (syrup of ipecacuanha) as a means of gastric emptying is falling out of favour and being replaced by greater use of activated charcoal (see below).

Gastric aspiration and lavage

This technique is difficult and distressing in children and is indicated only in serious cases, usually where the patient is unconscious. In adults it is much better tolerated and is often used in patients who are unconscious (providing an endotracheal tube is in place). The patient should be placed on a trolley in the left lateral position with the head end tilted slightly downwards. A wide bore (30 English gauge Jacques) tube is passed into the stomach and the contents are aspirated using a syringe and lowering the tube below the level of the patient's bed to allow drainage by gravity. A sample of aspirate should be taken and kept in a fridge for possible toxicological analysis. After aspiration, lukewarm water is instilled (200–300 ml at 38°C) into the stomach over a period of 2–3 min, and is left in place for approximately 1 min. Gravity drainage is allowed for a further 3 or 4 min. The procedure should be continued until the aspirate becomes clear or until approximately 6–8 l of water have been used. Again evidence for the effectiveness of this treatment is limited, even after widespread usage for many years. As with ipecacuanha

the trend is for gastric lavage to be used less frequently.

Adsorbents and cathartics

Many substances including some foods are capable of adsorbing drugs or poisons and thus reducing their absorption. In practice, however, only activated charcoal is widely used as a treatment for poisoning. It is formulated as a fine powder that can be suspended in water and either taken as a drink or administered via an orogastric or nasogastric tube. The term 'activated' is merely an indication that the charcoal meets required standards for adsorbents. It is capable of adsorbing most toxic substances and can also be administered after the use of an emetic or gastric lavage. In general 10 g of charcoal combine 1 g of the toxin and the usual single dose is 50–100 g.

Table 23.3 lists those substances not adsorbed by activated charcoal.

There is also evidence that repeated doses of activated charcoal (10–25 g, 2- to 4-hourly) can enhance the clearance of drugs which have already been absorbed. This is thought to occur by interruption of the enterohepatic circulation and by back diffusion of the drug across the gut mucosa. Repeated doses are therefore used for drugs with long half-lives and active metabolites, examples of which are given in Table 23.3.

The use of cathartics may be expected to speed up gastrointestinal transit and thus to reduce the time during which absorption of the poison can occur. In practice there is little evidence to support such treatment but

AGENTS NOT ABSORBED BY CHARCOAL	
Acids	Iron salts
Alcohols, e.g. ethanol, methanol	Glycols, e.g. ethylene glycol
Cyanide	Lead salts
DDT	Lithium salts
Organic solvents	Mercury salts

Table 23.3 Agents not absorbed by charcoal.

magnesium sulphate (Epsom salts) may be useful in reducing drug absorption when the overdose involved a sustained release formulation.

Whole bowel irrigation

This is a newer method of gut decontamination. It involves the administration of polyethylene glycol/electrolyte solutions orally or via a nasogastric tube, until the effluent resembles the irrigating solution (usually 2–6 h). It is currently most widely used for gut decontamination of body packers and overdoses of drugs poorly absorbed by activated charcoal or formulated for sustained release.

Enhancement of drug elimination

If a drug or its active metabolite is excreted in the urine, it is theoretically possible to increase elimination by increasing glomerular filtration and/or decreasing tubular reabsorption. In practice, such treatments are clinically useful for only a small number of drugs and in most patients treatment should aim simply to maintain normal renal function by adjusting the fluid intake and administering the diuretic furosemide. Forced diuresis refers to the administration of large volumes of intravenous fluid to promote increased urine production and this may be supported by the administration of drugs to render the urine alkaline (sodium bicarbonate) or acid (ammonium chloride). Such procedures are not without risk, because there is a danger of precipitating both fluid overload and electrolyte imbalance, notably hypokalaemia. Alteration of the urine pH is made in accordance with the pKa of the drug in order to ensure that the drug in the urine is ionized and therefore not reabsorbed. Thus for phenobarbitone and salicylate, both of which have acidic pKa values, an alkaline urine is required. In theory, an acid urine pH could increase the excretion of drugs with an alkaline pKa, but there are no useful examples. Currently the use of alkaline diuresis is restricted mainly to the treatment of salicylate poisoning and the recommended regime places greater emphasis on alkalinization of the urine, rather than on the volume of urine produced.

Haemodialysis haemoperfusion (passage of blood over an adsorbent)

In practice, these extra corporal techniques are usually used in the management of poisoned patients, primarily to support renal function. Although it can be shown that they are efficient in clearing a drug from the circulating blood volume, the amount of drug thus removed is small in most cases, because the drug is distributed more widely throughout the body. Significant active elimination of the drug is likely only for drugs with a low volume of distribution and the presence of high plasma drug concentrations. Haemodialysis, on the one hand, is effective only for removal of relatively small molecules (less than 350 Da molecular weight) such as ethanol, methanol, ethylene glycol and salicylate; haemoperfusion, on the other, can remove much larger molecules because there is no membrane between the blood and the adsorbent. These treatments are not without risk (e.g. infection or haemorrhage) and should be used only when the criteria listed above are accompanied by evidence of severe poisoning or a deteriorating clinical state in spite of good supportive care.

Specific treatment (antidotes)

An antidote can be defined as a therapeutic agent used to counteract the toxic effects of a xenobiotic (to cover both natural and manufactured poisons). Thus, activated charcoal and other drugs used in supportive care could be considered as antidotes. It is useful, however, to consider separately those antidotes with more specific indications, bearing in mind that they have varied mechanisms of action (Table 23.4) and that many are used only rarely. In some cases, such as snake antivenom, they are held only by small numbers of centres whilst in others the antidotes have to be considered still under investigations. A

ANTIDOTES

Poisons	Antidotes	Mechanism of action
Anticholinergic agents	Physostigmine	Cholinesterase inhibitor
Anticoagulants (Warfarin type)	Vitamin K (phytomenadione)	Cofactor for synthesis of clotting factors
Beta-adrenergic blockers	Isoprenaline	Competitive agonist at beta-receptor
	Glucagon	Stimulates myocardial adenyl cyclase
Carbon monoxide	Oxygen (normo or hyperbaric)	Competitive displacement of carbon monoxide from haemoglobin molecule
Cyanide	Dicobalt edetate Sodium nitrate	Chelating agent. Forms methaemoglobin which combines with cyanide
	Sodium thiosulphate Hydroxocobalamin	Acclerates detoxification of cyanide Combines with cyanide to form cyanocobalamin
Digoxin and digitoxin	Fab antidote fragments	Antidote forms an inert complex with poison
Ethylene glycol or methanol	Ethanol	Competitive substrate for alcohol dehydrogenase, slows toxic metabolite production
Benzodiazepines	Flumazenil	Competitive antagonist at benzodiazepine receptors
Heavy metals (lead, mercury, arsenic)	DMSA (2,3-dimercaptosuccinic acid)	Chelating agent
	DMPS (2,3-dimercaptopropane-1-sulphonate)	Chelating agent
	Sodium calcium edetate	Chelating agent
	Dimercaprol	Chelating agent
Hydrofluoric acid	Calcium gluconate	Forms an inert complex (calcium fluoride)
Iron salts	Desferrioxamine	Chelating agent
Narcotics (dextropropoxyphene, heroin, co-proxamol, etc.)	Naloxone	Competitive antagonist at opioid receptors
Organophosphates	Atropine	Competitive antagonist at acetylcholine receptor
	Pralidoxime	Cholinesterase reactivator
Paracetamol	Acetylcysteine Methionine	Accelerate detoxification of potentially toxic metabolite (glutathione precursor and SH donor)
Thallium	Berlin Blue	Chelating agent

Table 23.4 List of antidotes and their mechanism of action.

POISONS INFORMATION SERVICES

Belfast	028 9024 0503
Birmingham	0121 507 5588/9
Cardiff	029 2070 9901
Edinburgh	0131 229 2477 (or)
	0131 228 2441 (viewdata)
Leeds	0113 243 0715 (or)
	0113 292 3547
London	0207 635 9191 (or)
	0207 955 5095
Newcastle	0191 232 5131

Table 23.5 Poisons information services.

Poisons Information Centre can advise on both how to obtain supplies of antidotes and on their correct usage (see Table 23.5).

23.3 Psychiatric social assessment

This is needed in all cases of deliberate overdosage but it is no longer considered essential for all cases to be referred to a psychiatrist. It is the responsibility of the medical team to make the first assessment and to refer the patients as appropriate.

23.4 Special features of common drug overdose

While it is safe to assume that sooner or later most drugs will be taken in overdose, it is practical for most doctors to attempt to learn only about those which occur most frequently. This section discusses the clinical features and management of some of the most common drug overdoses. In so doing it takes note of advances in therapeutics that have relegated some toxic drugs to the history books (e.g. the hypnotic barbiturates, glutethemide and methaqualone), introduced safer alternatives (e.g. the newer antidepressants and over-the-counter ibuprofen), and of the improved safety associated with child resistant closures.

The drugs discussed have been grouped into antidepressants and sedatives, analgesics, metals and miscellaneous.

Even for these drugs, the management of the individual case may be complicated by several variables, including: mixed or repeated overdosage, underlying disease, and delay before reaching medical attention. For all the more unusual forms of poisoning, it is important to know how to obtain information and advice from a Poisons Information Centre.

Antidepressant drugs

Monoamine oxidase inhibitors
Poisoning with this group of drugs is becoming less common, as other antidepressant drugs have largely replaced them.

Mechanism of action. These drugs prevent the breakdown of endogenous monoamines and this is the basis of the hypertension that is their most important toxic effect.

Clinical features. Severe hypertension may result if a patient on a monoamine oxidase inhibitor takes food with a high content of sympathomimetic amines such as tyramine.

Overdose may present a complex picture, including tachycardia and either hypertension or hypotension. The basis for the latter is not clear. Severe cases may be complicated by muscle spasms, hyperpyrexia, rhabdomyolosis, acute renal failure, DIC, and coma.

Management. Gastric lavage (GL) and/or activated charcoal (AC) if the patient presents within 2 h of ingestion. Otherwise treatment is directed at the particular toxic effects which are prominent in individual patients.

Tricyclic antidepressants

Mechanism of action. These drugs inhibit noradrenaline reuptake into central and peripheral neurones, and serotonin reuptake into central neurones. They also block parasympathetic muscarinic receptors, and have an effect on the heart similar to that of class Ia antiarrhythmic agents (membrane stabilization).

Clinical features. In mild cases the anticholinergic effects predominate: dry mouth, dilated pupils, sinus tachycardia, drowsiness, and urinary retention. More severe cases may show signs of cerebral toxicity: convulsions, coma, respiratory depression, and of cardiac toxicity: ectopic beats, broad QRS complexes, arrhythmias including ventricular tachycardia and ventricular fibrillation, and hypotension as a result of a negative inotropic effect.

Laboratory investigation. Hypokalaemia and metabolic acidosis are common.

Management. GL followed by AC is indicated for significant amounts (>300 mg). In unconscious patients this may be useful up to 4 h post-ingestion. A further dose of activated charcoal may be helpful, especially in large overdoses or when a sustained release preparation has been taken. Electrocardiogram (ECG) monitoring should be instituted, pH and electrolytes must be checked and if necessary corrected. Severe arrhythmias with hypotension may respond to correction of potassium and pH; otherwise phenytoin or atenolol may be helpful.

Comment
1 Disopyramide, lidocaine, quinidine, procainamide, atropine and cholinesterase inhibitors are contraindicated.

2 Prolonged external cardiac massage may be effective in maintaining cardiac output for many hours with full recovery.

Newer antidepressants

These include the selective serotonin reuptake inhibitors (SSRIs): paroxetine, sertraline and fluoxetine, and the related drugs: Moclobemide, venlafaxime and nefazodone.

Mechanism of action. SSRIs prevent the reuptake of serotonin into nerve endings, thus increasing the synaptic concentration of serotonin. Some also have beta-adrenoreceptor effects, and paroxetine has weak muscarinic effects.

Venlafaxine, nefazodone and moclobemide have effects that are distinct from each other and from the SSRIs, but in overdose the dangers are similar.

Clinical features. These are usually mild and transient when taken alone in lower doses, and include mild gastrointestinal, central nervous system and cardiovascular disturbances. Higher doses may lead to convulsions, coma or death.

The serotonin syndrome occurs when an SSRI is ingested in combination with another drug that increases the availability of serotonin (e.g. monoamine oxidase inhibitors (MAOIs), tryptophan). It is potentially fatal. Clinical features include myoclinic jerking, hyperreflexia, hyperthermia, rhabdomyolysis, renal failure and disseminated intravascular coagulation.

Management. GL and AC are indicated for significant overdoses. Otherwise management is symptomatic and supportive.

Sedatives

Benzodiazepines
Mechanism of action. Benzodiazepines enhance the effect of the inhibitory neurotransmitter gamma-aminobutyric acid (GABA). The resulting generalized depression of the

reticular activating system and other neuronal systems leads to coma and respiratory arrest.

Preparations vary widely in potency and duration of action. In general they are of low acute toxicity when taken alone. However, toxicity is enhanced with the concomitant ingestion of alcohol or other CNS depressant drugs. Newer potent short-acting agents carry a higher risk of complications. Children, the elderly and those with pre-existing respiratory disorders are particularly susceptible.

Clinical features. Confusion, slurred speech, ataxia, drowsiness progressing to coma, hyporeflexia, hypotension, respiratory depression.

Investigations
1 Arterial blood gas.
2 Pulse oximetry.
3 Blood glucose.

Management. Treatment is mainly symptomatic and supportive with particular attention to blood pressure (BP) and respiration. Patients who have ingested a significant amount and present within two hours of ingestion should undergo GL and receive AC. The airway must be protected at all times and endotracheal intubation and mechanical ventilation may be necessary. Flumazenil is an antidote with a relatively short half-life. Currently it is administered only to reverse the effects of benzodiazepines used in anaesthesia. It is not licensed for the use in benzodiazepine overdosage and might precipitate convulsions and acute withdrawal symptoms in dependant patients.

Newer sedatives

Zopiclone
Mechanism of action. Zopiclone acts on the central GABA–benzodiazepine–chloride channel receptor complex, but at a site distinct from that of the benzodiazepines.

Clinical features. Relatively few cases of overdose have been reported, as this is a new drug. Drowsiness, ataxia and headache may occur, but no serious adverse effects (including hypotension and respiratory depression) have so far been notified.

Management. GL and AC are indicated for large overdoses. Management is otherwise symptomatic and supportive.

Zolpidem

Mechanism of action. Zolpidem is structurally unrelated to the benzodiazepines (BZs), but binds to one of the central benzodiazepine receptor subtypes.

Clinical features. Again, few cases of overdose have been reported, and most of these were relatively benign. In the majority, drowsiness was the only symptom, and it required no specific therapeutic measures.

Management. Larger overdoses should be treated with GL and AC. Subsequently management is symptomatic and supportive.

Analgesics

Salicylates
Mechanism of action. In overdose salicylates stimulate the respiratory centre, causing hyperventilation and respiratory alkalosis. The body compensates by excreting bicarbonate, sodium, and potassium ions and water in the urine, resulting in electrolyte imbalance, dehydration and a decrease in the buffering capacity of the body. This allows the development of a high anion gap metabolic acidosis, which enhances transfer of the salicylate ion across the blood–brain barrier. Only in severe overdoses does aspirin cause CNS depression. A severely poisoned patient may be alert, garrulous and even aggressive. It is very easy to underestimate the severity of salicylate poisoning on clinical grounds.

Clinical features. Mild or moderate overdose: nausea, vomiting, epigastric pain, tinnitus, flushing, sweating, hyperventilation, dehydration, tremor and respiratory alkalosis with metabolic acidosis.

Severe overdose: hypo- or hyperglycaemia, hypokalaemia, hypo- or hypernatraemia, hypoprothrombinaemia, confusion, drowsiness, delirium and coma.

CNS effects are usually relieved if acidosis is corrected.

Investigations
1 Salicylate level 4 h post-ingestion and then every 3 h until peak level achieved.
2 Arterial pH.
3 Renal function.
4 Blood glucose.
5 Prothrombin time.

Management. Gastric lavage and activated charcoal is administered up to 12 h post-ingestion because salicylates in large amounts form concretions in the stomach. This is followed by repeated doses of AC. Rehydrate with oral or intravenous fluids. In severe overdoses with high salicylate levels urinary alkalization is very effective as the rate of aspirin excretion may be increased by a factor of 20. This should be considered when plasma salicylate levels are higher than 600 mg/l (4.32 mmol/l) in adults or 450 mg/l (3.24 mmol/l) in children and the elderly. Indications for haemodialysis are persistently high salicylate concentrations unresponsive to urinary alkalization, renal failure, non-cardiogenic pulmonary oedoma, convulsions, CNS effects not resolved by correction of acidosis, and acid–base or electrolyte imbalance.

Non-steroidal anti-inflammatory drugs (NSAIDS)
Fatal poisoning is rare.

Ibuprofen
With the increasing use of ibuprofen as an over-the-counter medicine, it is now taken frequently in overdose. However, in contrast to aspirin and paracetamol it is considered to be of low toxicity. Ingestion of very high doses can cause marked toxicity and it may enhance salicylate toxicity when co-ingested with aspirin.

Clinical features. Often with small or moderate overdose there are no symptoms. However, a few cause nausea, vomiting, epigastric pain, tinnitus, headaches, ataxia and drowsiness. In severe overdoses haematemesis, hypotension, convulsions, coma and apnoea have been reported.

Management. GL and AC if more than 100 mg/kg has been ingested. Encourage adequate fluids to maintain good urine output.

Mefenamic acid
Overdose occurs most frequently in young women prescribed the drug for dysmenorrhoea. There is a high incidence of convulsions that are usually brief and short-lived and responsive to diazepam. In massive overdoses intractable fitting can occur which requires paralysis and artificial ventilation.

Other NSAIDs, although widely used, are seen in overdose only infrequently.

Paracetamol
The main problem is hepatotoxicity. Paracetamol overdose is common and potentially fatal.

Mechanism of action. Paracetamol is metabolized in the liver. At therapeutic concentrations the major products are glucuronide and sulphate conjugates. A much smaller proportion is metabolized by the microsomal mixed function oxidases, with the product of this pathway being detoxified by combination with glutathione. However, in overdose, greatly increased amounts of paracetamol are metabolized by this secondary pathway, which exhausts glutathione stores and leaves an excess of a toxic metabolite. This then combines covalently with protein macromolecules in the liver to produce hepatic necrosis with a centrolobular pattern. If the patient survives coma normal liver function is usually restored in a few months.

Susceptibility to paracetamol overdose varies. There are various 'high risk' groups who may be susceptible to paracetamol at lower plasma paracetamol levels. They include:

1 Malnourished/anorexic patients.
2 HIV positive patients.
3 Patients with pre-existing liver disease or induced liver enzymes, e.g. chronic alcoholics.
4 Patients taking enzyme inducing drugs such as carbamazepine, phenytoin, barbiturates, primidone, rifampicin.

Clinical features. Initially there may be no symptoms despite a potential lethal overdose. Alternatively there may be nausea, vomiting, abdominal pain, pallor and very rarely drowsiness, coma and metabolic acidosis when very large amounts have been taken.

If coma is present care should be taken to exclude any other causes.

By 16–24 h postingestion prothrombin time, transaminase and bilirubin levels start to rise. By 72–120 h peak hepatotoxicity occurs with jaundice, coagulation abnormalities, hepatic failure, renal failure, hypoglycaemia, encephalopathy or coma if the patient is untreated.

Investigations
1 Paracetamol level 4 h post-ingestion.
2 Prothrombin time.
3 Renal function.
4 Arterial pH.
5 Blood glucose.
6 Liver function test.

Management. The best guide to the likelihood of the development of hepatic necrosis is the plasma level of paracetamol and the rate of decline, i.e. the half-life of the drug. A half-life of more than 4 h indicates saturation of the major routes of conjugation and potential toxicity. To wait for this information, however, requires a delay of more than 4 h from the patient's presentation before therapy is commenced. In practice, as a level of more than

150 mg/l (1 mmol/l) 4 h or more after ingestion suggests that hepatic necrosis is likely, treatment should be given.

Figure 23.2 gives a guide to the management of paracetamol poisoning determined by plasma level and time after ingestion. In the high risk groups treatment should be commenced if the plasma concentration of paracetamol is half of the level normally considered toxic, i.e. on or above a line joining 100 mg/l (0.66 mmol/l) at 4 h post-ingestion and 25 mg/l (0.17 mmol/l) at 12 h post-ingestion. To be effective, treatment should begin as early as possible. It consists of either methionine given orally or N-acetyl cysteine given intravenously. Methionine enhances glutathione synthesis by the donation of thiol groups, while N-acetyl cysteine is hydrolysed *in vivo* to cysteine, a glutathione precursor. Thus, additional glutathione is made available to combine with the toxic metabolite and thus prevent binding to liver cells.

Drowsiness, confusion and a deteriorating level of consciousness indicate the development of encephalopathy and progression to fulminant hepatic failure. A specialist liver centre should be contacted if the INR is:

1 >2 at 24 h.
2 >4 at 48 h.
3 >6 at 72 h.

or if the patient has any of the following: an elevated plasma creatinine, evidence of acidosis, hypoglycaemia, renal failure, hypotension or encephalopathy, as they are all indications of severe hepatotoxicity.

Oral methionine is effective if given within 8 h of the overdose and providing the patient is not vomiting. Acetylcysteine is given intravenously and is useful up to 72 h after ingestion. Nevertheless, it is important not to delay treatment.

Metal poisoning

Iron

Mechanism of action. Iron is corrosive and initially produces gastritis, which may be erosive or haemorrhagic. Perforation can occur

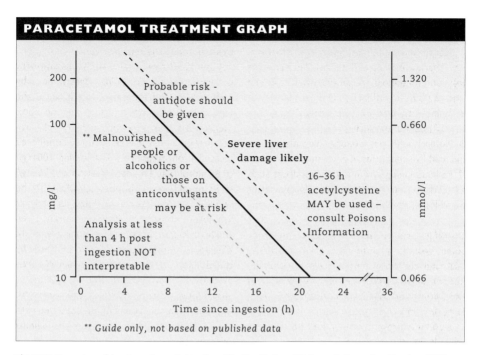

PARACETAMOL TREATMENT GRAPH

Probable risk - antidote should be given

** Malnourished people or alcoholics or those on anticonvulsants may be at risk

Severe liver damage likely

16–36 h acetylcysteine MAY be used – consult Poisons Information

Analysis at less than 4 h post ingestion NOT interpretable

Time since ingestion (h)

** Guide only, not based on published data

Fig. 23.2 Paracetamol treatment graph (produced by the National Poisons Information Service, 1991).

and fluid or blood loss may be substantial. Following an overdose the mucosal barrier becomes overwhelmed and large amounts of iron rapidly enter the circulation, saturating transferrin. Unbound iron then circulates freely and is taken up by parenchymal cells, particularly in the liver. It causes mitochondrial damage, interfering with cellular respiration and resulting in metabolic acidosis and ultimately cell death. Hepatic failure with hypoglycaemia and coagulopathy may develop. Multi-organ failure ensues and is often fatal.

Clinical features. The clinical course of iron poisoning may be divided into four phases; the timescale is variable and can be given only as a guide.

Phase 1: 30 min–6 h post-ingestion: vomiting, haematemesis, diarrhoea, drowsiness, coma, convulsion, metabolic acidosis, shock, gastro-intestinal haemorrhage.

Phase 2: 6–24 h: clinical effects usually abate and the patient recovers or moves onto the next phase.

Phase 3: 12–48 h: relapse with severe lethargy, coma, convulsions, hepatic failure, metabolic acidosis, cardiovascular collapse, pulmonary oedema, renal failure.

Phase 4: 2–5 weeks: stricture formation, small bowel obstruction.

Investigations
1 Plain abdominal radiograph.
2 Serum iron level 4 h post-ingestion.
3 Blood glucose.
4 White cell count.
5 Arterial blood gas.
6 Liver function tests.
7 Renal function.

Management. If the amount of ingested iron exceeds 30 mg/kg body weight or the patient is symptomatic an abdominal X-ray should be performed. Undissolved iron tablets are radio-paque; if any are visible in the stomach on X-ray then GL should be undertaken. AC is not effective as it does not bind iron. Repeated lavage may be required to remove all the tablets observed on X-ray. A high blood iron level might be indicative of severe toxicity but it is essential to interpret the level in the light of the patient's clinical condition and an accurate patient history.

Desferrioxamine is a specific antidote chelating free iron to form ferrioxamine. It is believed to remove iron from cellular binding sites and hence prevent tissue damage. The decision to use desferrioxamine should be based on the patient's clinical condition and the iron blood level. It is administered by slow intravenous infusion to a maximum of 80 mg/kg body weight a day. Hypotension and pulmonary damage (acute respiratory distress syndrome, ARDS) are rare side effects. The chelate complex usually imparts a pink–brown colour to the urine. The duration of treatment is controversial and depends on the clinical condition.

Lead

Most cases of lead toxicity result from long-term occupational or environmental exposure. Children are at particular risk from repeated ingestion of lead contaminated house dust, yard soil, or paint chips.

Mechanism of action. The multisystem toxicity of lead is mediated by inhibition of enzymatic processes and by interaction with essential cations, such as calcium, zinc and iron. The primary organ systems affected are the nervous system, the kidneys and the reproductive and haematopoietic systems.

Clinical features. Acute poisoning may cause anorexia, metallic taste, vomiting, abdominal pain, diarrhoea, muscle weakness and cramps. CNS symptoms include headache, insomnia, drowsiness, coma and convulsions.

Chronic poisoning can result in gastrointestinal disturbances with abdominal pain and tenderness. Nephropathy, anaemia and neuromuscular dysfunction with paralysis of the extensor muscles of the wrist and ankles occurs. Encephalopathy is mainly seen in children and chronic low level exposure is linked with decreased intelligence and learning and behaviour disorders.

Investigations
1 Blood lead level.
2 Plain abdominal radiograph.
3 X-ray of long bones ('lead lines').
4 Haemoglobin and blood film (basophilic stippling).
5 Iron studies, ferritin and calcium (deficits facilitate lead absorption).
6 Occupational and environmental history.

Management. GL should be performed if the abdominal X-ray shows radiopaque material in the stomach. The gut must be cleared before chelation therapy is commenced. The decision to administer a chelating agent depends on the blood lead level and clinical presentation. Lead encephalopathy is a medical emergency and requires prompt treatment. Sodium calcium EDTA and meso 2,3-dimercaptosuccinic acid (DMSA) are chelating agents useful in the treatment of acute or chronic lead poisoning. Prevention of further exposure is of utmost importance.

Mercury

Dental amalgam fillings have been reported to release mercury vapour into the oral cavity. The chronic inhalation exposure has been associated with non-specific vegetative and neuropsychiatric symptoms, and a characteristic fine tremor.

23.5 Miscellaneous drugs

3,4-Methylenedioxymethamfetamine (MDMA, 'Ecstasy')

Mechanism of action. MDMA is an amfetamine derivative. Some effects are a consequence of serotonin and dopamine release in the CNS, while others are the result of central and peripheral sympathetic stimulation of alpha- and beta-adrenergic receptors. Animal experiments have shown that MDMA causes irreversible destruction of serotonergic nerve terminals.

Clinical features.
Mild: nausea, vomiting, abdominal pain, increased muscle tone, muscle pain, trismus (jaw clenching), dilated pupils, sweating, agitation, anxiety, hypertension, tachycardia.
Moderate: hypertonia, hyperreflexia, hypotension, visual hallucinations.
Severe: delirium, coma, convulsion, hyponatraemic encephalopathy, intracerebral haemorrhage, cardiac arrhythmias, hyperthermic syndrome leading to rhabdomyolysis, renal failure, DIC, metabolic acidosis and cardiovascular collapse.

Investigations
1 Urea and electrolytes, white cell count (WCC), platelets, creatine kinase (CK), coagulation screen.
2 ECG.
3 Chest X-ray.
4 Urine for myoglobin.

Management. The treatment is symptomatic and supportive. Observe all cases for at least 6 h. Give oral activated charcoal (AC) up to 2 h post-ingestion. Monitor BP, pulse, body temperature and ECG. Anxiety and agitation may respond to diazepam or chlorpromazine. Tachycardia and hypertension should be treated with beta- and/or alpha-blockers. Symptomatic hyponatraemia and hyperthermia require aggressive treatment in an intensive care environment, including fluid and electrolyte replacement, the use of dentrolene as a muscle relaxant and even paralysis and ventilation.

Lithium

Lithium is used for the treatment of bipolar depression and other psychiatric disorders.

Serious toxicity is most commonly caused by chronic overmedication in patients with renal impairment. Acute overdose, in contrast, is generally less severe.

Clinical effects. These include nausea, vomiting, diarrhoea, blurred vision, ataxia, nystagmus, slurred speech, confusion, drowsiness, hyperreflexia, muscle fasciculations and polyuria. In severe cases coma, convulsions, dysrhythmias and renal failure can occur.

Investigations
1 Lithium level.
2 Renal function.
3 ECG.

Management. Includes adequate hydration with oral or intravenous fluids. Lithium levels should be measured 6–8 hourly to monitor excretion. Haemodialysis is indicated where:
1 Moderate or severe clinical effects are present.
2 Lithium levels are not falling as it indicates poor renal excretion.
3 Renal failure.
Haemodialysis should be continued until serum lithium level falls below 1 mmol/l, but levels should continue to be monitored as redistribution from the tissues often results in a rebound increase in levels over the following 6–12 h necessitating repeat dialysis.

Theophyllines

Mechanism of action. These drugs inhibit the enzyme phosphodiesterase, antagonize adenosine receptors and cause the release of endogenous catecholamines.

Clinical features. These may be delayed with sustained-release preparations. Nausea, vomiting, tremor, hyperventilation and tachycardia are usual. In severe cases convulsions, respiratory depression, hypotension, and cardiac arrhythmias may occur.

Laboratory investigation. Hypokalaemia, hyperglycaemia and metabolic acidosis may occur.

Management. Administer antiemetics for vomiting. Give repeated doses of AC until it appears in the stools. Correct pH and electrolytes. Measure theophylline levels. Charcoal haemoperfusion may be life saving in severe cases.

CHAPTER 24

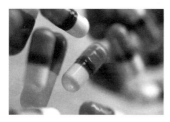

Drug Prescription: Legal and Practical Aspects

Although a medicine and its active drug constituents can have a powerful effect in the treatment of disease and the alleviation of symptoms, the inappropriate choice of drug or the incorrect dose of an appropriate drug could lead to serious morbidity or even mortality. The choice of therapeutic agent must be based on information gained from clinical history, examination and any necessary further investigations. Other factors that influence the choice are the age of the patient and associated pathology (renal or hepatic disease).

Once the decision has been made, the patient must be supplied with the medicine or treatment. The importance of this stage has often been ignored both in practice and in the training of doctors. Poor communication by the medical practitioner is a major factor in poor compliance of the patient with instructions. Clear, unambiguous instructions to the patient are essential not only to indicate the dose and frequency with which the medicine is to be taken, but also to reinforce any additional advice about diet, smoking and the level of social and physical activity.

In most countries there are restrictions on the availability of drugs. In the UK medicines are classified into three categories:

1 General sales list preparations are medicines that can be supplied by most retailers in supermarkets, etc. Some simple analgesics, e.g. aspirin and antacids, are widely available for sale. These preparations may be used excessively or inappropriately and can contribute to drug-related morbidity either by direct toxicity or through drug interactions.

2 Pharmacy medicines, which may only be supplied by a registered pharmacist, can be supplied to a patient without a prescription from a registered medical practitioner. These preparations may cause adverse effects and interact with other prescribed drugs.

3 Prescription-only medicines can only be supplied by a pharmacist on the prescription of a registered medical (or dental) practitioner, although dental practitioners are required by their registration body to restrict their prescribing to areas in which they are competent. Nurse prescribers are also appropriate practitioners for prescription-only medicines listed in the *Nurse Prescribing Formulary*.

Comment. Details of legal requirements vary in different countries. The ethical and practical responsibilities are universal.

24.1 Legal aspects of prescribing in the UK

Prescribing of drugs in the UK is regulated by the Medicines Act of 1968, the Misuse of Drugs Act of 1971, the Poisons Act 1972, and the Misuse of Drugs Regulations of 1973 amended in 1985 together with a number of more recent European Directives, e.g. 92/26.

Controlled drugs

Under the Misuse of Drugs Regulations of 1985, drugs with a high abuse potential, drugs of addiction and others with non-therapeutic psychotropic activity are categorized as controlled drugs. These include narcotic analgesics, cocaine, barbiturates, anabolic steroids, amfetamines and related agents. Controlled drugs are divided into five schedules that are subject to varying legal requirements concerning safe custody, mandatory prescription details, handwriting requirements, etc. Relevant information can be found in the regulations.

Schedule 1 includes cannabis, hallucinogens and other non-medicinal drugs with an abuse potential and this section is not of therapeutic relevance.

Schedule 2 includes over 100 'controlled' drugs with greater or lesser medicinal uses such as opiates (diamorphine, morphine, pethidine, etc.), major stimulants such as the amfetamines and secobarbital (quinalbarbitone). There are limitations and conditions on the prescription of these drugs and the following specific legal guidelines must be followed:

1 The prescription must be written in the physician's own handwriting.

2 The prescription must include the name and address of the patient.

3 The medicine or drug, the dosage form, e.g. 'tablets', the strength of the preparation, the dose and the quantity to be supplied or the total number of doses should be stated in figures and words, e.g. 10 (ten) mg.

4 The prescription must be signed and dated by the practitioner and include his address.

Schedule 3 includes a small number of minor stimulant drugs such as diethylpropion, and other drugs not thought to be as likely to be misused as those in schedule 2, nor to be as harmful if misused. This includes most barbiturates, temazepam and the analgesics buprenorphine and pentazocine. Prescribing controls that apply to schedule 2 drugs also apply to drugs in this schedule with some exceptions. There are other differences relating to manufacture, possession and destruction but these are of no therapeutic relevance.

Schedule 4 is divided into two parts and includes most of the anabolic and androgenic steroids and growth hormones together with many benzodiazepines, which are increasingly recognized as having potential to be abused. At present there are no special limitations on prescription of these drugs.

Schedule 5 includes weak narcotic analgesics and dilute preparations of morphine such as mixture of kaolin and morphine BP used for symptomatic treatment of diarrhoea. No special prescription or possession restrictions apply.

The requirements of controlled drug prescription are the basis of good prescription writing and should be used as a model for all prescriptions. There are legal obligations on medical practitioners to report to the Home Office for registration any patient who is believed to be dependent or addicted to controlled drugs. The legal aspects of drug regulation and the control of drug abuse are further reviewed in the *British National Formulary*.

24.2 Practical aspects of prescribing

It is obvious that while appropriate drug therapy can be of great benefit, inappropriate therapy is not harmless. On all occasions, there should be a positive reason for prescribing a drug. Drug treatment should never become a routine. In hospital it is still not uncommon to find 'routine' prescriptions for hypnotics, analgesics and purgatives without any consideration of individual need. Many patients and doctors expect a consultation to result automatically in the prescription of a medicine. Both of these procedures are undesirable and bad prescribing practice.

When drug treatment is indicated, it is mandatory that the most appropriate agent is given in the correct dose and in a regimen that results in optimum treatment with minimum adverse effects.

When the treatment has been selected, the doctor communicates his wishes to the pharmacist and the patient by his prescription. Accurate communication with the pharmacist is essential if the patient is to receive the desired treatment.

Prescriptions for medicine should be written legibly either typewritten, computer generated or in ink (mandatory for controlled drugs) and clearly in English. There is no justification for writing illegible or unintelligible prescriptions. The use of Latin or Greek terms or obscure abbreviations is anachronistic and liable to be misunderstood by nursing staff and/or patients.

When writing prescriptions, practitioners should:

1 Specify the patient's full name, address, and age, although the legal requirement is 'age if under 12'.

2 Indicate clearly the drug or medicine. As discussed below, it is preferable to use the approved or generic name rather than the proprietary or brand name.

3 Specify precisely the strength of tablets, capsules or mixtures. It is good prescribing practice to indicate these in words and figures and mandatory for prescriptions of controlled drugs.

4 Indicate the dose frequency and total quantity to be supplied or the duration of treatment. Once again it is good practice to include these in words and figures as this is a legal requirement for controlled drugs.

5 Do not leave large blank spaces on the prescription, which may be filled in by forgery to obtain unauthorized supplies of drugs of abuse.

6 Sign the prescription, date it and indicate your name and address. Addition of a telephone number assists the pharmacist in contacting the prescriber in the case of a prescription for an unusual drug or dose regimen.

Approved (generic) or proprietary (brand) name prescribing?

Drugs available on prescription have approved or generic names. Individual manufacturers give their own preparations proprietary (brand or trade) names.

A drug that is not covered by patent rights may be available in several proprietary formulations of the same generic preparation. There are obvious commercial pressures to encourage proprietary prescription. Proprietary names are usually short, snappy and memorable. They do not, however, necessarily give any indication of the active ingredients of the medicine. All marketed preparations (including generic preparations) have passed basic standards of purity and safety. They may differ in their formulation and this may affect absorption and distribution. Although there have been a few examples where formulation differences have led to marked changes in effect and toxicity, on the vast majority of occasions the minor pharmaceutical differences between formulations are irrelevant in clinical practice. It is good prescribing practice to use the generic name of drugs unless there is a very compelling reason for using brand names, for example, when a combination tablet is being used or when a slow-release preparation of a drug with a narrow therapeutic range (e.g. theophylline) is being prescribed. In the UK, proprietary prescription in general practice legally compels the pharmacist to provide that particular brand with attendant inconvenience to the pharmacist and often delay to the patient. As proprietary preparations vary greatly in price, generic prescribing may result in the supply of a less expensive preparation with attendant savings in the overall cost of drug treatment. Comparative costs of equivalent preparations can be readily assessed from the British National Formulary.

The British National Formulary is published by the British Medical Association and the Royal Pharmaceutical Society of Great Britain twice a year and is provided free to practising doctors and medical students in the UK. All marketed medicines are listed systematically together with brief notes on adverse effects, contraindications and details of dosage. It is a practical pocket reference manual. It should be used in conjunction with textbooks and monographs that provide background information on the rational basis of treatment and guidance on the choice of drug from a list of preparations. It should also be used in conjunction with formularies compiled and published at a local hospital or general practice level. These formularies are now very common and essentially serve to indicate which drugs will be readily available to prescribers in a particular locality or hospital.

Good prescribing practice

1 Familiarize yourself with a limited number of well-established drugs with known effects and side effects. Do not chop and change amongst equivalent preparations on whim or fancy. Avoid trying out new preparations simply because of novelty or extensive commercial promotion. Always prescribe by generic or approved names.

2 Try to devise a treatment regimen that allows drugs to be given once or twice daily. Try to reduce the total number of drugs being given to a minimum and encourage patients to take medicines at a convenient time or place in their daily routine. Avoid vague terms like 'with food' or 'after meals' as the frequency of drug taking may depend on the number of meals taken each day. However, if it is intended that a medicine, such as a non-steroidal anti-inflammatory drug (NSAID), is taken with food, then state this and the frequency. Always avoid the use of 'as before' or 'as directed' and specify the dose and frequency. Do not prescribe 'as required' without stating the maximum daily dose and dose interval.

3 Check the dose carefully each time you prescribe. Do not trust to memory and be particularly careful when doses are in the microgram range or when prescribing for children and the elderly.

4 It is now routine practice in Britain to indicate the name of the dispensed medicine on the label.

5 Use compound preparations and combination tablets only when there is an established therapeutic need for all the constituents, and where the combination of two or more drugs aids compliance.

6 Finally, always review drug prescriptions regularly: every day in hospital patients or weekly or monthly as appropriate in outpatients or general practice. When reviewing prescriptions ask the questions:

(a) Is the drug treatment still necessary?

(b) Is the optimum dose regimen being followed?

(c) Is the desired effect being achieved?

(d) Are there any symptoms or adverse effects that could be secondary to drug treatment?

(e) In general practice, has a maximum of one month's supply been prescribed?

Do not continue treatment by repeating prescriptions over long periods of time without assessing the response in the patient, or worse still, without seeing the patient.

Comment. The basis of good prescribing is a sound training in clinical methods and pathophysiology, which together with an understanding of pharmacodynamic and pharmacokinetic properties of the drugs being used, permits maximum benefit to be achieved with the minimum risk of adverse effects. Prescriptions are legal documents. They should consist of clear, legible instructions to the pharmacist. Illegible, incomplete or ambiguous prescriptions are not only bad medicine, they are also illegal.

24.3 Evolution of a new drug

Drug development aims to produce a novel therapeutic agent that is superior in efficacy to existing remedies and which causes less frequent or less severe adverse effects.

The development of a new therapeutic agent involves many years of work by a multidisciplinary group. Formerly, drugs were extracted from natural plant and animal sources. Therapeutic use was empirical and based on traditional experience. Over the last 100 years an impressive number of drugs have been synthesized chemically. With the development of molecular biology and genetic engineering, it is likely that even more agents will be produced artificially.

Synthetic techniques have produced pure substances. This has led to increased specificity of action and, in some cases, greater efficacy and reduced toxicity. Unfortunately new drug development is expensive, and only a few substances (less than 1%) of those developed are actually marketed and used in practice.

The range of novel chemical entities developed has occasionally led to unexpected toxicity. As a consequence, most governments have established bodies to regulate drug marketing, e.g. Medicines Control Agency and the Committee on Safety of Medicines in Britain, and the Food and Drug Administration in the USA. These agencies supervise clinical research on new drugs and advise on licensing new products. Although they serve to protect the public and are seen to do so, the statutory procedures that must be followed in applying for a licence for a new drug add greatly to the costs and time of development.

24.4 Clinical evaluation of a new drug

New drugs can be given to humans only after animal studies have proved efficacy and toxicological studies have provided a measure of the possible risk. At this stage a further requirement is analytical evidence of chemical purity and pharmaceutical stability.

Evaluation in man can be considered in four phases. The relevance and extent of studies at these stages depends on the drug and its indications. Drugs for use in rare diseases, or in life-threatening and as yet untreatable states, may be evaluated in patient groups at an earlier stage than those with readily measurable effects on common diseases.

Phase 1

Phase 1 involves small-scale studies in normal volunteers. These studies should determine whether the drug can be given to humans without serious symptoms or toxicity, and whether it has the desired pharmacological effects. These studies often begin with a dose-ranging study, using 1/50–1/100 the effective dose in animals and increasing until the desired effect, or adverse effects, are seen. These studies should only be performed on volunteers who are informed about the implications of the tests, and who give their consent freely. Studies should include careful assessment of clinical, haematological and biochemical evidence before and after drug administration to identify pharmacological actions and adverse effects. Phase 1 studies should be performed only by experienced staff, under medical supervision, and in premises with appropriate resuscitative facilities and support.

Phase 2

Phase 2 studies determine whether the new drug has the desired effect on patients with the appropriate disease. In the UK these investigations can be performed only after submission of preclinical and phase 1 study results to the Committee on Safety of Medicines. This body issues either a clinical trial certificate (CTC) or authorizes limited clinical trials under an exemption procedure (CTX). Phase 2 studies initially may be open, uncontrolled, dose-ranging experiments but should include controlled studies under single or double blind conditions. They may involve comparisons with inactive placebo or known active agents.

Phase 3

If the results of therapeutic efficacy and safety justify it, the next step is progression to large-scale clinical trials to determine how the new drug compares in clinical practice with existing remedies, and to establish its profile of action and frequency of adverse effects.

After phase 3 studies the evidence from all stages of development is assembled and if the conclusions indicate a useful action, the drug may be submitted to the regulatory authorities with a request for a product licence.

Phase 4

A new drug is usually marketed after only a few hundred, or at the most a few thousand, patients have been exposed to it for a relatively short period (weeks or months). As discussed in Chapter 25[Q2], post-marketing surveillance is increasingly undertaken to assess efficacy and toxicity of new drugs on a larger scale. No uniform scheme for phase 4 supervision has yet been established, but few doubt the necessity of collecting this Information on low-frequency adverse effects.

24.5 Marketing and promotion

The rationale for the development of new drugs should be to provide *better* drugs; better in the sense of being more effective, safer or cheaper. Unfortunately, only a small proportion of 'new' drugs actually represents a truly novel development or application. More often, 'new' drugs at best incorporate modest molecular variations based on existing drugs, or pharmaceutical formulation changes that have a marginal effect on absorption, toxicity or efficacy. At worst they are copies of existing drugs or minor reformulations to extend patent rights and royalties.

Drug development is expensive. This is borne by the pharmaceutical industry, which justifiably expects to recoup the cost of development when the product is finally marketed. In some therapeutic areas where drugs are widely used—e.g. antibiotics, NSAIDs, analgesics and antihypertensives—heavy investment in marketing and promotion has led to the use of undistinguished new drugs appearing in place of equally effective, cheaper and established alternatives whose side-effect profile is well known. Therapeutic fads and fashions should be avoided and prescribing practices changed only when good evidence of improved efficacy or reduced toxicity is available.

The physician needs guidance on critical assessment of what represents an important advance. Unfortunately, his or her most accessible source of information is the representative of the pharmaceutical manufacturer who has been specially trained and briefed to promote a particular new product (indeed the representative's livelihood may depend on the ability to do so). Recently, health authorities in the UK have employed medical prescribing advisors to provide unbiased advice to local general practitioners on drug selection and utilization.

Practitioners must seek out sources of information from information pharmacists, specialist clinical colleagues, postgraduate meetings and publications in the scientific literature. Publications, in themselves, can be misleading. Evidence from a few controlled studies published in well-established journals subject to peer review are more reliable than bulky obscure proceedings of sponsored meetings to promote a particular drug.

Physicians should make an active attempt to determine in what way a new drug represents an improvement over existing therapy, and what the price is in terms of adverse effects and actual cost of the drug.

As new drugs may be marketed after studies in only a few hundred or thousand patients, special vigilance is required in the first few years of use to determine low frequency, but potentially serious, adverse effects.

Comments. New drug developments should be examined critically; objective evidence from several sources should be sought to highlight improved therapeutic efficacy and reduced toxicity in controlled comparison with established remedies.

24.6 Compliance with drug therapy

Approximately one-third of outpatients take their treatment as directed, one-third partly comply and one-third never comply. Poor 'compliance' is found in all socioeconomic and ethnic backgrounds and there is no satisfactory method of predicting who will fail to comply with treatment. However, compliance is likely to be decreased in certain circumstances:

1 The very young and the very old.
2 Patients requiring long-term treatment.
3 Failure to understand that treatment is beneficial or that the disease is potentially dangerous.
4 Complexity of treatment: prescription of too many drugs in different doses.
5 Difficulty of access to the drugs, for example when a patient with rheumatoid arthritis is faced with a childproof container.
6 Adverse effects: although if these are genuinely unavoidable they might be tolerated if the treatment is seen to be beneficial.
7 Expense: this is likely to be a factor in those countries where medicines are purchased at their full value.

Detection of poor compliance

This is not easy. Doctors in general believe that poor compliance happens to other doctors' patients. There are, however, certain simple procedures that can help in detecting poor compliance.

1 Ask the patient how he or she is getting on with the medication and whether they are finding it easy to take the treatment as prescribed. A friendly enquiry of this nature might reveal poor compliance and the reasons for it.
2 Assessment of pharmacological effect. This is clearly easier for some drugs than for others. A patient receiving a beta-blocker, for example, should have a relative bradycardia. In general terms failure to achieve a therapeutic goal should always raise the question of poor compliance.
3 Assessment of the rate of drug consumption. This has its limitations as medication can be disposed of easily, but two approaches can be tried. In general practice the actual and expected rate at which repeat prescriptions are requested might show a gross disparity, suggesting that the medication is not being taken at the expected rate. The other approach is to count the number of tablets in the drug container and to calculate the number used.
4 Drug level monitoring (see Chapter 2). Its most definitive role in determining compliance is the finding of unexpectedly low levels or no drug at all in the plasma. Levels that are merely subtherapeutic might be the result of poor compliance but could also reflect abnormally low bioavailability or high clearance. Quantitative assessment can be made of many drugs in saliva. As a simple screening manoeuvre it may be useful to perform qualitative tests for the presence or absence of drugs in urine.

Improving compliance

There is no absolutely reliable method of ensuring compliance with drug therapy. However, the following may be helpful:

1 Patient counselling. Explain clearly to the patient, or relative where appropriate, why treatment is necessary and what is likely to be achieved by the treatment.
2 Keep treatment regimen simple. Wherever possible use once- or twice-daily doses and try to avoid the need for a mid-day dose. Review drug treatment regularly to assess whether all treatment is still necessary.
3 Treatment schedule. Explain when the drugs should be taken and in what dose. In addition to explaining verbally, write it down as the patient may forget your instructions.
4 Outline possible adverse effects and encourage the patient to contact you before the next appointment if symptoms get worse rather than better.
5 Enquire at each follow-up about adverse effects and ask how your patient is getting on with the treatment in general. If adverse effects develop change the dose or the drug.
6 In elderly patients, or those disabled by arthritis, ensure that the drug is accessible and not in a childproof container.
7 If it is imperative that a drug be taken but there is a serious doubt about patient compliance then slow-release intramuscular depot

preparations are available. Examples include phenothiazines and progestogens.

8 Patients can become confused by the array of different medicines they collect over time. Encourage the patient or carer to dispose of all medicines no longer in use by returning them to a pharmacy.

Comment. There is little point in putting a lot of effort and money into reaching a diagnosis if the patient is not going to comply with the therapy. The natural history of the underlying disease is then the same as if you had never begun the diagnostic evaluation. Poor compliance should always be borne in mind and efforts made to ensure that treatment is taken as prescribed. Among the various methods for improving compliance, the one which is more important than all the others is patient counselling. Explain the reasons for drug therapy clearly to your patient and on subsequent review continue to ask sympathetically about the progress of treatment.

CHAPTER 25

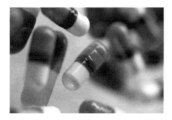

Adverse Drug Reactions

25.1 Definition and magnitude of the problem

An adverse drug reaction can be defined as 'any undesired or unintended effect of drug treatment'. This definition is intentionally very broad and includes such effects as an acute allergic reaction to penicillin, severe hypoglycaemia after excessive insulin administration, osteoporosis after long-term corticosteroid therapy, rebound hypertension after discontinuing clonidine and phocomelia in the children of mothers exposed to thalidomide during early pregnancy.

It has been estimated that an average hospital medical patient receives between five and 10 different drugs during a 10-day stay in hospital. During this time about 25% of patients experience one or more adverse drug effects, and 1% experience a life-threatening event due to drugs. Of these the majority are patients who have tumours and develop pancytopenia as a result of cancer chemotherapy. Approximately one in a thousand medical patients suffers a life-threatening adverse drug effect in which the risks of therapy seemed in retrospect to outweigh the potential benefits. The potential for adverse reaction is even greater in general practice. Some 25% of acute medical admissions to hospital can be attributed in whole or in part to the adverse effects of drug therapy.

Older age groups receive a disproportionately high number of prescriptions for drugs and adverse drug reactions are particularly common in this group for pharmacokinetic, pharmacodynamic and social reasons.

25.2 Predictable adverse reactions

Adverse drug effects can be classified in many ways. A useful approach to the problem is given in Table 25.1. In this scheme adverse effects are grouped into those that are predictable on the basis of the drug's known actions and those that are not. The former type usually occurs early in the course of treatment, is a common event that is dose related, and is either recognized as a possibility before clinical trials begin or very shortly thereafter. By contrast, the latter type is usually infrequent, rarely recognized until widespread use of the medicine has occurred, and need not necessarily be dose dependent.

Excessive pharmacological effects

Predictable adverse drug effects are due to excessive pharmacological activity of the drug in question. This arises particularly with central nervous system depressants, cardioactive, hypotensive and hypoglycaemic agents. Specific examples of this type of reaction are:

1 Respiratory depression in severe bronchitic patients given morphine or benzodiazepine hypnotics.

ADVERSE DRUG EFFECTS

Predictable reactions
Excess pharmacological activity
Rebound response upon discontinuation

Unpredictable reactions
Allergic effects
Genetically determined effects
Idiosyncratic effects

Table 25.1 Adverse drug effects.

2 Hypotension resulting in stroke, myocardial infarction or renal failure in patients receiving excessive doses of antihypertensive drugs.
3 Bradycardia in patients receiving excessive digoxin doses.

Less obvious but equally important are predictable adverse effects where the particular pharmacological effect involved is not the one for which the drug was initially administered. For example, a patient receiving an antihistamine for the prevention of motion sickness may become drowsy.

All patients are at risk of developing this type of reaction if enough high doses are given. However, certain subgroups are particularly susceptible (Chapters 3 and 4) and include those with renal disease, liver disease, the very young and the elderly.

Withdrawal symptoms or rebound responses after discontinuation of treatment

This type of reaction is unusual in that it occurs in the absence of the causative agent. The abrupt interruption of therapy is followed by a characteristic withdrawal syndrome:
1 Extreme agitation, tachycardia, confusion, delirium and convulsions may occur following the discontinuation of long-term central nervous system depressants such as barbiturates, benzodiazepines and alcohol.
2 Acute Addisonian crisis may be precipitated by the abrupt cessation of corticosteroid therapy.

3 Severe hypertension and symptoms of sympathetic overactivity may arise shortly after discontinuing clonidine therapy.
4 Withdrawal symptoms after narcotic analgesics.

25.3 Unpredictable adverse effects

In all these instances adaptation has occurred to the drug at the receptor level. This adaptation is usually associated with some tolerance to the effects of the drug, and a gradually increasing dose of drug may be necessary to sustain the initial effect. Withdrawal effects may be minimized by gradual withdrawal of the drugs involved with or without substitution with longer-acting or less potent agents and gradual withdrawal.

Allergic drug responses

Drug allergy and hypersensitivity are common adverse drug effects. Indeed some clinicians regard these types of response as the most frequent adverse drug effects. Such reactions are unpredictable and are often not dose related.

They occur only in a small proportion of the population exposed to the drug, and it is usually impossible to predict the individuals who will experience this response in advance. These reactions vary from mild erythematous skin reactions to major anaphylactic shock. An allergic adverse effect of a drug is characterized by the fact that:

1 The reaction does not resemble the expected pharmacological drug effect.

2 There is delay between first exposure to the drug and the development of a reaction.

3 The reaction recurs upon repeated exposure even to traces of the drug.

The drugs most frequently associated with allergic skin reactions are the penicillins, the sulphonamides and blood products.

Genetically determined effects

The major toxicity of some drugs is restricted to individuals with a particular genotype or genetic make-up. Thus patients with hereditary pseudocholinesterase deficiency are unable to metabolize the muscle relaxant succinylcholine and may develop prolonged paralysis and apnoea following its use (Chapter 18). Similarly, individuals with glucose-6-phosphate dehydrogenase deficiency are at substantial risk of developing acute haemolytic anaemia after exposure to the antimalarial drug primaquine and to sulphonamides and quinidine. Some of the most common types of genetic abnormalities that may lead to drug toxicity are shown in Table 25.2.

Genetically determined acetylator polymorphism affects responses and adverse effects to isoniazid, hydralazine and procainamide. Such drugs are metabolized in the liver by the enzyme N-acetyl transferase. There is a bimodal distribution of acetylator capacity in the population, with some individuals being slow and others fast acetylators (Chapter 1). Slow acetylators of isoniazid given standard doses are much more likely than fast acetylators to suffer from peripheral neuropathy. The drug-induced lupus syndrome is much more common in slow acetylators receiving hydralazine or procainamide. Adverse effects of hydralazine and also gold salts and D-penicillamine are linked to the specific histocompatibility antigens. In the future, tissue typing may help to predict susceptibility to drug toxicity.

Idiosyncratic drug reactions

The term idiosyncrasy is used primarily to cover unusual, unexpected or bizarre drug effects that cannot readily be explained or predicted in individual recipients.

Also included in this type of reaction are drug-induced fetal abnormalities such as phocomelia (limb deformity), which developed in the offspring of mothers receiving thalidomide in early pregnancy.

Drug-induced malignant disease is fortunately rare and may be considered an idiosyncratic drug effect:

GENETICALLY DETERMINED DRUG TOXICITY

Defect	Toxic drug	Symptoms
Pseudocholinesterase deficiency	Succinylcholine	Paralysis, apnoea
Glucose-6-phosphate dehydrogenase deficiency	Sulphonamides, quinidine, primaquine	Haemolysis
Acetylator polymorphism	Procainamide, hydralazine, isoniazid	Systemic lupus (in slow acetylators) Neuropathy (in slow acetylators)
Hepatic porphyria	Barbiturates	Symptomatic porphyria

Table 25.2 Some genetically determined types of drug toxicity.

1 Analgesic abuse may rarely cause cancer of the renal pelvis.

2 Long-term oestrogens without coincidental progestogens may induce uterine cancer.

3 Immunosuppressive drugs may induce lymphoid tumours.

4 Intramuscular iron preparations may cause sarcomata at the site of injection.

5 Thyroid cancer may develop in patients who have received ^{131}I-therapy in the past.

25.4 Discovery of drug-induced disease

Before a new drug is released for widespread use the manufacturer must obtain a licence from the appropriate government authority [Committee on Proprietary Medicinal Products (CPMP) in the European Community (EC), Food and Drug Administration in the USA, etc.]. It is likely that over 3000 healthy volunteers and patients will have received the drug in supervised trials before permission for general marketing is given, unless the drug is for a rare disease when experience may be much smaller. By this stage most of the pharmacological effects are known.

Adverse effects resulting from excess pharmacological activity may be well documented. Such is not the case for unpredictable toxicity, where adverse effects are often not identified until the drug has been subjected to much more widespread use. Only after several years was it recognized that the beta-receptor blocking drug practolol could cause an oculomucocutaneous syndrome when taken regularly over a long period. Likewise, thalidomide had been marketed for several years before its potential for causing severe limb deformities (phocomelia) in the offspring of mothers taking it in early pregnancy was appreciated.

In order to identify unexpected adverse drug effects several different approaches have been adopted: each involving careful observational study of patients.

1 Spontaneous report of suspected adverse drug reactions. This occurs when prescribers report suspected reactions to a central agency which investigates, collates and reviews the resulting information.

2 Cohort study. This is used when groups of drug recipients are followed to evaluate outcomes after drug exposure.

3 Case-control study. This is used when patients with suspected drug-induced disease are compared with a reference population to determine if there is indeed excessive drug use amongst the suspect disease patients.

4 Review of vital statistics. This occurs when epidemiologists review national or regional statistics to note any unusual epidemics of diseases or uncommon disorders.

Each approach has its strengths and weaknesses but the different types of study are complementary.

Spontaneous reports of suspected adverse drug reactions

In the USA, UK, Scandinavia and most Western European countries there are agencies that collect information about suspected adverse drug effects. For example, in the UK, the Committee on Safety of Medicines has an adverse reaction subcommittee, which encourages physicians to report suspected adverse drug reactions on a standard form. The resulting information is analysed regularly to determine whether or not any unusual patterns of reports are emerging. Unfortunately it has a relatively low response rate, particularly from hospital-based physicians.

Spontaneous reporting has been useful in confirming whether or not a newly suspected reaction is widespread in the community. This approach, however, only assesses the number of suspected reactions. There is no estimate of the frequency of reactions because it gives no details of the numbers exposed to the drug in the population from which the reports were received.

Cohort studies

These generally allow the detection of events occurring with a frequency of greater than 1 per 500 exposed. Various types of cohort study have been conducted to detect and quantify drug toxicity. Duration of follow-up varies from weeks to decades.

Short-term randomized, controlled clinical trials

These are expensive to conduct and time consuming. They are usually carried out early in the lifetime of a drug and are confined to patients who have no disorders other than those relevant to the drug in question. Thus the approach is useful only in detecting and quantitating common acute adverse drug effects in otherwise healthy subjects.

Long-term randomized, controlled clinical trials

These are formidable undertakings and are rarely conducted. They are expensive to organize and maintain. They are confined to medications that are used on a long-term basis, e.g. oral contraceptives, antidiabetic drugs and antihypertensive drugs. When successful they give useful information both on acute and delayed effects of drug treatment. However, there are often problems in maintaining the integrity of the study cohort, in demonstrating that satisfactory randomization of the treated and control groups has been carried out, and in showing that no new differences other than drug exposure have arisen after randomization.

Post-marketing surveillance of established drugs: non-randomized and often uncontrolled

Studies in which a group of recipients is identified and observed for possible adverse effects are now being conducted more frequently. The periods of observation are usually brief (days or weeks) and the size of the cohorts small (rarely more than 2000). Such studies are useful for quantifying known acute effects after short-term exposure to drugs and for identifying subgroups of the population who are at greatest risk of toxicity, e.g. elderly, those with renal impairment, liver disease, etc.

Post-marketing surveillance of new drugs: non-randomized and often uncontrolled

This approach is relatively new. It aims to review a large cohort of 10 000 or more recipients of a drug newly released onto the market and to follow such individuals for a substantial period of at least one and preferably several years. When successful, such studies have the potential for detecting both acute and delayed toxicity following short- or long-term exposure. Once again a major problem is to maintain the integrity of the study cohort. Although less expensive to conduct than a long-term clinical trial, such studies are nevertheless likely to be confined to those new drugs used for prolonged periods in large numbers of patients.

These studies give not only an indication of what reactions may occur but also some idea of the frequency with which they may be expected.

Case-control studies

The drug consuming habits of patients with a suspected drug-induced disease are compared with those of a reference population who do not have the suspect disease. This approach is increasingly being used to detect and quantify drug-related disease. It is particularly useful in showing associations between drug use and rare diseases where the risks of developing the disease are less than 1 in 500 persons exposed. Under those circumstances, it would be prohibitively expensive and complex to attempt to follow a cohort of recipients, and it is easier to start at the suspected disease and work back to the drug exposure.

In case-control studies the results are expressed as relative risks: that is, for example, the risk of being a cigarette smoker in a series of patients with lung cancer compared to the risk in reference patients without lung cancer. This information is insufficient to assess the actual risk of getting lung cancer if one is a smoker. Calculating such a risk requires additional information not usually available to those conducting the case-control study.

There are major limitations to case-control studies.

1 While they may show associations between diseases and drug use, they do not prove that these associations are causal.

2 They are difficult to conduct in practice because they can be subject to bias as a result either of the type of reference population studied or of foreknowledge of the hypothesis under review by the interviewer.

3 It is important to confine interest to newly diagnosed cases in order to avoid distortion of drug-consuming habits as a consequence of awareness of the presence of a significant disease. For example, when assessing the association between chronic renal failure and analgesic abuse, it would not be advisable to look at previously diagnosed cases of renal failure since such patients are likely to have been advised to avoid drugs in general and analgesics in particular. A case-control study that included previously diagnosed cases of renal failure amongst the cases could therefore produce a result which did not show any drug association with analgesic abuse even if, in reality, analgesic abuse was indeed associated with significant risk of chronic renal failure.

Using these techniques it is likely that the ability to detect serious drug-related toxicity will greatly improve in the coming decades. Provided that these limitations are appreciated and the resulting information is handled intelligently, this approach has much to offer particularly when dealing with rare or delayed drug effects.

Because of the expense and difficulty of collecting and maintaining a cohort of recipients to study, or a group of disease sufferers to investigate, increasing use is being made of record linkage studies to facilitate these studies. This approach involves linking pre-recorded data sets from defined populations, often general practices. Records of prescriptions issued and hospital referrals (with resulting diagnoses) are linked to provide a study resource with which to conduct cohort and case-control studies. Such studies can be used to test hypotheses arising from reports in the literature or to generate hypotheses from within the data set.

Vital statistics

In theory, a review of national or regional health-care statistics should be a useful way of detecting an unsuspected epidemic of an unusual condition or a marked increase in prevalence of a common condition. This might prove to be so if the collection of such statistics was sufficiently accurate and data processing and review were undertaken sufficiently rapidly. At present this approach is not practical. In the western USA an epidemic of uterine cancer occurred during the 1970s. This was well documented in the regional statistics but no one appreciated its significance until isolated reports linking long-term oestrogen use to uterine cancer were published. By then the major epidemic was already under way. Efficient and informed review of the vital statistics could well have led to the discovery of this problem 2 or 3 years earlier. Regular perusal of accurate regional vital statistics could indicate those conditions that showed an unexpected increase in frequency and which might, therefore, be drug induced.

25.5 Reduction of the risk of adverse effects

Many powerful drugs are now available. It is hardly surprising that untoward effects are produced occasionally. With a better knowledge of the pharmacological mechanisms by which drugs exert their effects, their toxicity, and the pathophysiology of diseases, it is likely that in the future drug therapy may become safer. The risks of developing adverse drug effects can be reduced by observing several simple rules:

1 Always include a detailed drug history as part of the clinical history or consultation.

2 Only use drug treatment when there is a clear indication for it and there is no non-pharmacological alternative.

3 Avoid multiple drug regimens and combination tablets whenever possible.

4 Pay particular attention to drug dose and response in the young, the old and those with coexisting renal, hepatic or cardiac disease.

5 Review the need for continuing treatment regularly and stop drugs that are no longer necessary.

Index

Page numbers in *italic* refer to Figures and those in **bold** refer to Tables.